Infections in Urology

Editor

MICHAEL H. HSIEH

UROLOGIC CLINICS
OF NORTH AMERICA

www.urologic.theclinics.com

Editor-in-Chief
KEVIN R. LOUGHLIN

November 2024 • Volume 51 • Number 4

ELSEVIER

1600 John F. Kennedy Boulevard • Suite 1800 • Philadelphia, Pennsylvania, 19103-2899

http://www.theclinics.com

UROLOGIC CLINICS OF NORTH AMERICA Volume 51, Number 4
November 2024 ISSN 0094-0143, ISBN-13: 978-0-443-29494-5

Editor: Kerry Holland
Developmental Editor: Nitesh Barthwal

Urologic Clinics of North America (ISSN 0094-0143) is published quarterly by Elsevier Inc., 360 Park Avenue South, New York, NY 10010-1710. Months of issue are February, May, August, and November. Business and Editorial Offices: 1600 John F. Kennedy Blvd., Suite 1800, Philadelphia, PA 19103-2899. Periodicals postage paid at New York, NY and additional mailing offices. Subscription prices are $427.00 per year (US individuals), $100.00 per year (US students and residents), $483.00 per year (Canadian individuals), $100.00 per year (Canadian students/residents), $557.00 per year (foreign individuals), and $240.00 per year (foreign students/residents). For institutional access pricing please contact Customer Service via the contact information below. Foreign air speed delivery is included in all *Clinics* subscription prices. All prices are subject to change without notice. Orders, claims, and journal inquiries: Please visit our Support Hub page https://service.elsevier.com for assistance.

Reprints. For copies of 100 or more, of articles in this publication, please contact the Commercial Reprints Department, Elsevier Inc., 360 Park Avenue South, New York, New York 10010-1710. Tel.: 212-633-3874; Fax: 212-633-3820; E-mail: reprints@elsevier.com.

Urologic Clinics of North America is covered in MEDLINE/PubMed (*Index Medicus*), *Excerpta Medica, Current Contents/Clinical Medicine, Science Citation Index,* and *ISI/BIOMED*.

Contributors

EDITOR-IN-CHIEF

KEVIN R. LOUGHLIN, MD, MBA
Emeritus Professor of Surgery (Urology), Harvard Medical School, Visiting Scientist, Vascular Biology Research Program at Boston Children's Hospital, Boston, Massachusetts, USA

EDITOR

MICHAEL H. HSIEH, MD, PhD
Professor of Urology, The George Washington University, Director of Research, Division of Urology, Children's National Hospital, Washington, DC, USA

AUTHORS

A. LENORE ACKERMAN, MD, PhD
Director of Research, Division of Pelvic Medicine and Reconstructive Surgery, Assistant Professor of Urology and Obstetrics and Gynecology, Department of Urology, David Geffen School of Medicine at UCLA, Los Angeles, California, USA

OLUWAFOLAJIMI ADESANYA, MD
Clinical Research Associate, Department of Urology, James Buchanan Brady Urological Institute, Johns Hopkins University School of Medicine, Baltimore, Maryland, USA

MUHAMMAD SALMAN ASHRAF, MBBS, FIDSA
Associate Professor of Medicine, Division of Infectious Diseases, University of Nebraska Medical Center, Omaha; Medical Director of Healthcare-Associated Infections and Antimicrobial Resistance Program, Division of Public Health, Nebraska Department of Health and Human Services, Lincoln, Nebraska, USA

GINA M. BADALATO, MD
Vice Chair of Education, Faculty Affairs, Associate Professor, Department of Urology, Columbia University Medical Center, New York, New York, USA

KETTY BAI, BS
Medical Student, Department of Urology, New York, New York, USA

NICOLE A. BELKO, MD
Fellow, Division of Urology, Children's National Medical Center, Washington, DC, USA

KRISTY BORAWSKI, MD
Professor, Department of Urology, University of North Carolina School of Medicine, The University of North Carolina at Chapel Hill, Chapel Hill, North Carolina, USA

NICK BOWLER, MD
Resident, Department of Urology, George Washington University Hospital, Washington, DC, USA

AMANDIP S. CHEEMA, MD, MHS
Urology Resident, Department of Urology, Loyola University Medical Center, Maywood, Illinois, USA

BEN CHEW, MD
Associate Professor, Department of Urologic Sciences, The Stone Centre at Vancouver General Hospital, University of British Columbia, Vancouver, British Columbia, Canada

ZOË COHEN, MD
Urology Resident, Department of Urology, Columbia University Irving Medical Center, New York, New York, USA

KIMBERLY L. COOPER, MD
Associate Professor, Department of Urology, Columbia University Irving Medical Center, New York, New York, USA

ALANNA CRUZ-BENDEZU, MD
Resident, Department of Urology, George Washington University Hospital, Washington, DC, USA

MARC DALL'ERA, MD
Professor and Interim Chair, Department of Urologic Surgery, University of California, Davis, Sacramento, California, USA

RAHUL DUTTA, MD
Urologist, Division of Pelvic Medicine and Reconstructive Surgery, Department of Urology, David Geffen School of Medicine at UCLA, Los Angeles, California, USA

AHMAD M. EL-ARABI, MD
Assistant Professor, Department of Urology, Loyola University Medical Center, Maywood, Illinois, USA

CATHERINE S. FORSTER, MD, MS, FAAP
Assistant Professor, Department of Pediatrics, UPMC Children's Hospital of Pittsburgh, Pittsburgh, Pennsylvania, USA

BRIANA GODDARD, MD
Resident Physician, Department of Urology, George Washington University Hospital, Washington, DC, USA

CHRISTOPHER M. GONZALEZ, MD, MBA, FACS
Chair, Albert J. Jr. and Claire R. Speh Professor, Department of Urology, Loyola University Medical Center, Maywood, Illinois, USA

ALLISON GRANT, MD
Urology Resident, Department of Urology, Columbia University Irving Medical Center, New York, New York, USA

SARAH HANSTOCK, BSc
PhD Student, Department of Urologic Sciences, The Stone Centre at Vancouver General Hospital, University of British Columbia, Vancouver, British Columbia, Canada

MICHAEL H. HSIEH, MD, PhD
Professor of Urology, The George Washington University, Director of Research, Division of Urology, Children's National Hospital, Washington, DC, USA

NICOLAI HUBNER, MD
Visiting Assistant Professor, Department of Urologic Surgery, University of California, Davis, Sacramento, California, USA

DIRK LANGE, PhD
Associate Professor, Department of Urologic Sciences, The Stone Centre at Vancouver General Hospital, University of British Columbia, Vancouver, British Columbia, Canada

JOANNA ORZEL, MD
Resident Physician, Department of Urology, University of Iowa Hospitals and Clinics, University of Iowa, Iowa City, Iowa, USA

MILAN K. PATEL, MD
Urologist, Department of Urology, Loyola University Medical Center, Maywood, Illinois, USA

HANS G. POHL, MD
Chief, Division of Urology, Children's National Medical Center, Professor, Department of Urology and Pediatrics, George Washington University School of Medicine and Health Sciences, Washington, DC, USA

JUAN TERAN PLASENCIA, MD
Assistant Professor of Medicine, Division of Infectious Diseases, University of Nebraska Medical Center, Omaha, Nebraska, USA

SHERRY S. ROSS, MD
Associate Professor, Department of Urology, Division Director of Pediatric Urology, University of North Carolina Chapel Hill School of Medicine, The University of North Carolina at Chapel Hill, Chapel Hill, North Carolina, USA

MATTHEW P. RUTMAN, MD
Director of Clinical Operations, Chief of
Urology at Allen Hospital NYP, Director of
Voiding Dysfunction and Female Urology,
Associate Professor, Department of Urology,
New York, New York, USA

DANIEL STEIN, MD, MHS
Assistant Professor, Department of Urology,
George Washington University Hospital,
Washington, DC, USA

LYNN STOTHERS, MD
Professor, Division of Pelvic Medicine and
Reconstructive Surgery, Department of
Urology, David Geffen School of Medicine at
UCLA, Los Angeles, California, USA

REID A. STUBBEE, MD
Resident Physician, Department of Urology,
University of Iowa Hospitals and Clinics,
University of Iowa, Iowa City, Iowa, USA

SEAN TAFURI, MD
Resident, Department of Urology, George
Washington University Hospital, Washington,
DC, USA

CHAD R. TRACY, MD
Clinical Professor, Department of Urology,
University of Iowa Hospitals and Clinics,
University of Iowa, Iowa City, Iowa,
USA

GLENN T. WERNEBURG, MD, PhD
Resident Physician, Department of Urology,
Glickman Urological and Kidney Institute,
Cleveland Clinic Foundation, Cleveland, Ohio,
USA

MICHAEL J. WHALEN, MD
Associate Professor and Vice-Chair,
Department of Urology, George Washington
University School of Medicine, Washington,
DC, USA

Contents

Prostate biopsies are commonly performed for the early detection of prostate cancer and yet are associated with risks of life-threatening infections. Drug-resistant strains of *Escherichia coli* are the most common etiologic agents. Multiple maneuvers can reduce the risk of postbiopsy infections and sepsis during transrectal prostate biopsy including periprocedural empiric or targeted prophylactic antibiotics (based on previous rectal culture) and prebiopsy rectal cleansing with a povidone-iodine solution. The transperineal approach is associated with a very low risk of infection without requiring antibiotic prophylaxis.

Surgical site infections (SSIs) represent a major source of postoperative complications adversely impacting morbidity and mortality indices in surgical care. The discovery of antibiotics in the mid-20th century, and their ensuing use for preoperative antimicrobial bowel preparation and prophylaxis, drastically reduced the occurrence of SSIs providing a major tool to surgeons of various specialties, including urology. Because, the appropriate use of these antimicrobials is critical for their continued safety and efficacy, an understanding of the recommendations guiding their application is essential for all surgeons. Here, we comprehensively review these recommendations with a focus on open and laparoscopic urologic surgeries.

Prosthetic joint infection (PJI) and prosthetic valve endocarditis (PVE) are uncommon but serious complications. According to current best practice statements, prior to a genitourinary procedure, patients with prosthetic joints should receive antibiotic prophylaxis if they are within 2 years of arthroplasty, if they are high risk for infection due to their individual comorbidities, or if the procedure poses a high risk for bacteremia. Patients with prosthetic valves should not receive antibiotic prophylaxis for the sole purpose of prevention of endocarditis. *Enterococcus* species are the uropathogens most often associated with PJI and PVE. Antibiotic selection should take into account local resistance patterns.

Microbiome dysbiosis is closely related to the etiology of kidney stone disease (KSD) and influences a multitude of pathways. Due to our knowledge gaps on this topic, it is still unclear if microbiome interventions can be translated to demonstrate clinical efficacy. Current evidence suggests that the enhancement of butyrate-producing pathways should be the next step for KSD research. While we are not yet at a point where we can make clinical recommendations for KSD, there are many simple dietary or supplement-based approaches that could be applied in the future for prophylaxis or treatment of KSD.

Fungal pathogens within the urine, specifically *Candida* species, are a common finding amongst hospitalized patients. Risk factors for the development of candiduria involve patients with indwelling urinary drainage devices, surgical patients, patients undergoing urologic instrumentation, and diabetic patients. Candiduria often presents with an asymptomatic course but can also be a severe life-threatening process. This article will review the epidemiology and risk factors associated with fungal urinary tract infections, and the diagnosis and categorization of these infections along with a review of current medical and surgical treatments for this condition.

The urine culture is imperfect, and a series of alternative approaches are in development to assist in diagnosis, treatment, and prevention of urinary tract infection (UTI). Culture-independent approaches typically do not distinguish between viable and nonviable bacteria, and are generally not included in current clinical guidance. Next-generation sequencing may play an important future role in precise targeting of antibiotic treatment of asymptomatic bacteriuria prior to endourologic surgery or in pregnancy. Future studies are needed to determine whether microbiota modulation could prevent UTI. Possible modulation mechanisms may include fecal microbiota transplant, application of topical vaginal estrogen or probiotics, and bacteriophage therapy.

Prosthetic urology can substantially enhance the quality of life for patients. However, it is not without challenges. Infections of penile prostheses and artificial urinary sphincters are often difficult to diagnose, manage, and treat. Over time, device improvements, refined surgical methods, better understanding of microbiology, and biofilms in combination with higher sterility standards and protocols, have significantly reduced the rates of infection. Here, the authors offer a comprehensive overview of prosthetic urologic infections and their management in the current era.

Transgender and gender-diverse individuals experience disproportionately high rates of sexually transmitted infections (STIs). In this review, the authors discuss the epidemiology, screening recommendations, and treatment guidelines for STIs in transgender and gender-diverse people.

Although antibiotics remain the mainstay of urinary tract infection treatment, many affected women can be caught in a vicious cycle in which antibiotics given to eradicate one infection predispose them to develop another. This effect is primarily mediated by disturbances in the gut microbiome that both directly enrich for uropathogenic overgrowth and induce systemic alterations in inflammation, tissue permeability, and metabolism that also decrease host resistance to infection recurrences. Here, we discuss nonantibiotic approaches to manipulating the gut microbiome to reverse the systemic consequences of antibiotics, including cranberry supplementation and other dietary approaches, probiotic administration, and fecal microbiota transplantation.

Urinary tract infection (UTI) is frequent in the first year of life with bowel and bladder dysfunction, GU tract abnormalities, neurogenic bladder, and the intact prepuce conveying an increased risk. Urine culture is the gold standard for diagnosis. Antibiotics are tailored to resistance patterns. Guidelines have been established to direct the evaluation for GU anomalies but differ significantly. Bladder and bowel dysfunction is important to screen for and treat in potty-trained patients. Circumcised boys with febrile UTIs are more likely to have anatomic abnormalities than uncircumcised boys.

Urinary tract infections (UTIs) are the most common infection in patients with neurogenic bladder. Diagnosis is fraught with challenges since there is no globally accepted definition for UTI and symptoms can vary widely. Due to the increased risk of morbidity, it is important to have a thorough understanding of the risk of UTI, diagnostic criteria, and to treat aggressively when UTI is confirmed. Prevention of UTI is optimal but more studies are needed to identify the best methods to prevent UTIs in this population.

Understanding the management of asymptomatic bacteriuria (ASB) is important given the prevalence of the condition, associated risks in certain patient populations, and the risks associated with inappropriate antibiotic administration. Generally, screening and treatment is only recommended in pregnant women and in those undergoing urologic procedures that will violate the urothelium. Knowing the appropriate time to screen and treat ASB is critical for managing high-risk patients and preventing the growth of antibiotic resistance. Recent research into the protective nature of avirulent strains of *Escherichia coli* might offer a new approach to management of ASB.

UROLOGIC CLINICS OF NORTH AMERICA

SERIES OF RELATED INTEREST
Surgical Clinics of North America
https://www.surgical.theclinics.com/

Foreword

Infections in Urology: The Gathering Storm of Antibiotic Resistance

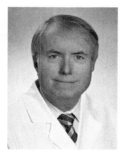

Kevin R. Loughlin, MD, MBA
Editor-in-Chief

Treating and preventing infections of the urinary tract is an essential part of urologic practice. In this issue of *Urologic Clinics*, Doctor Michael Hsieh has assembled experts with diverse backgrounds to provide a comprehensive review of the current management and prevention of urinary tract infections.

The importance of correct diagnosis and management of urinary tract infections cannot be over-emphasized. It is estimated that about 10 in 25 women and 3 in 25 men will have symptoms of a urinary tract infection during their lifetime.[1]

Beyond the clinical challenge of the prevalence of urinary tract infections is the increasing problem of antibiotic drug resistance. This is due to a combination of factors, including the overuse of antibiotics in both humans and animals, misuse of antibiotics, spontaneous resistance, and transmitted resistance.[2]

The World Health Organization estimates that bacterial antimicrobial resistance (AMR) was directly responsible for 1.27 million global deaths in 2019 and contributed to 4.95 million deaths.[3] The World Bank estimates that AMR could result in $1 trillion to $3.4 trillion gross domestic product losses per year by 2030.[4]

Our goal as urologists should be to treat documented infections when they exist and to prophylax with antibiotics to prevent infections when appropriate. This issue of *Urologic Clinics* should serve as a useful adjunct for urologists to achieve these goals.

Kevin R. Loughlin, MD, MBA
Vascular Biology Research Laboratory
Boston Children's Hospital
300 Longwood Avenue
Boston, MA 02115, USA

E-mail address:
kloughlin@partners.org

REFERENCES

1. Understanding UTIs across the lifespan. Urology Care Foundation. Available at: Urologyhealth.org/healthy-living/urology. Accessed August 11, 2024.
2. Available at: my.clevelandclinic.org/health/activities/21655-antibiotic-resistance. Accessed.
3. Antimicrobial Resistance Collaborators. Global burden of bacterial antimicrobial resistance in 2019: a systematic analysis. Lancet 2022;399(10325):629–55.
4. Drug-resistant infections: a threat to our economic future (2027). Available at: https://www.worldbank.org/en/topic/health/publication/drugresistant-infections-a-threat-to our-economic-future. Accessed.

Urol Clin N Am 51 (2024) xiii
https://doi.org/10.1016/j.ucl.2024.08.002
0094-0143/24/© 2024 Published by Elsevier Inc.

Preface
Infections in Urology

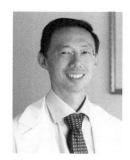

Michael H. Hsieh, MD, PhD
Editor

The challenge to tailor antibiotic choices to the individual patient as well as the specific procedure is ever increasing in the modern era of multidrug-resistant organisms and increasingly complex patients and surgeries. The urologist faces decisions every day in both clinical practice and the operating room setting on how to effectively utilize antibiotics while taking into account individual patient factors as well as procedural factors. The goals of minimizing the incidence of infections and limiting morbidity from infections are shared by clinicians across the specialties ranging from Cardiology, to Orthopedics, to Infectious Disease, to Obstetrics, to Pediatrics, to Internal Medicine. Collaboration on the part of the physicians is key to managing individual patients with infections that require treatment and in procedures that necessitate prophylaxis. Judicious use of antibiotics in the appropriate doses for the indicated duration helps to limit the development of resistant organisms and to maintain the efficacy of broad-spectrum antibiotics for the continued treatment of patients in the future.

In this issue of *Urologic Clinics*, we focus on antibiotic management in cases specific to the urologist, including penile prosthesis and artificial urinary sphincters, prostate biopsy, and stone treatment, as well as general open and laparoscopic urologic surgeries. We also address the emerging role of the microbiome in urologic care, antibiotic management for urologic infections in

multiple specific patient scenarios, including UTI in pregnancy, UTI in patients with neurogenic bladder, and infections in the elderly, as well as the workup of pediatric UTI. Sexually transmitted infections and fungal infections are also covered in detail. Our goal is for this issue to provide guidance to physicians in urology as well as in other specialties as we all work to effectively treat urologic infections and provide appropriate prophylaxis prior to procedures in order to minimize incidence of infections. Maintaining efficacy of antibiotics, minimizing morbidity from infection, and managing complex patients in the setting of increasingly resistant organisms are challenges best met by a multidisciplinary approach.

Thank you to all who contributed their time and expertise to this issue. We appreciate all the work that went into assembling this comprehensive review and anticipate that it will serve as a guide for clinicians across the specialties as they manage urologic infections in the modern era.

Michael H. Hsieh, MD, PhD
Division of Urology
Children's National Hospital
111 Michigan Avenue Northwest, 4th Floor
West Wing, Urology
Washington, DC 20010, USA

E-mail address:
mhsieh@childrensnational.org

Urol Clin N Am 51 (2024) xv
https://doi.org/10.1016/j.ucl.2024.08.001
0094-0143/24/© 2024 Published by Elsevier Inc.

Preventing Infections After Prostate Biopsy
Prophylactic Antibiotics, Prebiopsy Rectal Culture, and Biopsy Approach

Nicolai Hubner, MD, Marc Dall'Era, MD*

KEYWORDS

- Prostate biopsy • Infection • Sepsis • Rectal enema • Transrectal • Transperineal
- Antibiotic prophylaxis

KEY POINTS

- Rectal povidone-iodine cleansing can reduce the risk of infection after transrectal prostate biopsy.
- Augmented or targeted antibiotic prophylaxis (based on rectal culture) is safest for transrectal prostate biopsy.
- Transperineal prostate biopsy is associated with a very low risk for postbiopsy infections without the need for prophylactic antibiotics compared to the transrectal approach and should be preferred when feasible.

BACKGROUND

Despite advances in diagnostic evaluation such as multiparametric MRI and prostate-specific membrane antigen-targeted PET, prostate biopsy remains a necessary step in the diagnosis of prostate cancer. With widespread availability of high-quality transrectal ultrasound (TRUS) machines and PSA screening starting in the early 1990s, rates of prostate biopsy increased dramatically. While improved imaging, biomarker use, and risk stratification can reduce the number of men undergoing unnecessary procedures, it is estimated that greater than 1 million prostate biopsies are performed in the United States each year. In addition, with rising acceptance of active surveillance for low-risk prostate cancer as well as focal therapy, many men require multiple biopsy sessions over time.

Historically, prostate biopsy has been performed through the rectal mucosa with TRUS guidance. This approach, while anatomically convenient, is associated with the risk of serious infections as bacteria within the rectum are seeded into the prostate and blood stream during the procedure. Post-prostate biopsy infections, some of which are life threatening, are the most concerning risk of this procedure. Contemporary series report infectious complications after prostate biopsy of 2% to 5%. The Prostate, Lung, Colorectal and Ovarian Cancer Screening trial reported a rate of 7.8 infectious complications per 1000 biopsies but no additional deaths.[1] In the European randomized prostate cancer screening trial, fever was noted in 4.2% of men after biopsy with 0.8% hospital admission rate.[2] Analyzing data from a Surveillance, Epidemiology, and End Results dataset linked to Medicare outcomes, Shoag and colleagues[3] reported rising infection rates between 2001 and 2007, which then leveled off through 2015.

Patients typically present with fever and flu-like symptoms to more serious findings including hypotension, tachycardia, and mental status changes. While patients presenting with these

Department of Urologic Surgery, University of California, Davis, 4860 Y Street, Suite 3500, Sacramento, CA 95817, USA
* Corresponding author.
E-mail address: mdallera@ucdavis.edu

Urol Clin N Am 51 (2024) 439–444
https://doi.org/10.1016/j.ucl.2024.06.001
0094-0143/24/© 2024 Elsevier Inc. All rights reserved, including those for text and data mining, AI training, and similar technologies.

urologic.theclinics.com

symptoms after a prostate biopsy need to be evaluated by a physician immediately, many require hospital admission, systemic intravenous antibiotics, and supportive therapy such as intravenous (IV) fluid resuscitation and intensive care monitoring. Serious forms of bacteremia and septicemia can have a fatal outcome.[2]

The rectal microbiome is exceptionally diverse with both gram-positive and gram-negative organisms. *Escherichia coli* is responsible for most infectious complications after prostate biopsy. While most urinary tract or prostate infections can be treated with oral antibiotics, systemic infections require IV antibiotics. More concerning is rising incidence of multidrug-resistant and extended-spectrum beta lactamase-producing strains globally.[4] As quinolones were the preferred agents for antibiotic prophylaxis during transrectal (TR) biopsy,[5] the risk of postbiopsy infections has increased with rising rates of quinolone resistance in the community. In a series of 1000 men undergoing prostate biopsy, postbiopsy sepsis occurred in 1.2%, and fluoroquinolone-resistant *E coli* (FREC) accounted for 75% of these serious infections.[6] Multiple techniques have been evaluated to reduce the risk from prostate biopsy, such as augmented prophylaxis (with 2 or more agents), targeted prophylaxis after rectal swabs, and iodine rectal cleaning and enemas, yet the data supporting each of these are of mediocre quality and benefits are unclear.

Recently, the TR approach has been abandoned in favor of the transperineal (TP) route, which offers very low risk for infection and postbiopsy sepsis, with better antibiotic stewardship as this approach requires reduced or even no antibiotic prophylaxis. Perceived barriers to TP biopsy include more time and expensive as well as patient pain and anxiety. While most international societies recommend the TP approach to be the preferred one,[5] TR biopsy remains an option. The American Urological Association guidelines on prostate cancer early detection do not make a preference for biopsy approach.[7] The aim of this article is to discuss and summarize the options to reduce the risk of infectious complications from prostate biopsy.

Prebiopsy Evaluation and Antibiotics in Transrectal Prostate Biopsy

Baseline patient factors can contribute to the risk of infections after prostate biopsy and should be carefully assessed. Common comorbid conditions such as diabetes, cancer, immunosuppression, previous exposure to antibiotics, or previous infection after biopsy can all increase the risk and should be taken into account. Recent exposure to fluoroquinolones may put patients at additional risk for harboring resistant *E coli* strains.

Antibiotic Prophylaxis

The American Urological Association white paper on preventing complications after prostate biopsy recommends fluoroquinolone or first, second, or third-generation cephalosporins prior to the procedure. Fluoroquinolone antibiotics have been the first choice for periprocedural antibiotic prophylaxis for TR prostate biopsy, for many years due to their positive pharmacokinetics, allowing for high tissue penetration. Reports of serious toxicities with fluoroquinolone use including tendon rupture have caused their use to be more regulated globally and even suspended in some countries (EMA/795349/2018).[8] Fosfomycin trometamol has been suggested as an alternative for single-agent prophylaxis before prostate biopsy as it showed fewer infectious complications than standard fluoroquinolones in 2 recent meta-analysis (relative risk [RR] 0.49, 95%confidence interval [CI] 0.27–0.87).[9,10] However, the use of fosfomycin trometamol as periprocedural prophylaxis is not licensed in many countries, and higher rates of complications have been shown in other studies.[11] Other possible alternatives for empiric single-agent prophylaxis include cephalosporins and aminoglycosides.[12,13] It is important to understand local resistance patterns of uropathogens to determine best prophylaxis, as local resistance patterns may vary. Additionally, new antibiotics are being developed. Gepotidacin is a new first-in-class antibiotic of the triazaacenaphthylene group. It has been evaluated in phase 2 trials for urinary tract infection and gonorrhea,[14,15] and phase III trials are currently ongoing. Penetration of prostate tissue is specifically being investigated (NCT04484740).

Augmented prophylaxis, using 2 empiric antibiotic agents instead of a single agent, has also been shown to reduce the number of infectious complications in a meta-analysis of 9 studies including 2597 patients (RR for single agent 2.10, 95%CI 1.53–2.88).[9] Multiple combinations have been used in trials including ciprofloxacin and gentamicin, ciprofloxacin and metronidazole, and levofloxacin and amikacin.[16–18] The use of augmented prophylaxis has shown benefit in most trials and is used in many centers. The AUA white paper suggests intramuscular gentamicin or ceftriaxone can be used and need to be given at least 1 hour before biopsy for adequate tissue and serum levels. Gentamicin should be dosed based on patient weight to maximize utility while minimizing potential toxicity. Use of multiple antibiotics, however, can contribute rising bacterial resistance to these antibiotics.

Targeted prophylaxis has been described as another option to further reduce infectious complications after prostate biopsy. For this, a rectal swab culture is performed prior to biopsy, and antibiotic prophylaxis is then selected based on the culture results. If no resistant bacteria are present, the standard empiric regimen can be used. In a meta-analysis including 6 studies and 1511 patients regarding this endpoint, the use of targeted over empiric prophylaxis significantly reduced the risk for infectious complications (RR for empiric prophylaxis 1.81, 95%CI 1.28–2.55). Interestingly, one of the larger prospective trials included in this meta-analysis of 496 patients randomized to receive empiric, augmented, or targeted prophylaxis showed higher rates of infections in the targeted prophylaxis group. This study, however, utilized a single dose of targeted prophylaxis, which may have contributed to these findings.[16] A retrospective study including 13 Southern California Kaiser Permanente clinics and over 15,000 patients also found no significant difference in postbiopsy sepsis rates comparing empiric antibiotic to targeted antibiotic use. While the overall rate of sepsis was low (0.64%), further analyses showed that augmented prophylaxis was better than either the targeted or the single-agent empiric approach.[19] Time and cost constraints may limit the utility of a targeted prophylaxis approach for prostate biopsy. A recent study, from the Netherlands randomized 636 patients to receive targeted prophylaxis after rectal swab culture or empiric fluoroquinolone (ciprofloxacin) prophylaxis, found that targeted prophylaxis was associated with significantly increased health care costs over the empiric approach.[20] As found in other studies, FREC on rectal swab was the greatest risk factor for infectious complication after TR prostate biopsy, which was found in 15.4% of cases. A sensitivity analysis showed that an FREC incidence rate of 40% was necessary for the targeted prophylaxis approach to be cost effective. Local resistance patterns should be evaluated before selecting the best infection prevention strategy for an individual practice.

Biopsy Needle Disinfection and Rectal Preparation

Several investigators have evaluated the protective effect of biopsy needle disinfection between each sample core being taken. Formalin (10% solution) needle disinfection was associated with a very low postbiopsy infection or sepsis rate compared with historical controls in a single institution, nonrandomized study.[21] Abughosh and colleagues performed a randomized trial comparing rectal cleansing with povidone-iodine versus no preparation prior to transrectal prostate biopsy. Although they noted a 46% percent relative risk reduction (2.6% vs 4.5%) in favor of rectal cleansing, the difference was not statistically significant. On multivariate analysis, ciprofloxacin resistance or recent history of taking ciprofloxacin was an independent risk factor for infection.[22] A more recent meta-analysis of 90 randomized controlled trials including 16,941 patients evaluated multiple risk factors and interventions in the setting of prostate biopsy regarding their association with infectious complications.[23] The authors showed that, other than use of the TP approach, rectal preparation using povidone-iodine had a statistically significant impact on reducing the risk infectious complications by 50% (RR 0.50, 95%CI 0.38–0.65; $P > .001$). Rectal preparation with povidone-iodine also significantly reduced hospitalization rates after biopsy (RR 0.38, 95%CI 0.21–0.69; $P = .002$). No other modifiable factors such as number of biopsy cores, periprostatic nerve-block, number of injections for periprostatic nerve block, needle guide type, needle type, and rectal enema were associated with infections. The authors note, however, that the overall rating of evidence was low for all the interventions mentioned earlier. The individual studies included into the metanalysis showed similar results in regards to the positive effect of povidone-iodine rectal preparation.[24] This benefit was improved if done prior to biopsy as opposed to after biopsy.[25] The most recent European Association of Urology (EAU) guidelines recommend the use of povidone-iodine rectal preparation in addition to antibiotic prophylaxis prior to transrectal prostate biopsy.

Transperineal Prostate Biopsy

TP prostate biopsy offers an alternative approach to preventing infections after prostate biopsy while limiting antibiotic overuse. In recent years, TP prostate biopsy has become the preferred approach when feasible as recommended in the most recent EAU guidelines. With this technique, the prostate is still visualized using TRUS; however, needle placement is done through the perineal skin. Povidone-iodine disinfection of the skin should be used to achieve a sterile field and both the perineal skin and prostate are anesthetized with lidocaine. Currently, single-agent empiric antibiotic prophylaxis with a first-generation cephalosporin is still used in most centers; however, prospective trials suggest this may not be necessary. Jacewicz and colleagues had showed that with TP biopsy, there was no significant difference in postbiopsy infections or sepsis with or without antibiotic prophylaxis. Overall, 555 patients were randomized to receive either 1.5 g of cefuroxime or not, prior to TP biopsy. Within their cohort, no patients in either group suffered from postprocedure infection or sepsis requiring hospitalization (difference 0%, 95%CI −1.37 to 1.37).[26]

While TP prostate biopsy outcomes have been reported in multiple retrospective series, 2 recent randomized, prospective trials compared TR with TP biopsy and reported on infectious complications and cancer detection with each approach. Hu and colleagues[27] compared TP biopsy without antibiotics versus TR biopsy with targeted prophylaxis (ie, prior rectal swab culture and antibiotic prophylaxis according to findings) in 658 patients in the PREVENT clinical trial. The primary endpoint was an infectious complication within 7 days of the biopsy with zero infections reported after TP biopsy and 4 (1.4%) infections after TR biopsy. The difference between groups of 1.4% was not statistically significant (95% CI −3.2% to 0.3%; $P = .059$). The secondary endpoint of cancer detection showed a similar rates of clinically significant prostate cancer (csPCa) in both arms (53% vs 50%). Similarly, Mian and colleagues[28] randomized 763 men to undergo TR versus TP prostate biopsy under local anesthetic and found no difference in infectious complications between the groups, and no patients developed sepsis after biopsy. It is important to note that in both studies, the TP approach allowed patients to avoid taking any antibiotic prophylaxis. A third randomized trial by Ploussard and colleagues compared TP versus TR biopsy with the primary endpoint being the detection of csPCa, defined as Gleason Grade Group 2 or greater and secondary endpoint of grade 2 or greater adverse events. Overall, 270 patients were randomized to receive MRI-targeted TP versus TR biopsy and csPCA was found in 47.2% for TP and 54.2% for TR patients.[29] Overall detection rates of any cancer were also comparable with 71.3% and 64.1% for TP versus TR, respectively. There was no significant difference in adverse events between the groups, and only one patient (0.8%), from the TR group, experienced grade 3 sepsis. Unfortunately, there was no clear information on the periprocedural antibiotics used in this study.

With multiple prospective randomized trials now confirming favorable outcomes regarding infectious complications even when omitting antibiotic prophylaxis, the TP approach appears to offer a safe approach to prostate biopsy with similar cancer detection and better antibiotic stewardship for the world.[30]

SUMMARY

While uncommon, infections after prostate biopsy can be associated with considerable risk of morbidity and rarely mortality. Rectal cleansing with povidone-iodine and augmented antibiotic prophylaxis can reduce the risk of infection after TR prostate biopsy. Overall, the use of TP biopsy minimizes the risk of infection while optimizing antibiotic stewardship. The TR approach can achieve equally low rates of infection as with TP biopsy, although with substantially more intense antibiotic regimens. Local antibiotic resistance patterns and costs should also be considered when choosing the optimal approach to infection prevention for individual practices.

CLINICS CARE POINTS

- If TR biopsy is performed, the safest antibiotic regimen is a targeted antibiotic prophylaxis, after performing rectal swab culture.
- Locoregional resistance patterns, especially for *E coli* bacteria, should be considered when deciding on empiric prophylaxis.
- Rectal povidone-iodine cleansing or enemas can reduce the risk of infectious complications after TR prostate biopsy.
- The TP prostate biopsy is associated with a very low risk for postbiopsy infections without the need for prophylactic antibiotics compared to the TR approach and should be preferred when feasible.

DISCLOSURE

The authors have nothing to disclose.

REFERENCES

1. Pinsky PF, Parnes HL, Andriole G. Mortality and complications after prostate biopsy in the Prostate, Lung, Colorectal and Ovarian Cancer Screening (PLCO) trial. BJU Int 2014;113(2):254–9.
2. Loeb S, van den Heuvel S, Zhu X, et al. Infectious complications and hospital admissions after prostate biopsy in a European randomized trial. Eur Urol 2012;61(6):1110–4.
3. Shoag JE, Gaffney C, Pantuck M, et al. Risk factors for infection after prostate biopsy in the United States. Urology 2020;138:113–8.
4. MacKinnon MC, McEwen SA, Pearl DL, et al. Increasing incidence and antimicrobial resistance

in Escherichia coli bloodstream infections: a multinational population-based cohort study. Antimicrob Resist Infect Control 2021;10(1):131.

5. Mottet N, Bellmunt J, Bolla M, et al. EAU-ESTRO-SIOG guidelines on prostate cancer. part 1: screening, diagnosis, and local treatment with curative intent. Eur Urol 2017;71(4):618–29.

6. Pinkhasov GI, Lin Y-K, Palmerola R, et al. Complications following prostate needle biopsy requiring hospital admission or emergency department visits - experience from 1000 consecutive cases. BJU Int 2012;110(3):369–74.

7. Wei JT, Barocas D, Carlsson S, et al. Early detection of prostate cancer: AUA/SUO Guideline Part II: considerations for a prostate biopsy. J Urol 2023;210(1): 54–63.

8. Bonkat G, Pilatz A, Wagenlehner F. Time to adapt our practice? the european commission has restricted the use of fluoroquinolones since March 2019. Eur Urol 2019;76(3):273–5. Switzerland.

9. Pilatz A, Dimitropoulos K, Veeratterapillay R, et al. Antibiotic prophylaxis for the prevention of infectious complications following prostate biopsy: a systematic review and meta-analysis. J Urol 2020;204(2): 224–30.

10. Noreikaite J, Jones P, Fitzpatrick J, et al. Fosfomycin vs. quinolone-based antibiotic prophylaxis for transrectal ultrasound-guided biopsy of the prostate: a systematic review and meta-analysis. Prostate Cancer Prostatic Dis 2018;21(2): 153–60.

11. Carignan A, Sabbagh R, Masse V, et al. Effectiveness of fosfomycin tromethamine prophylaxis in preventing infection following transrectal ultrasound-guided prostate needle biopsy: Results from a large Canadian cohort. J Glob Antimicrob Resist 2019;17:112–6.

12. Cam K, Kayikci A, Akman Y, et al. Prospective assessment of the efficacy of single dose versus traditional 3-day antimicrobial prophylaxis in 12-core transrectal prostate biopsy. Int J Urol Off J Japanese Urol Assoc 2008;15(11):997–1001.

13. Chazan B, Zelichenko G, Shental Y, et al. Antimicrobial prophylaxis for transrectal ultrasound guided biopsy of prostate: a comparative study between single dose of Gentamicin vs. Ofloxacin. Int J Infect Dis 2010;14:e199–200.

14. Overcash JS, Tiffany CA, Scangarella-Oman NE, et al. Phase 2a pharmacokinetic, safety, and exploratory efficacy evaluation of oral gepotidacin (GSK2140944) in female participants with uncomplicated urinary tract infection (acute uncomplicated cystitis). Antimicrob Agents Chemother 2020;64(7). https://doi.org/10.1128/AAC.00199-20.

15. Watkins RR, Thapaliya D, Lemonovich TL, et al. Gepotidacin: a novel, oral, 'first-in-class' triazaacenaphthylene antibiotic for the treatment of uncomplicated urinary tract infections and urogenital gonorrhoea. J Antimicrob Chemother 2023;78(5):1137–42.

16. Elshal AM, Atwa AM, El-Nahas AR, et al. Chemoprophylaxis during transrectal prostate needle biopsy: critical analysis through randomized clinical trial. World J Urol 2018;36:1845–52.

17. Miyazaki Y, Akamatsu S, Kanamaru S, et al. A prospective randomized trial comparing a combined regimen of amikacin and levofloxacin to levofloxacin alone as prophylaxis in transrectal prostate needle biopsy. Urol J 2016;13(1):2533–40.

18. Izadpanahi M-H, Nouri-Mahdavi K, Majidi SM, et al. Clinical study addition of ceftriaxone and amikacin to a ciprofloxacin plus metronidazole regimen for preventing infectious complications of transrectal ultrasound-guided prostate biopsy: a randomized controlled trial. Adv Urol 2017;2017(1):4635386.

19. Jiang P, Liss MA, Szabo RJ. Targeted antimicrobial prophylaxis does not always prevent sepsis after transrectal prostate biopsy. J Urol 2018;200(2): 361–8.

20. Tops SCM, Kolwijck E, Koldewijn EL, et al. Cost effectiveness of rectal culture-based antibiotic prophylaxis in transrectal prostate biopsy: the results from a randomized, nonblinded, multicenter trial. Eur Urol Open Sci 2023;50:70–7.

21. Issa MM, Al-Qassab UA, Hall J, et al. Formalin disinfection of biopsy needle minimizes the risk of sepsis following prostate biopsy. J Urol 2013;190(5): 1769–75.

22. Abughosh Z, Margolick J, Goldenberg SL, et al. A prospective randomized trial of povidone-iodine prophylactic cleansing of the rectum before transrectal ultrasound guided prostate biopsy. J Urol 2013;189(4):1326–31.

23. Pradere B, Veeratterapillay R, Dimitropoulos K, et al. Nonantibiotic Strategies for the prevention of infectious complications following prostate biopsy: a systematic review and meta-analysis. J Urol 2021; 205(3):653–63.

24. Ergani B, Çetin T, Yalçın MY, et al. Effect of rectal mucosa cleansing on acute prostatitis during prostate biopsy: A randomized prospective study. Turkish J Urol 2020;46(2):159–64.

25. Yu L, Ma L, Yu H. [Impact of insertion timing of iodophor cotton ball on the control of infection complications after transrectal ultrasound guided prostate biopsy]. Zhonghua Yixue Zazhi 2014;94(8): 609–11.

26. Jacewicz M, Günzel K, Rud E, et al. Antibiotic prophylaxis versus no antibiotic prophylaxis in transperineal prostate biopsies (NORAPP): a randomised, open-label, non-inferiority trial. Lancet Infect Dis 2022;22(10):1465–71.

27. Hu JC, Assel M, Allaf ME, et al. Transperineal versus transrectal magnetic resonance imaging-targeted and systematic prostate biopsy to prevent infectious

complications: the PREVENT randomized trial. Eur Urol 2024. https://doi.org/10.1016/j.eururo.2023.12.015.

28. Mian BM, Feustel PJ, Aziz A, et al. Complications following transrectal and transperineal prostate biopsy: results of the probe-pc randomized clinical trial. J Urol 2024;211(2):205–13.

29. Ploussard G, Barret E, Fiard G, et al. Transperineal versus transrectal magnetic resonance imaging-targeted biopsies for prostate cancer diagnosis: final results of the randomized PERFECT trial (CCAFU-PR1). Eur Urol Oncol 2024. https://doi.org/10.1016/j.euo.2024.01.019.

30. Liss MA, Ehdaie B, Loeb S, et al. An update of the American Urological Association white paper on the prevention and treatment of the more common complications related to prostate biopsy. J Urol 2017;198(2):329–34.

Advances in Bowel Preparation and Antimicrobial Prophylaxis for Open and Laparoscopic Urologic Surgery

Oluwafolajimi Adesanya, MD[a], Nick Bowler, MD[b], Sean Tafuri, MD[b], Alanna Cruz-Bendezu, MD[b], Michael J. Whalen, MD[c],*

KEYWORDS

- Bowel preparation • Antimicrobial prophylaxis • Robotic surgery • Laparoscopic surgery • Urology

KEY POINTS

- Oral mechanical bowel preparation is recommended for open, laparoscopic or robotic urologic surgeries requiring manipulation of the colorectal bowel segment.
- Preoperative antibiotic bowel preparation remains a mainstay of clean-contaminated open, laparoscopic or robotic urologic surgeries with bowel manipulation.
- Enhanced Recovery After Surgery protocols have been implemented successfully for radical cystectomy and robot-assisted laparoscopic prostatectomy.
- Preoperative antibiotic prophylaxis is indicated in clean open, laparoscopic or robotic urologic surgeries only during prosthesis implantation or when inguinal/perineal incision is necessary.
- Antibiotics for preoperative prophylaxis are often administered within 1 hour of skin incision and discontinued within 24 hours post-procedure.

BOWEL PREPARATION IN SURGERY: HISTORY, PRINCIPLES, AND EVOLUTION

The gastrointestinal tract houses over 35,000 bacterial species, with up to 10^{12} bacteria per gram of fecal content.[1] It is no surprise therefore, that bowel surgeries have the highest rates of surgical site infections (SSIs), ranging from 5.5% to 23.2%,[2] portending a significant risk to postoperative patient outcomes, morbidity and even mortality rates.[3] Bowel preparation involves the cleansing of the bowel lumen, through the oral, rectal or a combined oral and rectal approach, and has been in use for several decades as a preoperative strategy to reduce the risk of SSI following gastrointestinal (GI) tract surgery. Mechanical bowel preparation (MBP) using an osmotically active agent to decompress the bowel prior to surgery, was the standard approach utilized in the early years, despite a lack of explicit evidence of its benefits in reducing surgical morbidity.[4] In 1971, Nichols and Condon reported a new approach which combined MBP, with prophylactic oral antibiotics neomycin and erythromycin.[5,6] They explain that the MBP served to cleanse the gut of fecal matter, while facilitating the action of the oral antibiotics to decrease the gut burden of

a Department of Urology, James Buchanan Brady Urological Institute, Johns Hopkins University School of Medicine, Baltimore, MD 21287-2101, USA; b Department of Urology, George Washington University Hospital, Washington, DC 20037, USA; c Department of Urology, George Washington University School of Medicine, Washington, DC 20037, USA
* Corresponding author.
E-mail address: mwhalen@mfa.gwu.edu

Urol Clin N Am 51 (2024) 445–465
https://doi.org/10.1016/j.ucl.2024.06.005
0094-0143/24/© 2024 Elsevier Inc. All rights are reserved, including those for text and data mining, AI training, and similar technologies.

bacteria. Thus, the subsequent years saw an increased adoption of this combined approach, which was aided by new meta-analytic evidence reported by Baum and colleagues, in 1981.[7] Soon, intravenous antibiotics began to replace oral agents within bowel preparation regimens, due to their relative convenience with respect to perioperative dosing and obviating the need for preoperative patient prescriptions and proper patient education. In 1990, Smith and colleagues demonstrated the benefit of combined preoperative oral and perioperative intravenous antibiotic administration, over either approach alone in reducing rates of postoperative SSIs.[8]

In spite of this evidence, the use of oral antibiotics within bowel preparation regimens continued to decline, and by 2010, Markell and colleagues showed that only 39% of surveyed North American surgeons routinely administered preoperative oral antibiotics,[9] a notable decline when compared to 1990. However, subsequent meta-analyses by Ross and colleagues, in 2013 and Nelson and colleagues, in 2014, demonstrated an up-to 44% reduction in risk of SSIs following a combined use of oral and intravenous antibiotics, compared to using each approach alone,[10,11] thus, heralding the resurgence of this approach by 2015, with its re-introduction within several clinical practice guidelines.[12–14] However, the choice of antibiotic remained a controversy as the various clinical trials utilized different agents, nevertheless, it was believed that the appropriate antibiotic agent for bowel preparation would possess aerobic and/or aneorbic coverage, as needed, to be effective.[10] The most commonly-used agents are 1g oral neomycin and 1g oral metronidazole, taken 12 hourly on the day prior to surgery, and a single-dose amikacin/metronidazole administered intravenously at surgery.[15] The currently-accepted methodology of preoperative MBP (when justified by the specific surgical procedure; see below) involves using an oral lavage of a large volume (4L) or small volume (2L) of polyethylene glycol (PEG), an osmotically-balanced electrolyte solution, with bisacodyl, a laxative. The PEG solution cleanses the colon by mechanical washout while bisacodyl promotes colonic peristalsis to aid bowel decompression and reduce volume-related discomfort including bloating and cramping induced by the PEG solution.[16,17] Common alternatives include osmotically-active phosphate, picophosphate or magnesium-based salt solutions, which have the benefit of requiring less volume, compared to PEG-based solutions, but come with an increased risk of precipitating electrolyte imbalance with deleterious impact on renal function.[18]

RELEVANCE OF MECHANICAL BOWEL PREPARATION: EVIDENCE AND GUIDELINES

While several Randomized Controlled Trials (RCTs) and meta-analyses had established the benefits of preoperative oral and perioperative intravenous antibiotic administration, MBP has remained the more controversial aspect of bowel preparation, as no study has investigated the benefit of MBP alone to SSI reduction postoperatively. Rather, studies emerged questioning the usefulness of MBP.[19] In a prospective RCT, Contant and colleagues, showed no significant difference in colonic anastomotic leak rates, between patients who received MBP and those who did not.[20] Another retrospective study reported similar results suggesting the omission of MBP prior to colorectal surgery did not significantly impact outcomes.[21] Further, Bucher and colleagues, demonstrated a significant association between preoperative MBP and postoperative complications including erosion of superficial bowel mucosa, and inflammatory lymphocytic and polymorphonuclear infiltrates in the colonic surface.[22] Several other RCTs[23–25] and meta-analyses[26–29] have been conducted, none of which provide conclusive evidence of the benefits of MBP alone regarding the improvement of postoperative outcomes following elective colorectal surgery. While the 2-day preoperative administration oral MBP remains recommended in combination with preoperative oral antibiotics, per the most recent ACS bowel preparation and SSI prevention practice guidelines,[12,17] the evidence in support of this recommendation remains moderate, thus, encouraging the consideration of an alternative approach termed limited bowel preparation (LBP), which excludes the extensive use of oral MBP prior to surgery.

BOWEL PREPARATION IN UROLOGIC SURGERY: EVOLUTION AND EVIDENCE

Radical cystectomy has emerged as the standard-of-care for muscle-invasive bladder cancer.[30] Urinary diversion in this procedure is accomplished through the reconstruction of the native bowel. While several approaches for urinary diversion exist, the most common technique involves ureteral anastomosis to a distal segment of the ileum, which acts as a conduit for urine flow to a cutaneous stoma.[31] However, the bowel manipulation involved in this reconstructive step creates an avenue for bacterial contamination of the peritoneum. Preoperative bowel preparation with a combination of MBP and antibiotic prophylaxis has been routinely used to mitigate bacterial contamination and associated morbidity following urinary diversion;[32,33] however, while preoperative antibiotic prophylaxis had been established as a critical component of this process, several studies failed to prove a similar benefit for oral MBP. This has called the practice into question among colorectal surgeons, and more recently, among urologic surgeons as well. Tabibi and colleagues, reported results from a single institution prospective clinical trial, in which there were no significant differences in postoperative anastomotic leak, enterocutaneous fistula, wound infection and dehiscence among 30 patients who underwent standard 3-day oral MBP and 32 patients who obtained LBP with soft diet and no oral intake 8 hours prior to ileal urinary diversion surgery.[34] A subsequent clinical trial by Large and colleagues, and meta-analyses by Yang and colleagues, and Deng and colleagues, yielded similar findings, failing to demonstrate the benefit comprehensive oral MBP on bowel leak, bowel obstruction, and overall mortality indices, following urinary diversion using the ileal bowel segment.[35–37] A more recent meta-analysis of 6 clinical trials, by Feng and colleagues, demonstrated significantly reduced time to first bowel activity (SMD -0.77, 95% CI -1.47 to −0.07), risk of fever (RR 0.53, 95% CI 0.33–0.85), time to first flatus (SMD -1.06, 95% CI -2.02 to −0.10) and risk of wound healing disorders (RR 0.65, 95% CI 0.44–0.95) in patients who received LBP, compared with those who received comprehensive bowel preparation (CBP) prior to ileal urinary diversion surgery.[38] In line with the evidence, the American Urologic Association (AUA) recommends no bowel preparation prior to urinary diversion surgery if a small bowel segment is used;[39] however, CBP with MBP and oral antibiotics is recommended if a colorectal segment is to be used, in line with the current recommendations from the American Society of Colon and Rectal Surgeons (ASCRS).[40] This may be a result of the higher microbial burden of the colorectal bowel compared with the small bowel.[41]

ENHANCED RECOVERY AFTER SURGERY PATHWAYS: IN UROLOGY AND BEYOND

Enhanced Recovery After Surgery (ERAS) is a patient-centered, multimodal surgical care pathway, aimed at fast-tracking patient postoperative recovery by reducing the body's overall reaction to the stress of surgery.[42] The ERAS protocol involves implementing care strategies that optimize patient nutritional status, preoperative patient counseling, promote the use of non-opioid analgesia, standardize anesthetic regimens, and encourage trials of early postoperative oral feeding and ambulation, all aimed to reduce the incidence of postoperative ileus which translates into prolonged postoperative length-of-stay (LOS) and higher overall cost-of-care.[40,43] First proposed in 1997, by a group of surgeons in Northern Europe, for patients undergoing colorectal surgery, the principles of ERAS quickly spread to involve surgeons all over the world and from other surgical specialties, aided primarily by significant success in its early years.[44,45] At their core, ERAS protocols aim to achieve early recovery of bowel function, a critical factor influencing postoperative LOS. In the modern era, this objective is achieved primarily via the administration of alvimopan, an oral, peripherally-acting μ-opioid antagonist, which acts by minimizing the effects of opioid analgesics on bowel function.[40,46] Significant level one evidence via RCTs and even meta-analyses have provided irrefutable proof of alvimopan's ability to accelerate recovery of bowel function, reduce postoperative LOS and cost-of-care in patient undergoing open GI surgery.[47–56] Following their success in open colorectal surgery, ERAS protocols were implemented in urologic surgery, with a focus on radical cystectomy patients (**Fig. 1**), and with alvimopan being offered to these patients as early as 2011.[57] By 2012, Vora and colleagues,

Preoperative	Intraoperative	Postoperative
• Preoperative patient counseling • Nutritional counseling • Self training on abdominal stoma care • Preoperative carbohydrate loading • Preoperative medical optimization • Smoking cessation advice • Anemia correction • Omitting preoperative oral mechanical bowel preparation	• Regional (epidural) anesthesia • Antimicrobial prophylaxis • Antiseptic skin preparation • Thromboembolic prophylaxis • Preventing intraoperative hypothermia • Restrictive perioperative fluid management • Remove nasogastric tube at end of surgery • Minimally invasive surgery • Urinary drainage	• Prevention of postoperative ileus using alvimopan or MgO • Prevention of postoperative nausea and vomitting • Postoperative non-opioid analgesia e.g., celecoxib • Early mobilization beginning 3h postop • Early oral diet with clear fluid 3h postop • Postoperative physiotherapy form postop day 1

Fig. 1. An Enhanced Recovery After Surgery protocol for radical cystectomy with urinary diversion and neobladder reconstruction, focusing on limited bowel preparation and utilizing a standardized feeding and analgesia regimen. Original image with data from Nakamura and colleagues[66] postop: postoperative.

reported results from the first RCT of alvimopan in radical cystectomy patients, demonstrating significantly reduced postoperative time to first flatus (3.1 vs 5.6 days, $P<.001$), bowel movement (3.8 vs 6.0 days, $P<.001$), initiation of liquid diet (4.1 vs 6.3 days, $P<.001$), initiation of regular diet (5.7 vs 7.3 days, $P = .023$), LOS (7.4 vs 9.5 days, $P = .04$) and frequency of postoperative ileus (0% vs 25.9%, $P = .012$).[58] Similar results were obtained from multiple other RCTs,[59–61] and meta-analyses,[62–65] firmly establishing the safety and efficacy of alvimopan specifically, and ERAS pathways in general, in patients undergoing major urologic surgery including radical cystectomy and even radical prostatectomy.

Bowel Preparation for Open, Laparoscopic, and Robotic Urologic Surgery: Current Recommendations

With a focus on laparoscopic and open urologic surgery, we present the current guideline recommendations on the use of bowel preparation across the different classes of surgical wounds (summarized in **Table 1**) below. A summary of these recommendations is presented in **Table 2**.

CLEAN CASES

Preoperative bowel preparation is only indicated for urologic surgeries involving manipulation of a bowel segment, which could be ileal or colorectal.

Bowel preparation is thus not necessary for most clean procedures as they do not fulfill this criterion, and they may unnecessarily expose patients to the adverse effects of MBP including metabolic disturbances and microbiota alterations.[67,68] The role of oral laxatives and/or osmotic agents like PEG or magnesium citrate for "colonic decompression" is not evidence-based, although still implemented by practicing surgeons (see below).

CLEAN-CONTAMINATED CASES WITHOUT BOWEL MANIPULATION

The need for MBP in clean-contaminated open and laparoscopic cases such as robot-assisted laparoscopic prostatectomy or robotic nephrectomy has been questioned. Recent studies have failed to demonstrate evidence of the benefit of MBP prior to laparoscopic/robotic prostatectomy or nephrectomy.[69–71] MBP can likely be omitted in these cases, however, expert opinion suggests that bowel preparation may improve visualization during surgery, thus, LBP with a clear liquid diet the day before surgery, and a half dose of magnesium citrate may be considered in these patients.[72]

CONTAMINATED CASES WITH BOWEL MANIPULATION

The AUA currently recommends the use of CBP with oral antibiotics and MBP for contaminated

Table 1
National research council wound classification criteria

Classification	Postoperative Risk of Infection	Criteria
Clean (Class I)	1%–5%	Elective (not urgent or emergency) procedure; closed; no inflammation; no entry into the gastrointestinal, genitourinary, oropharyngeal, biliary, or tracheobronchial tracts; no sterile technique break (eg, adrenalectomy, lymphadenectomy)
Clean-contaminated (Class II)	3%–11%	Urgent or emergency; elective; controlled entry into the gastrointestinal, genitourinary, oropharyngeal, biliary, or tracheobronchial tracts; minimal spillage; minor sterile technique break (eg, ureterectomy, pyeloplasty, radical prostatectomy, partial cystectomy)
Contaminated (Class III)	10%–17%	Acute and non-purulent inflammation; major spillage from hollow viscera; major break in sterile technique; penetrating trauma less than 4 hours old (eg, transrectal prostate biopsy, ureteroscopy)
Dirty (Class IV)	27%–40%	Purulent; preoperative perforation of the gastrointestinal, genitourinary, oropharyngeal, biliary, or tracheobronchial tracts; penetrating trauma more than 4 hours old

Table 2
Bowel preparation recommendations for open, laparoscopic and robotic urologic surgery

Procedure Classification	Procedure Examples	Recommended Bowel Preparation	Bowel Preparation of Choice (if Indicated)
Class I (clean procedures)	Adrenalectomy; lymphadenectomy; prosthetic device implantation (AUS, IPP, sacral neuromodulators); groin and perineal procedures for example, vasectomy, orchiectomy, hydrocelectomy, varicocelectomy.	No bowel preparation indicated	n/a
Class II (clean-contaminated procedures)	Nephrectomy; ureterectomy; radical prostatectomy; cystectomy; urinary diversion with small bowel conduit; PCN; Vaginal surgery for example, fistula repair, urethral sling for stress incontinence	No bowel preparation indicated	n/a or LBP with a clear liquid diet the day before surgery, and a half dose of magnesium citrate
Class III (contaminated procedures)	Urinary diversion with large bowel conduit	Bowel preparation not indicated for cases utilizing ileum Cases utilizing a colorectal segment should undergo mechanical bowel preparation in addition to an oral antibiotic regimen Patients should undergo routine colonoscopy prior to utilization of colon for urinary diversion	Consider 238 g of PEG-3350 mixed with 1.9 L of Gatorade, starting 8 PM the night before surgery patients should consume 8 ounces of the solution every 10 minutes–15 minutes until completion plus 1g oral neomycin and 1g oral erythromycin administered at 2 PM, 3 PM and 10 PM the day before surgery, 500 mg doses of metronidazole may be substituted for erythromycin

urologic cases involving the manipulation of the colorectal segment, while such procedures involving use of an ileal segment do not require bowel preparation prior to surgery.[39] This is supported by numerous studies showing that MBP is not necessary prior to radical cystectomy with ileal urinary diversion,[36,73] and is echoed by other practice guidelines from the European Association of Urology and the ERAS society.[74,75] While there is no recommendation regarding a specific gent for MBP, 238 g of PEG-3350 mixed with 1.9 L of Gatorade was found to be well tolerated by patients.[76] The PEG mixture should be commenced at 8 PM on the day prior to surgery at a dose of 8 ounces every 10 minutes to 15 minutes until completion.[76] Similarly, while no specific guideline recommendation has been made on the optimal choice of antibiotic for bowel preparation, a combination of 1g oral neomycin and 1g oral erythromycin administered at 2 PM, 3 PM and 10 PM on the day prior to surgery, is widely used. Erythromycin may be replaced with 500 mg of metronidazole for improved tolerability.[17,77] Of note, in additional to pharmacologic bowel preparation, it is advisable to have routine colonoscopy performed by gastroenterology or colorectal surgery to screen for colorectal cancer prior to utilization of colon for urinary diversion.

Complications of Bowel Preparation

Metabolic disturbances

Although bowel preparation is generally well-tolerated when performed appropriately, mild complications including nausea, vomiting, bloating, and abdominal discomfort have been associated with the use of oral MBP solutions.[67] Sodium phosphate (NaP)-based solutions have particularly been linked to severe complications such as ileus and significant electrolyte disturbances including hyponatremia, hyperphosphatemia, hypocalcemia, and hypokalemia, with the latter being the most feared of these disturbances.[78–80] NaP-induced hyperphosphatemia is exacerbated by the ability of NaP to decrease serum creatinine clearance time, raising major concerns for its use in patients with impaired renal function.[81] Further, NaP has been found to significantly decrease blood pH levels, leading to metabolic acidosis and seizures, particularly in the elderly and in dehydrated patients.[81,82] Alternatively, PEG-based oral MBP solutions are iso-osmotic with serum plasma, and do not cause electrolyte imbalance. Thus, PEG-based oral MBP solutions are preferred in elderly patients and patients with impaired renal function, heart failure or inflammatory bowel disease.[83]

Microbiota alterations

MBP has also been associated with significant alterations in bowel microbiota population, and erosion of the colonic mucosa, leading to increased bacterial translocation across the bowel wall.[22,84] This effect has been reported to be transient, with studies indicating a return to baseline microbiota composition within 14 days post-bowel preparation.[68] While the use of probiotics has been proposed to reduce gut microbiota disruptions and shorten time to recovery following MBP,[85] there are insufficient data at this time to validate the efficacy of this approach.

PREOPERATIVE ANTIMICROBIAL PROPHYLAXIS: HISTORY AND EVOLUTION

Prior to the discovery of antibiotics, surgical procedures were fraught with high postoperative infection rates, with deleterious and often fatal consequences on patient outcomes. Following the discovery of the first antibiotics, penicillin, mid-20th century surgeons now had a revolutionary tool for managing and preventing SSIs, resulting in a precipitous fall in postoperative infection rates and widespread improvement in patient outcomes. Hughes and colleagues, reported that prophylaxis with penicillin alone, lowered postoperative infection rates following abdominal surgery by 15%,[86] while an analysis of 9 clinical trials conducted between 1960 and 1980, reported reduced postoperative infection rates in patients receiving antibiotic prophylaxis compared to patients who did not (48% vs 26%).[87] These profound benefits resulted in a wide swing of the pendulum toward disseminated, haphazard, and unregulated preoperative administration of antibiotics, often determined solely by the surgeon's discretion. Such unguided approach precipitated the acute rise of antibiotic-resistant infections, such that by the late 1960s, over 80% of community and hospital-acquired *Staphylococcus aureus* strains were penicillin-resistant,[88] and by the late 1980s, methicillin-resistance had become endemic in the United States, affecting a third of hospitalized *S. aureus*-infected patients.[89] This informed an urgent need for guidance on antibiotic prophylaxis in surgical contexts, with several national health care organizations and professional societies including the Center for Disease Control (CDC),[90] the American College of Surgeons (ACS)[91] and the American Society of Health System Pharmacists (ASHP)[92] responding by releasing the first of such practice guidelines over the course of the next decade. These guidelines provided much needed clarity on several controversial aspects of pre-operative antibiotic prophylaxis administration including patient risk stratification, indications, and procedure-specific recommendations; however, the following decades would witness continued debate among surgeons on topics such as the most appropriate choice of antibiotic for preoperative prophylaxis, timing, as well as route of antibiotic administration, to maximize efficacy and minimize adverse events.

Choosing the Right Antibiotic: Principles and Determinants

The choice of antibiotic for preoperative prophylactic use depends on several factors including procedure type, procedure location, likely organism(s) to be encountered, patient's clinical profile including history of prior antibiotic use or antibiotic-resistant infection, drug adverse effect, and cost concerns.[93] The original surgical wound classification system developed by the National Academy of Science and the National Research Council defines 4 classes of surgical wounds—clean (Class I), clean-contaminated (Class II), contaminated (Class III), and dirty wounds (Class IV), with risk of infection of less than 2%, less than 10%, 20% and 40%, respectively (see Table 1).[94,95] Early guidelines on preoperative antibiotic prophylaxis focused on its use in Class II and some Class III surgical procedures, with a recognition that its use in most other contaminated (Class III) and dirty (Class IV) procedures, was largely therapeutic rather than prophylactic, as

SSIs have either already been or would likely be established in these cases, by definition.[91]

The use of preoperative prophylaxis in Class I surgeries, however, remained controversial, due to the inherently low risk of infection in these procedures, which may pale in comparison with the potential adverse effect of antibiotic use, with resistance development being of principle concern. Thus, antibiotic prophylaxis was highly restricted in clean procedures, with consideration only for those clean procedures in which even minor infections would portend dire consequences on patient outcomes, as is often the case in major cardiovascular surgeries, as well as during the insertion or replacement of prosthetic devices including artificial joints, implants, and heart valves.[91,96]

As a general principle, early guidelines widely recommended cefazolin, a first-generation cephalosporin, as the preferred antibiotic for most clean-contaminated procedures requiring prophylaxis, as it met most of the requisite criteria including efficacy against commonly encountered gram-negative enterics of the GI and genitourinary (GU) tract, long duration of action allowing for infrequent dosing, low risk of adverse events, and relatively low cost.[91,92] A review of the most recent ASHP guideline indicates that these general recommendations have remained largely unchanged, comprising the use of cefazolin or other suitable cephalosporin, as first line prophylactic agent, with clindamycin, vancomycin or a fluoroquinolone being suitable alternatives in patients with life-threatening ß-lactam allergy.[12,97]

Route of Administration: Topical or Systemic

Early guidelines focused on the use of intravenous and oral antibiotics as the primary routes for administering preoperative antibiotic prophylaxis, with limited utilization of topical agents, except in ophthalmic procedures, in which topical administration was the primary route.[92] Topical agents were mainly used in antibiotic irrigations or instillations prior to skin incision and at wound closure, and while there were concerns about inefficacy and insufficient added benefit of topical antibiotics,[98] there was evidence supporting the non-inferiority of topical antibiotics when compared with systemic agents under specific contexts. Sarr and colleagues, randomized patients undergoing high-risk biliary surgery into 3 groups, each receiving either topical, systemic or combination of topical and systemic agents, and found no difference in infective complications among the groups.[99] However, a recent meta-analysis of 13 RCT found no reduction in incidence of SSIs following topical antibiotic administration overall, and among sub-groups of

patients undergoing dermatologic (RR 0.77, 95% CI 0.39–1.55), ophthalmic (RR 0.08, 95% CI 0.00–1.52), spinal (RR 1.34, 95% CI 0.65–2.77), orthopedic (RR 0.69, 95% CI 0.37–1.29), or cardiothoracic surgeries (RR 1.60, 95% CI 0.79–3.25).[100] Thus, recent practice guidelines largely overlap with early versions, with topical antibiotics not being recommended on account of contradicting evidence and ambiguity regarding their safety and efficacy, except in ophthalmic procedures, where preoperative antisepsis with povidone-iodine, as well as topical neomycin, polymyxin B, gentamicin or fluoroquinolone is recommended.[97] It is worth noting that regardless of administration route, all antibiotic agents act either by direct killing of bacteria (bactericidal) or inhibiting bacterial growth (bacteriostatic), which help to reduce bacterial load, and prevent bacteria spread.[101]

Antiseptic Skin Preparation: State of the Evidence

Topical agents like aqueous or alcohol-based povidone-iodine and chlorhexidine solutions are not antibiotics but are antiseptic agents with bactericidal or bacteriostatic properties usually applied topically prior to skin incision Darouiche and colleagues, demonstrated the superior efficacy of alcohol-based chlorhexidine over aqueous povidone-iodine for reducing rates of SSIs among patients undergoing clean-contaminated abdominal surgery.[102] This result was corroborated by a recent meta-analysis by Wade and colleagues, reporting that alcohol-based chlorhexidine solution was twice as effective as alcohol-based or aqueous povidone-iodine solution, in reducing the risk of postoperative SSI (RR: 0.49, 95% CI: 0.24–1.02).[103] In fact, a more recent retrospective study of patients undergoing penile prosthesis implantation found that intraoperative use of betadine irrigation was associated with a 9-fold increase in risk of postoperative penile prosthesis infection.[104] In line with this evidence, the National Institute for Health and Care Excellence (NICE) guidelines recommend the use of 0.5% alcohol-based chlorhexidine for antisepsis in skin locations away from mucosal membranes, but not on locations near mucous membranes.[105] This is because of the increased risk of mucosal irritation and desquamation associated with the use of alcohol-based chlorhexidine solutions.[106,107] Recommended alternatives in this case include 4% aqueous chlorhexidine (Hibiclens) or 7.5% aqueous povidone-iodine (Betadine) solution.[105,108]

Antibiotic Prophylaxis in Urology

The use of antibiotic prophylaxis in urologic procedures was a controversial subject in its early years, a debate fueled by contradictory findings on its efficacy by early investigators, who either recommended,[109,110] or found no benefits to its use.[111–114] Following a review by Chodak and Plaut,[115] who identified significant flaws in the design of earlier prospective trials on the efficacy of antibiotic prophylaxis in urology patients, subsequent better-designed studies reported significant reductions in rates of postoperative bacteriuria and urinary tract infections (UTI) following transurethral resection of the prostate (TURP) and retropubic prostatectomy.[116–120] The use of pre-operative antibiotic prophylaxis in urology patients was initially dictated by the practice guidelines released by the ACS[91] and ASHP,[92] and generally involved the use of oral trimethoprim-sulfamethoxazole (TMP-SMX), fluoroquinolone or IV cefazolin, in patients at high risk of postoperative bacteriuria. The use of these non-urology-specific practice guidelines and their subsequent updates continued until 2008, when the AUA released its first best practice policy statement (BPPS) on urologic surgery antimicrobial prophylaxis,[121] in which fluoroquinolones, TMP-SMX or cephalosporins were recommended as first-line options, depending on the procedure type, convenience, safety, and cost considerations, with clindamycin, metronidazole and aztreonams being suitable alternatives.[121] The usefulness of preoperative antiseptic skin preparation has also been demonstrated, with Yeung and colleagues, reporting the efficacy and superiority of alcohol-based chlorhexidine solution over povidone-iodine, for reducing skin flora at the surgical site prior to penile prosthesis implantation surgery.[122]

Antibiotic Prophylaxis for Open, Laparoscopic, and Robotic Urologic Surgery: Current Recommendations

With a focus on open, laparoscopic and robotic urologic procedures, in this review, we present the most recent recommendations from the AUA BPPS on antimicrobial prophylaxis below and summarized in **Table 3**.[39]

Clean cases
The use of antibiotic prophylaxis covering for normal skin flora for clean procedures has long been debated.[123] Recent studies on outpatient class I procedures including laparoscopic surgeries for renal and adrenal tumors,[124] graft creation and arteriovenous fistula repair,[125] have failed to demonstrate significant benefits of antibiotic prophylaxis. Thus, the AUA recommends that single-dose antibiotic prophylaxis for usual skin flora, may not be necessary for clean procedures, except

in individual cases classified as higher risk, such as procedures involving the incision of the groin or perineum and for the implantation of a prosthesis device.[39] In such cases, the guidelines recommend single dose cefazolin or clindamycin administered within 1 hour of skin incision.[39] The use of preoperative antiseptic skin preparation with alcohol-based chlorhexidine is also recommended for urologic prosthesis implantation surgeries, based on previously-discussed evidence.[122]

Clean-contaminated cases
The risk of postoperative SSIs for clean-contaminated procedures varies considerably, even with the use of appropriate antibiotic prophylaxis covering the most likely pathogens, a phenomenon reflective of the inherent differences in baseline infection risk among the procedures categorized under the clean-contaminated class. For example, while the SSI rates associated with outpatient cystoscopy, a class II procedure by definition, are reliably low, warranting a case-by-case consideration of the need for antibiotic prophylaxis as reported by Gregg and colleagues,[126] and others[127–129]; the infection risk following a TURP, another class II procedure by definition, is considerably higher.[130] Thus, the AUA recommend the use of single-dose antibiotic prophylaxis for patients undergoing specific clean-contaminated procedures, with notable exceptions being patients without pre-existing infections undergoing routine cystoscopy and urodynamic studies.[39] While the decision to implement antibiotic prophylaxis for class II procedures ultimately depends on the procedure type, the choice of antibiotic would depend on patient-specific risk factors, local facility antibiogram, and preoperative urine culture results, with adequate preoperative treatment of any confirmed UTIs prior to instrumentation. Currently recommended first line agents include single-dose cefazolin or TMP/SMX administered within an hour of skin incision. Alternative agents include (a) ampicillin/sulbactam; (b) combination of metronidazole with an aminoglycoside or aztreonam; (c) combination of clindamycin with an aminoglycoside or aztreonam. Antifungal coverage with fluconazole may be considered for vaginal procedures, in high-risk patients.[39]

Contaminated cases
Class III/contaminated surgeries are characterized by a significant post-procedural risk of SSIs, with a similarly significant demonstrated risk reduction from 39% to 13% following the appropriate use of selected antibiotic prophylaxis.[10] Thus, antibiotic prophylaxis is highly recommended for most urologic contaminated surgeries including

Table 3
Antibiotic prophylaxis recommendations for open, laparoscopic and robotic urologic surgery[39]

Procedure Classification	Procedure Examples	Probable Infectious Organisms	Condition for Antibiotic Prophylaxis	First Line Antibiotics	Alternative choice(s) Antibiotics	Duration of Therapy
Class I (clean procedures)	Adrenalectomy Lymphadenectomy	Skin flora including *Staphylococcus aureus*	Consider on a case-by-case basis but generally indicated for prosthesis implantation and in procedures requiring groin or perineal incisions	Cefazolin	Clindamycin	Single dose
	Prosthetic device implantation (AUS, IPP, sacral neuromodulators)	Gram-negative rods including *E. coli, Proteus sp., Klebsiella* and *Enterococcus, S aureus*, anerobic and fungal organisms		Aminoglycoside + 1st/2nd generation cephalosporin or Aminoglycoside + vancomycin or Aztreonam + vancomycin or Aztreonam + 1st/2nd generation cephalosporin	Aminopenicillin + β-lactamase inhibitor (Ampicillin/ Sulbactam or Piperacillin/ Tazobactam)	≤24 hours
	Groin and perineal procedures for example, vasectomy, orchiectomy, hydrocelectomy, varicocelectomy	Gram-negative rods including *E coli, Proteus sp., Klebsiella* and *Enterococcus, S aureus*		Cefazolin	Ampicillin/Sulbactam	Single dose
Class II (clean-contaminated procedures)	Nephrectomy Ureterectomy Radical prostatectomy Cystectomy	Gram negative rods for example, *E coli, Enterococci*	Indicated for all cases	Cefazolin or TMP-SMX	Ampicillin/Sulbactam or Aminoglycoside + Metronidazole or Aminoglycoside + Clindamycin or Aztreonam + Metronidazole or Aztreonam + Clindamycin	Single Dose
	Transurethral procedures for example, TURP and TURBT				Amoxicillin/ Clavulanate or Aminoglycoside + Ampicillin or	

(continued on next page)

Table 3
(continued)

Procedure Classification	Procedure Examples	Probable Infectious Organisms	Condition for Antibiotic Prophylaxis	First Line Antibiotics	Alternative choice(s) Antibiotics	Duration of Therapy
	Urinary diversion with small bowel conduit Uretero-pelvic junction repair	Skin flora, *S aureus*, gram negative rods, *Enterococci*		Cefazolin	Aztreonam + Ampicillin Aminoglycoside + Clindamycin or Cefuroxime or Aminopenicillin/ß-lactamase inhibitor + Metronidazole	
	Urinary diversion with large bowel conduits	Gram negative rods, anerobes		(Cefazolin or Cefoxitin or Cefotetan or Ceftriaxone) + Metronidazole or Ertapenem	Ampicillin/Sulbactam or Piperacillin/Tazobactam	
	Percutaneous renal surgery for example, PCNL			1st/2nd generation Cephalosporin or Aminoglycoside + Metronidazole or Aminoglycoside + Clindamycin or Aztreonam + Metronidazole or Aztreonam + Clindamycin		
	Vaginal surgery for example, fistula repair, urethral sling for stress incontinence	Skin flora, *S aureus*, vaginal anerobes, *Enterococci*		2nd generation cephalosporin for example, Cefoxitin, Cefotetan, for anerobic coverage	Aminoglycoside + Metronidazole or Aminoglycoside + Clindamycin or Aztreonam + Metronidazole or Aztreonam + Clindamycin	
Class III (contaminated procedures)	Prostate brachytherapy	Skin flora, gram negative rods and *S aureus*	Indicated for all cases	Cefazolin	Clindamycin	Single Dose

transrectal prostate biopsy, radical cystectomy with urinary diversion or bowel augmentation, and penetrating trauma with resulting perforation of the GI or GU tract. For urologic surgeries involving manipulation of the non-obstructed small bowel, single-dose cefazolin is recommended, as the microbial burden of the small bowel is relatively lower; while for urologic procedures involving manipulation of the colon and rectum, coverage for both aerobic and anerobic microbes is essential, for which cefazolin has been shown to be insufficient.[131] For these cases the AUA recommends a single parenteral dose of metronidazole in combination with cefazolin or other suitable cephalosporin or ertapenem. Alternative agents include a combination of aminopenicillin and a ß-lactamase inhibitor.[39] Of note, the AUA no longer recommends the use of fluoroquinolones as antibiotic prophylaxis for contaminated cases. The AUA recommends single-dose antifungal prophylaxis with oral fluconazole or intravenous amphotericin B, for patients with asymptomatic funguria, undergoing class II/III laparoscopic, robotic or open surgeries of the urinary tract. While a longer course is recommended for neutropenic patients with funguria, due to the high risk of fungemia, with Candida being the most common agent. Symptomatic funguria requires preoperative treatment, regardless of procedure type.[39]

Special Considerations in Pre-operative Antibiotic Prophylaxis in Urologic Surgery

Case 1: use of urologic prosthesis including artificial urinary sphincter and implantable penile prosthesis

Placement of a urologic device including the implantation of an artificial urinary sphincter, penile prosthesis or sacral neuromodulators is considered a clean procedure (Class I), with an intermediate risk of SSI according to the most recent AUA urologic procedure-associated risk probability of SSI framework.[39] However, while the risk is intermediate, occurrence of an SSI in this setting could be devastating on patient outcomes with significant associated morbidity,[132] which warrants the need for antibiotic prophylaxis in these procedure. The appropriate antibiotic agent for these surgeries would cover for the skin commensals including coagulase-negative *Staphylococcus* as well as biofilm-forming gram-negative enteric of the GU system including *Pseudomonas*.[130,133] More recently, there has been an increase in incidence of methicillin-resistant *Staphylococcus aureus* (MRSA) and fungal infections cultured from explanted infected prosthesis devices.[134] For these procedures, the AUA recommends the use of an aminoglycoside or 1st/2nd generation cephalosporin as first-line antibiotic of choice, which may be combined together or used separately in combination with either vancomycin (for aminoglycosides) or aztreonam (for cephalosporin), beginning pre-operatively and lasting for 24 hours or less post-operatively. Alternative agents include combination of penicillin with ß-lactamase inhibitor.[39]

Case 2: patient with history of antibiotic-resistant infection

The patient's current microbiome and previous history of drug-resistant infection are major considerations in the choice of antibiotics to be used for preoperative antimicrobial prophylaxis. Patients with an index case, or a previous history of a multi-drug resistant (MDR) infection such as MRSA or vancomycin resistant Enterococcus, may require additional antibiotics with coverage for these infections. Screening for MRSA remains a controversial subject, while the AUA BPPS does not directly recommend MRSA screening and decolonization,[39] the most recent clinical practice guidelines from the ASHP does recommend MRSA screening with nasal mupirocin decolonization for MRSA-infected patients prior to cardiovascular surgery and total joint replacement.[97] Ultimately, the decision to implement MRSA screening and decolonization in urology patients should depend on the individual patient's history, baseline SSI status, and facility MRSA infection rates. While no consensus decolonization protocol has been adopted in literature, possible options include nasal mupirocin alone or in combination with chlorhexidine gluconate bath, either of which should be completed close to the date of surgery.[12] MRSA bundles including screening, decolonization, hand hygiene, and contact precautions need to be closely followed to be effective.[12]

Case 3: patient with history of bacterial colonization in bladder

The indications for preoperative antibiotic prophylaxis in a patient with a previous history of bladder colonization depend on the results of urine culture prior to surgery. A positive urine culture in a symptomatic patient represents an active UTI which should be treated appropriately prior to surgery. A positive urine culture in an asymptomatic patient represents asymptomatic bacteriuria (ASB), which commonly occurs in the elderly, in patients with prior urinary diversions or bowel manipulation, and in those with intermittent or prolonged catheterization, and the treatment of which depends on both patient and procedure-associated risk factors.[39] The AUA recommends treatment of ASB prior to urinary tract manipulation/instrumentation as part of open/laparoscopic/robotic surgery by using single-dose oral or intravenous antibiotics in high risk patients, including pregnant women, the elderly and immunocompromised, and in patients undergoing procedures with a high-risk probability for developing SSIs.[39]

Complications of Preoperative Antibiotic Prophylaxis

Antimicrobial resistance

Postoperative SSIs and antimicrobial resistance (AMR) are inextricably linked. *Staphylococcus aureus* and *Escherichia coli* represent the 2 top pathogens implicated in antibiotic resistant infections and are coincidentally the most common bacterial strains isolated from postoperative SSIs, for which up to 60% of surgical patients receive antibiotic prophylaxis. At least 50% of these patients are discharged home on antibiotic therapy.[135] Aiken and colleagues, demonstrated that the establishment of a postoperative SSI diagnosis increased antibiotic use by 7-fold in a tertiary health care setting.[136] A recent multicenter prospective study reported that between 16.6% to 36% of SSIs diagnosed following GI surgery were caused by a bacterial strain resistant to the surgical antibiotic prophylaxis previously administered to the patient.[137] While practice guidelines exist on the appropriate use of preoperative surgical prophylaxis, adherence remains suboptimal, often manifesting, for example, in the routine use of vancomycin for non-MRSA infections, or the prolonged use of antibiotic prophylaxis beyond stipulated timelines.[138,139] Such inappropriate use of preoperative antibiotic prophylaxis has been highlighted as a major driver of the emergence of MDR bacterial strains, representing a significant threat to the continued capacity of health care systems in both low and high-income countries, to deliver safe surgical care. MRSA and extended spectrum ß-lactamase (ESBL)-producing *Enterobacteriaceae* have both been linked to poor post-operative outcomes including prolonged LOS and increased 90-day mortality in affected patients.[140,141] Recent efforts have focused on development of predictive nomograms, leveraging evidence-based risk factors to predict the occurrence of postoperative SSIs.[142–144] These validated models would facilitate early identification of high-risk patients for institution of antibiotic prophylactic measures.

Clostridium difficile infection

Clostridium difficile is an anerobic, gram-positive rod transmitted via the feco-oral route.[145] While *C difficile* usually lives in balance with the colonic normal flora, alterations in the bacterial component of the colonic microbiota, most commonly caused by antibiotic use, can trigger changes in flora population, which encourages the overgrowth of *C difficile*, and induces its pathogenic characteristics.[87,146] Several reports have firmly established the risk of *Clostridium difficile* infection (CDI) following preoperative antibiotic use,[147–151] and while almost any antibiotic can precipitate CDI, the most commonly-linked agents include clindamycin, carbapenems, penicillin combinations and 3rd/4th-generation cephalosporins, all of which are recommended antibiotic agents for preoperative prophylaxis.[152] TMP-SMX on the other hand has been shown to possess the lowest risk of CDI.[152] Other risk factors linked to postoperative CDI include use of proton pump inhibitors, steroids, smoking and lower body mas index (BMI).[153] Postoperative CDI has been associated with prolonged hospital LOS, and higher rate of emergency department (ED) readmission within 30 days post-procedure.[154] Several organization have released practice guidelines proposing effective measures for the prevention and treatment of CDI in surgical patients.[155,156] The ASCRS practice guideline strongly recommends implementing an evidence-based antibiotic stewardship program, with the goal of promoting appropriate antibiotic use with respect to the choice and duration of administration of prophylactic antibiotics in surgical settings.[155] They also recommend the use of probiotics, which are microbial organisms capable of adjusting the colonic bacterial milieu to restore balance to altered colonic flora population. While these organisms are generally safe, data on their efficacy have often times been contradictory, with early RCTs indicating no benefit to their use.[157,158] However, more recent meta-analyses indicate that they are effective prophylactic but poor therapeutic agents against CDI.[159,160] While several probiotics including *Lactobacillus acidophilus* CL1285, *Lactobacillus casei* LBC80 R and *Saccharomyces boulardii,* have been trialed,[159,161] questions remain about the appropriate combination, optimal dosing strategies and duration of administration for effective CDI prophylaxis.[162] Oral vancomycin or fidaxomicin are the recommended first line antibiotic agents for treatment of initial CDI, and while they have also been administered as prophylactic strategies, this practice is only recommended in high-risk patients.[156] In recent time, efforts to develop an effective vaccine have been made; however, a phase 3 RCT for a bivalent *C difficile* toxoid vaccine was recently terminated for lack of efficacy.[163]

Allergic reactions to antibiotic prophylaxis

ß-lactam antibiotics including penicillins and cephalosporins are first-choice antibiotics used for preoperative prophylaxis; however, in patients with penicillin allergy, choice of antibiotic prophylaxis becomes less straightforward. Penicillin allergy currently affects about 10% of the United States population, with the estimated prevalence of clinically-significant IgE or T-lymphocyte-mediated penicillin allergy being 5%.[164] Current antibiotic prophylaxis guidelines recommend against the use of ß-lactam antibiotics including both penicillins and cephalosporins in patients with penicillin allergy,[12,39,97] due to the occurrence of significant immunologic cross-reactivity between penicillins and cephalosporins, and the risk of precipitating an allergic response including anaphylaxis, fatal bronchospasms, urticaria, and other cutaneous eruptions.[165] Cross-reactivity of penicillin and cephalosporins occurs in about 2% of American population, and approximately 40% of patients with a history of penicillin anaphylaxis will have cross-reactivity to cephalosporins.[164] This cross-reactivity is due to the similarities in the chemical structure of both agents, with cefazolin being a notable exception as a result of its unique side chain.[166] Thus, cefazolin does not cross-react significant with other ß-lactams and is safe to administer in patients with penicillin allergy.[166] Alternative agents recommended for use as prophylactic antibiotics in patients with penicillin allergy include vancomycin and clindamycin,[40] both of which increase the risk of CDI infections.[167] Of note, vancomycin is specifically associated with the development of red man syndrome,[168] a pseudo-allergic reaction, characterized by the drug-induced, IgE-independent degranulation of mast cells.[168] It presents as a pruritic, erythematous rash over the face, neck and torso, and its emergence is directly proportional to the infusion rate of intravenous vancomycin. Symptoms typically resolve following discontinuation of vancomycin administration, with subsequent replacement by an alternative agent, or reduction of drug infusion rate.[169] Other notable antibiotic-associated allergic reactions include Steven-Johnson syndrome, and Toxic Epidermal Necrolysis are characterized by a delayed hypersensitivity reactions to TMP-SMX, fluoroquinolones and penicillins, with resulting desquamation of the epidermal keratinocytes.[170]

FUTURE DIRECTIONS

While the principles and practice of bowel preparation and preoperative antibiotic prophylaxis in surgery generally, and in urology more specifically, have evolved considerably over the years, there is a need for continued research to ensure evidence-based practices, which maximize benefit and limit adverse effects on urologic patient care.

Notable knowledge gaps can be seen in the scant nature of the body of evidence supporting the continued recommendation of CBP for urinary diversion procedures involving colorectal bowel segment; the appropriate combination, dose and duration of administration of probiotics for *Clostridium difficile* infection prophylaxis; and the benefits of preoperative MRSA screening and decolonization in patients with a prior history of MRSA infection. These represent opportunities for future research to advance knowledge in the field with potential implications for current guideline recommendations. The design of RCTs that test currently validated predictive nomograms for antimicrobial resistant infections in urology patients, are needed, as these will provide an additional tool to aid in clinical decision-making while preserving the efficacy of currently-available antibiotic agents in urology practice.

SUMMARY

Oral MBP is not recommended for clean, clean-contaminated, as well as contaminated open, laparoscopic and robotic urologic surgeries involving manipulation of a small bowel segment. It is recommended for contaminated urologic surgeries requiring manipulation of a colorectal bowel segment. ERAS protocols have been successfully applied in urology, for radical cystectomy and robot-assisted radical prostatectomy. Preoperative antibiotic prophylaxis is widely used in a number of open, laparoscopic or robotic urologic procedures. Generally, it is recommended for all clean-contaminated and contaminated procedures but is recommended only for clean procedures involving prosthesis implantation or skin incision of the groin or perineum; clean-contaminated.

CLINICS CARE POINTS

- Oral MBP is not recommended for urinary diversion procedure utilizing an ileal bowel segment.
- Antibiotic bowel preparation is recommended for open, laparoscopic or robotic urologic surgeries requiring bowel manipulation.
- Antimicrobial prophylaxis is recommended for clean urologic procedures involving a prosthesis device.
- Preoperative antimicrobial skin preparation with alcohol-based chlorhexidine solution is recommended except for mucosal surfaces.

DISCLOSURE

The authors have none to declare.

REFERENCES

1. Jandhyala SM, Talukdar R, Subramanyam C, et al. Role of the normal gut microbiota. World J Gastroenterol WJG 2015;21(29):8787–803. https://doi.org/10.3748/wjg.v21.i29.8787.
2. Young H, Knepper B, Moore EE, et al. Surgical site infection after colon surgery: National Healthcare Safety Network risk factors and modeled rates compared with published risk factors and rates. J Am Coll Surg 2012;214(5):852–9. https://doi.org/10.1016/j.jamcollsurg.2012.01.041.
3. Sciuto A, Merola G, De Palma GD, et al. Predictive factors for anastomotic leakage after laparoscopic colorectal surgery. World J Gastroenterol 2018; 24(21):2247–60. https://doi.org/10.3748/wjg.v24.i21.2247.
4. Hughes ES. Asepsis in large-bowel surgery. Ann R Coll Surg Engl 1972;51(6):347–56.
5. Nichols RL, Condon RE. Preoperative preparation of the colon. Surg Gynecol Obstet 1971;132(2):323–37.
6. Nichols RL, Condon RE, Gorbach SL, et al. Efficacy of preoperative antimicrobial preparation of the bowel. Ann Surg 1972;176(2):227–32.
7. Baum ML, Anish DS, Chalmers TC, et al. A survey of clinical trials of antibiotic prophylaxis in colon surgery: evidence against further use of no-treatment controls. N Engl J Med 1981;305(14):795–9. https://doi.org/10.1056/NEJM198110013051404.
8. Smith MB, Goradia VK, Holmes JW, et al. Suppression of the human mucosal-related colonic microflora with prophylactic parenteral and/or oral antibiotics. World J Surg 1990;14(5):636–41. https://doi.org/10.1007/BF01658812.
9. Markell KW, Hunt BM, Charron PD, et al. Prophylaxis and management of wound infections after elective colorectal surgery: a survey of the American Society of Colon and Rectal Surgeons membership. J Gastrointest Surg 2010;14(7):1090–8. https://doi.org/10.1007/s11605-010-1218-7.
10. Nelson RL, Gladman E, Barbateskovic M. Antimicrobial prophylaxis for colorectal surgery. Cochrane Database Syst Rev 2014;2014(5):CD001181. https://doi.org/10.1002/14651858.CD001181.pub4.
11. Roos D, Dijksman LM, Tijssen JG, et al. Systematic review of perioperative selective decontamination of the digestive tract in elective gastrointestinal surgery. Br J Surg 2013;100(12):1579–88. https://doi.org/10.1002/bjs.9254.
12. Ban KA, Minei JP, Laronga C, et al. American College of Surgeons and Surgical Infection Society: Surgical Site Infection Guidelines, 2016 Update. J Am Coll Surg 2017;224(1):59–74. https://doi.org/10.1016/j.jamcollsurg.2016.10.029.
13. Berian JR, Hyman N. The evolution of bowel preparation for gastrointestinal surgery. Semin Colon Rectal Surg 2018;29(1):8–11. https://doi.org/10.1053/j.scrs.2017.09.002.
14. Kiran RP, Murray ACA, Chiuzan C, et al. Combined preoperative mechanical bowel preparation with oral antibiotics significantly reduces surgical site infection, anastomotic leak, and ileus after colorectal surgery. Ann Surg 2015;262(3):416–25. https://doi.org/10.1097/SLA.0000000000001416. discussion 423-425.
15. Alverdy JC, Hyman N. Bowel preparation under siege. Br J Surg 2020;107(3):167–70. https://doi.org/10.1002/bjs.11454.
16. Koskenvuo L, Lunkka P, Varpe P, et al. Mechanical bowel preparation and oral antibiotics versus mechanical bowel preparation only prior rectal surgery (MOBILE2): a multicentre, double-blinded, randomised controlled trial-study protocol. BMJ Open 2021;11(7):e051269. https://doi.org/10.1136/bmjopen-2021-051269.
17. Migaly J, Bafford AC, Francone TD, et al. The American Society of Colon and Rectal Surgeons Clinical Practice Guidelines for the Use of Bowel Preparation in Elective Colon and Rectal Surgery. Dis Colon Rectum 2019;62(1):3–8. https://doi.org/10.1097/DCR.0000000000001238.
18. Connor A, Tolan D, Hughes S, et al. Consensus guidelines for the safe prescription and administration of oral bowel-cleansing agents. Gut 2012; 61(11):1525–32. https://doi.org/10.1136/gutjnl-2011-300861.
19. Zmora O, Mahajna A, Bar-Zakai B, et al. Colon and rectal surgery without mechanical bowel preparation: a randomized prospective trial. Ann Surg 2003;237(3):363–7. https://doi.org/10.1097/01.SLA.0000055222.90581.59.
20. Contant CME, Hop WCJ, van't Sant HP, et al. Mechanical bowel preparation for elective colorectal surgery: a multicentre randomised trial. Lancet Lond Engl 2007;370(9605):2112–7. https://doi.org/10.1016/S0140-6736(07)61905-9.
21. Jung B, Påhlman L, Nyström PO, et al. Mechanical Bowel Preparation Study Group. Multicentre randomized clinical trial of mechanical bowel preparation in elective colonic resection. Br J Surg 2007; 94(6):689–95. https://doi.org/10.1002/bjs.5816.
22. Bucher P, Gervaz P, Egger JF, et al. Morphologic alterations associated with mechanical bowel preparation before elective colorectal surgery: a randomized trial. Dis Colon Rectum 2006;49(1):109–12. https://doi.org/10.1007/s10350-005-0215-5.
23. Ram E, Sherman Y, Weil R, et al. Is mechanical bowel preparation mandatory for elective colon surgery? A prospective randomized study. Arch

Surg Chic III 1960 2005;140(3):285–8. https://doi.org/10.1001/archsurg.140.3.285.

24. Miettinen RP, Laitinen ST, Mäkelä JT, et al. Bowel preparation with oral polyethylene glycol electrolyte solution vs. no preparation in elective open colorectal surgery: prospective, randomized study. Dis Colon Rectum 2000;43(5):669–75. https://doi.org/10.1007/BF02235585. discussion 675-677.

25. Fa-Si-Oen P, Roumen R, Buitenweg J, et al. Mechanical bowel preparation or not? Outcome of a multicenter, randomized trial in elective open colon surgery. Dis Colon Rectum 2005;48(8):1509–16. https://doi.org/10.1007/s10350-005-0068-y.

26. Dahabreh IJ, Steele DW, Shah N, et al. Oral Mechanical Bowel Preparation for Colorectal Surgery: Systematic Review and Meta-Analysis. Dis Colon Rectum 2015;58(7):698–707. https://doi.org/10.1097/DCR.0000000000000375.

27. Pineda CE, Shelton AA, Hernandez-Boussard T, et al. Mechanical bowel preparation in intestinal surgery: a meta-analysis and review of the literature. J Gastrointest Surg 2008;12(11):2037–44. https://doi.org/10.1007/s11605-008-0594-8.

28. Rollins KE, Javanmard-Emamghissi H, Lobo DN. Impact of mechanical bowel preparation in elective colorectal surgery: A meta-analysis. World J Gastroenterol 2018;24(4):519–36. https://doi.org/10.3748/wjg.v24.i4.519.

29. Slim K, Vicaut E, Launay-Savary MV, et al. Updated systematic review and meta-analysis of randomized clinical trials on the role of mechanical bowel preparation before colorectal surgery. Ann Surg 2009;249(2):203–9. https://doi.org/10.1097/SLA.0b013e318193425a.

30. Maffezzini M, Audisio R, Pavone-Macaluso M, et al. Bladder cancer. Crit Rev Oncol Hematol 1998;27(2):151–3. https://doi.org/10.1016/S1040-8428(97)10026-9.

31. Shergill AK, Wang DC, Thipphavong S, et al. Comprehensive Imaging and Surgical Review of Urinary Diversions: What the Radiologist Needs to Know. Curr Probl Diagn Radiol 2019;48(2):161–71. https://doi.org/10.1067/j.cpradiol.2018.02.001.

32. Freiha FS. Preoperative bowel preparation in urologic surgery. J Urol 1977;118(6):955–6. https://doi.org/10.1016/s0022-5347(17)58262-2.

33. Ackermann D, Suter P, Studer UE. Preoperative preparation of the bowel for urological surgery: a review. Eur Urol 1986;12(5):289–93. https://doi.org/10.1159/000472641.

34. Tabibi A, Simforoosh N, Basiri A, et al. Bowel preparation versus no preparation before ileal urinary diversion. Urology 2007;70(4):654–8. https://doi.org/10.1016/j.urology.2007.06.1107.

35. Yang L, Chen HS, Welk B, et al. Does using comprehensive preoperative bowel preparation offer any advantage for urinary diversion using ileum? A meta-analysis. Int Urol Nephrol 2013;45(1):25–31. https://doi.org/10.1007/s11255-012-0319-5.

36. Deng S, Dong Q, Wang J, et al. The role of mechanical bowel preparation before ileal urinary diversion: a systematic review and meta-analysis. Urol Int 2014;92(3):339–48. https://doi.org/10.1159/000354326.

37. Large MC, Kiriluk KJ, DeCastro GJ, et al. The impact of mechanical bowel preparation on postoperative complications for patients undergoing cystectomy and urinary diversion. J Urol 2012;188(5):1801–5. https://doi.org/10.1016/j.juro.2012.07.039.

38. Feng D, Li X, Liu S, et al. A comparison between limited bowel preparation and comprehensive bowel preparation in radical cystectomy with ileal urinary diversion: a systematic review and meta-analysis of randomized controlled trials. Int Urol Nephrol 2020;52(11):2005–14. https://doi.org/10.1007/s11255-020-02516-9.

39. Lightner DJ, Wymer K, Sanchez J, et al. Best Practice Statement on Urologic Procedures and Antimicrobial Prophylaxis. J Urol 2020;203(2):351–6. https://doi.org/10.1097/JU.0000000000000509.

40. Carmichael JC, Keller DS, Baldini G, et al. Clinical Practice Guidelines for Enhanced Recovery After Colon and Rectal Surgery From the American Society of Colon and Rectal Surgeons and Society of American Gastrointestinal and Endoscopic Surgeons. Dis Colon Rectum 2017;60(8):761–84. https://doi.org/10.1097/DCR.0000000000000883.

41. Gorbach SL. Microbiology of the Gastrointestinal Tract. In: Baron S, editor. Medical microbiology. 4th edition. University of Texas Medical Branch at Galveston; 1996. Available at: http://www.ncbi.nlm.nih.gov/books/NBK7670/. [Accessed 2 April 2024].

42. Taurchini M, Del Naja C, Tancredi A. Enhanced Recovery After Surgery: a patient centered process. J Vis Surg 2018;4:40. https://doi.org/10.21037/jovs.2018.01.20.

43. Wilmore DW, Kehlet H. Management of patients in fast track surgery. BMJ 2001;322(7284):473–6. https://doi.org/10.1136/bmj.322.7284.473.

44. Eskicioglu C, Forbes SS, Aarts MA, et al. Enhanced recovery after surgery (ERAS) programs for patients having colorectal surgery: a meta-analysis of randomized trials. J Gastrointest Surg 2009;13(12):2321–9. https://doi.org/10.1007/s11605-009-0927-2.

45. Lassen K, Soop M, Nygren J, et al. Consensus review of optimal perioperative care in colorectal surgery: Enhanced Recovery After Surgery (ERAS) Group recommendations. Arch Surg Chic III 1960 2009;144(10):961–9. https://doi.org/10.1001/archsurg.2009.170.

46. Irani JL, Hedrick TL, Miller TE, et al. Clinical practice guidelines for enhanced recovery after colon and rectal surgery from the American Society of Colon and Rectal Surgeons and the Society of American Gastrointestinal and Endoscopic Surgeons. Surg Endosc 2023;37(1):5–30. https://doi.org/10.1007/s00464-022-09758-x.

47. McNicol ED, Boyce D, Schumann R, et al. Mu-opioid antagonists for opioid-induced bowel dysfunction. Cochrane Database Syst Rev 2008;2:CD006332. https://doi.org/10.1002/14651858.CD006332.pub2.

48. Liu SS, Hodgson PS, Carpenter RL, et al. ADL 8-2698, a trans-3,4-dimethyl-4-(3-hydroxyphenyl) piperidine, prevents gastrointestinal effects of intravenous morphine without affecting analgesia. Clin Pharmacol Ther 2001;69(1):66–71. https://doi.org/10.1067/mcp.2001.112680.

49. Wolff BG, Michelassi F, Gerkin TM, et al. Alvimopan, a novel, peripherally acting mu opioid antagonist: results of a multicenter, randomized, double-blind, placebo-controlled, phase III trial of major abdominal surgery and postoperative ileus. Ann Surg 2004;240(4):728–34. https://doi.org/10.1097/01.sla.0000141158.27977.66. discussion 734-735.

50. Ludwig K, Enker WE, Delaney CP, et al. Gastrointestinal tract recovery in patients undergoing bowel resection: results of a randomized trial of alvimopan and placebo with a standardized accelerated postoperative care pathway. Arch Surg Chic Ill 1960 2008;143(11):1098–105. https://doi.org/10.1001/archsurg.143.11.1098.

51. Adam MA, Lee LM, Kim J, et al. Alvimopan Provides Additional Improvement in Outcomes and Cost Savings in Enhanced Recovery Colorectal Surgery. Ann Surg 2016;264(1):141–6. https://doi.org/10.1097/SLA.0000000000001428.

52. Absher RK, Gerkin TM, Banares LW. Alvimopan use in laparoscopic and open bowel resections: clinical results in a large community hospital system. Ann Pharmacother 2010;44(11):1701–8. https://doi.org/10.1345/aph.1P260.

53. Brown S, McLoughlin J, Russ A, et al. Alvimopan retains efficacy in patients undergoing colorectal surgery within an established ERAS program. Surg Endosc 2022;36(8):6129–37. https://doi.org/10.1007/s00464-021-08928-7.

54. Kaarto P, Westfall KM, Brockhaus K, et al. Alvimopan is associated with favorable outcomes in open and minimally invasive colorectal surgery: a regional database analysis. Surg Endosc 2023;37(8):6097–106. https://doi.org/10.1007/s00464-023-10098-7.

55. Xu LL, Zhou XQ, Yi PS, et al. Alvimopan combined with enhanced recovery strategy for managing postoperative ileus after open abdominal surgery: a systematic review and meta-analysis. J Surg Res 2016;203(1):211–21. https://doi.org/10.1016/j.jss.2016.01.027.

56. Vaughan-Shaw PG, Fecher IC, Harris S, et al. A meta-analysis of the effectiveness of the opioid receptor antagonist alvimopan in reducing hospital length of stay and time to GI recovery in patients enrolled in a standardized accelerated recovery program after abdominal surgery. Dis Colon Rectum 2012;55(5):611–20. https://doi.org/10.1097/DCR.0b013e318249fc78.

57. Melnyk M, Casey RG, Black P, et al. Enhanced recovery after surgery (ERAS) protocols: Time to change practice? Can Urol Assoc J 2011;5(5):342–8. https://doi.org/10.5489/cuaj.11002.

58. Vora AA, Harbin A, Rayson R, et al. Alvimopan provides rapid gastrointestinal recovery without nasogastric tube decompression after radical cystectomy and urinary diversion. Can J Urol 2012;19(3):6293–8.

59. Lee CT, Chang SS, Kamat AM, et al. Alvimopan accelerates gastrointestinal recovery after radical cystectomy: a multicenter randomized placebo-controlled trial. Eur Urol 2014;66(2):265–72. https://doi.org/10.1016/j.eururo.2014.02.036.

60. Hamilton Z, Parker W, Griffin J, et al. Alvimopan in an Enhanced Recovery Program Following Radical Cystectomy. Bladder Cancer 2015;1(2):137–42. https://doi.org/10.3233/BLC-150017.

61. Hanna P, Regmi S, Kalapara A, et al. Alvimopan as part of the Enhanced Recovery After Surgery protocol following radical cystectomy is associated with decreased hospital stay. Int J Urol 2021;28(6):696–701. https://doi.org/10.1111/iju.14546.

62. Cui Y, Chen H, Qi L, et al. Effect of alvimopan on accelerates gastrointestinal recovery after radical cystectomy: A systematic review and meta-analysis. Int J Surg Lond Engl 2016;25:1–6. https://doi.org/10.1016/j.ijsu.2015.11.013.

63. Azhar RA, Bochner B, Catto J, et al. Enhanced Recovery after Urological Surgery: A Contemporary Systematic Review of Outcomes, Key Elements, and Research Needs. Eur Urol 2016;70(1):176–87. https://doi.org/10.1016/j.eururo.2016.02.051.

64. Zhao Y, Zhang S, Liu B, et al. Clinical efficacy of enhanced recovery after surgery (ERAS) program in patients undergoing radical prostatectomy: a systematic review and meta-analysis. World J Surg Oncol 2020;18(1):131. https://doi.org/10.1186/s12957-020-01897-6.

65. Xing J, Wang J, Liu G, et al. Effects of enhanced recovery after surgery on robotic radical prostatectomy: a systematic review and meta-analysis. Gland Surg 2021;10(12):3264–71. https://doi.org/10.21037/gs-21-699.

66. Nakamura M, Tsuru I, Izumi T, et al. Advantages of enhanced recovery after surgery program in robot-assisted radical cystectomy. Sci Rep 2023;13(1):16237. https://doi.org/10.1038/s41598-023-43489-w.

67. Reumkens A, van der Zander Q, Winkens B, et al. Electrolyte disturbances after bowel preparation for colonoscopy: Systematic review and meta-analysis. Dig Endosc 2022;34(5):913–26. https://doi.org/10.1111/den.14237.

68. Nagata N, Tohya M, Fukuda S, et al. Effects of bowel preparation on the human gut microbiome and metabolome. Sci Rep 2019;9(1):4042. https://doi.org/10.1038/s41598-019-40182-9.

69. Sugihara T, Yasunaga H, Horiguchi H, et al. Does mechanical bowel preparation improve quality of laparoscopic nephrectomy? Propensity score-matched analysis in Japanese series. Urology 2013;81(1):74–9. https://doi.org/10.1016/j.urology.2012.09.032.

70. Sugihara T, Yasunaga H, Horiguchi H, et al. Does mechanical bowel preparation ameliorate damage from rectal injury in radical prostatectomy? Analysis of 151 rectal injury cases. Int J Urol 2014;21(6):566–70. https://doi.org/10.1111/iju.12368.

71. Sugihara T, Yasunaga H, Horiguchi H, et al. Is mechanical bowel preparation in laparoscopic radical prostatectomy beneficial? An analysis of a Japanese national database. BJU Int 2013;112(2):E76–81. https://doi.org/10.1111/j.1464-410X.2012.11725.x.

72. Chi AC, McGuire BB, Nadler RB. Modern Guidelines for Bowel Preparation and Antimicrobial Prophylaxis for Open and Laparoscopic Urologic Surgery. Urol Clin North Am 2015;42(4):429–40. https://doi.org/10.1016/j.ucl.2015.05.007.

73. Xu R, Zhao X, Zhong Z, et al. No advantage is gained by preoperative bowel preparation in radical cystectomy and ileal conduit: a randomized controlled trial of 86 patients. Int Urol Nephrol 2010;42(4):947–50. https://doi.org/10.1007/s11255-010-9732-9.

74. Witjes JA, Compérat E, Cowan NC, et al. EAU guidelines on muscle-invasive and metastatic bladder cancer: summary of the 2013 guidelines. Eur Urol 2014;65(4):778–92. https://doi.org/10.1016/j.eururo.2013.11.046.

75. Cerantola Y, Valerio M, Persson B, et al. Guidelines for perioperative care after radical cystectomy for bladder cancer: Enhanced Recovery After Surgery (ERAS(®)) society recommendations. Clin Nutr Edinb Scotl 2013;32(6):879–87. https://doi.org/10.1016/j.clnu.2013.09.014.

76. McKenna T, Macgill A, Porat G, et al. Colonoscopy preparation: polyethylene glycol with Gatorade is as safe and efficacious as four liters of polyethylene glycol with balanced electrolytes. Dig Dis Sci 2012;57(12):3098–105. https://doi.org/10.1007/s10620-012-2266-5.

77. Lewis RT. Oral versus systemic antibiotic prophylaxis in elective colon surgery: a randomized study and meta-analysis send a message from the 1990s. Can J Surg J Can Chir 2002;45(3):173–80.

78. Hookey LC, Depew WT, Vanner S. The safety profile of oral sodium phosphate for colonic cleansing before colonoscopy in adults. Gastrointest Endosc 2002;56(6):895–902. https://doi.org/10.1067/mge.2002.129522.

79. Ayus JC, Levine R, Arieff AI. Fatal dysnatraemia caused by elective colonoscopy. BMJ 2003;326(7385):382–4.

80. Costelha J, Dias R, Teixeira C, et al. Hyponatremic Coma after Bowel Preparation. Eur J Case Rep Intern Med 2019;6(9):001217. https://doi.org/10.12890/2019_001217.

81. Hayakawa Y, Tanaka Y, Funahashi H, et al. Hyperphosphatemia accelerates parathyroid cell proliferation and parathyroid hormone secretion in severe secondary parathyroid hyperplasia. Endocr J 1999;46(5):681–6. https://doi.org/10.1507/endocrj.46.681.

82. Mackey AC, Shaffer D, Prizont R. Seizure associated with the use of visicol for colonoscopy. N Engl J Med 2002;346(26):2095. https://doi.org/10.1056/NEJM200206273462619. author reply 2095.

83. Shapira Z, Feldman L, Lavy R, et al. Bowel preparation: comparing metabolic and electrolyte changes when using sodium phosphate/polyethylene glycol. Int J Surg Lond Engl 2010;8(5):356–8. https://doi.org/10.1016/j.ijsu.2010.04.009.

84. Jung B, Lannerstad O, Påhlman L, et al. Preoperative mechanical preparation of the colon: the patient's experience. BMC Surg 2007;7:5. https://doi.org/10.1186/1471-2482-7-5.

85. Son D, Choi YJ, Son MY, et al. Benefits of Probiotic Pretreatment on the Gut Microbiota and Minor Complications after Bowel Preparation for Colonoscopy: A Randomized Double-Blind, Placebo-Controlled Pilot Trial. Nutrients 2023;15(5):1141. https://doi.org/10.3390/nu15051141.

86. Hughes ES, Hardy KJ, Cuthbertson AM. Chemoprophylaxis in large bowel surgery. 3. Effect of antibiotics on incidence of local recurrence. Med J Aust 1970;1(8):369–71.

87. Bartlett SP, Burton RC. Effects of prophylactic antibiotics on wound infection after elective colon and rectal surgery: 1960 to 1980. Am J Surg 1983;145(2):300–9. https://doi.org/10.1016/0002-9610(83)90088-0.

88. Lowy FD. Antimicrobial resistance: the example of Staphylococcus aureus. J Clin Invest 2003;111(9):1265–73. https://doi.org/10.1172/JCI18535.

89. Panlilio AL, Culver DH, Gaynes RP, et al. Methicillin-resistant Staphylococcus aureus in U.S. hospitals, 1975-1991. Infect Control Hosp Epidemiol 1992;13(10):582–6. https://doi.org/10.1086/646432.

90. Antimicrobial prophylaxis in surgery. Med Lett Drugs Ther 1999;41(1060):75–9.

91. Page CP, Bohnen JM, Fletcher JR, et al. Antimicrobial prophylaxis for surgical wounds. Guidelines for

clinical care. Arch Surg Chic Ill 1960 1993;128(1):79–88. https://doi.org/10.1001/archsurg.1993.01420130087014.

92. ASHP Therapeutic Guidelines on Antimicrobial Prophylaxis in Surgery. American Society of Health-System Pharmacists. Am J Health-Syst Pharm AJHP 1999;56(18):1839–88. https://doi.org/10.1093/ajhp/56.18.1839.

93. Gagliardi AR, Fenech D, Eskicioglu C, et al. Factors influencing antibiotic prophylaxis for surgical site infection prevention in general surgery: a review of the literature. Can J Surg 2009;52(6):481–9.

94. Berard F, Gandon J. Postoperative wound infections: the influence of ultraviolet irradiation of the operating room and of various other factors. Ann Surg 1964;160(Suppl 2):1–192.

95. Cruse PJ, Foord R. A five-year prospective study of 23,649 surgical wounds. Arch Surg Chic Ill 1960 1973;107(2):206–10. https://doi.org/10.1001/archsurg.1973.01350200078018.

96. Westerman EL. Antibiotic prophylaxis in surgery: historical background, rationale, and relationship to prospective payment. Am J Infect Control 1984;12(6):339–43. https://doi.org/10.1016/0196-6553(84)90007-5.

97. Bratzler DW, Dellinger EP, Olsen KM, et al. Clinical practice guidelines for antimicrobial prophylaxis in surgery. Am J Health-Syst Pharm AJHP 2013;70(3):195–283. https://doi.org/10.2146/ajhp120568.

98. Raahave D, Hesselfeldt P, Pedersen T, et al. No effect of topical ampicillin prophylaxis in elective operations of the colon or rectum. Surg Gynecol Obstet 1989;168(2):112–4.

99. Sarr MG, Parikh KJ, Sanfey H, et al. Topical antibiotics in the high-risk biliary surgical patient. A prospective, randomized study. Am J Surg 1988;155(2):337–42. https://doi.org/10.1016/s0002-9610(88)80728-1.

100. Chen PJ, Hua YM, Toh HS, et al. Topical antibiotic prophylaxis for surgical wound infections in clean and clean-contaminated surgery: a systematic review and meta-analysis. BJS Open 2022;5(6):zrab125. https://doi.org/10.1093/bjsopen/zrab125.

101. Dhole S, Mahakalkar C, Kshirsagar S, et al. Antibiotic Prophylaxis in Surgery: Current Insights and Future Directions for Surgical Site Infection Prevention. Cureus 2023;15(10):e47858. https://doi.org/10.7759/cureus.47858.

102. Darouiche RO, Wall MJ, Itani KMF, et al. Chlorhexidine-Alcohol versus Povidone-Iodine for Surgical-Site Antisepsis. N Engl J Med 2010;362(1):18–26. https://doi.org/10.1056/NEJMoa0810988.

103. Wade RG, Burr NE, McCauley G, et al. The Comparative Efficacy of Chlorhexidine Gluconate and Povidone-iodine Antiseptics for the Prevention of Infection in Clean Surgery: A Systematic Review and Network Meta-analysis.

Ann Surg 2021;274(6):e481–8. https://doi.org/10.1097/SLA.0000000000004076.

104. Manka MG, Yang D, Andrews J, et al. Intraoperative use of betadine irrigation is associated with a 9-fold increased likelihood of penile prosthesis infection: results from a retrospective case-control study. Sex Med 2020;8(3):422–7. https://doi.org/10.1016/j.esxm.2020.05.010.

105. NICE. Surgical Site Infections: Prevention and Treatment. Vol NG125. NICE. 2019. Available at: https://www.nice.org.uk/guidance/ng125. [Accessed 1 April 2024].

106. Vucicevic Boras V, Brailo V, Andabak Rogulj A, et al. Oral adverse reactions caused by over-the-counter oral agents. Case Rep Dent 2015;2015:196292. https://doi.org/10.1155/2015/196292.

107. Charles D, Heal CF, Delpachitra M, et al. Alcoholic versus aqueous chlorhexidine for skin antisepsis: the AVALANCHE trial. CMAJ Can Med Assoc J 2017;189(31):E1008–16. https://doi.org/10.1503/cmaj.161460.

108. Vorherr H, Ulrich JA, Messer RH, et al. Antimicrobial effect of chlorhexidine on bacteria of groin, perineum and vagina. J Reprod Med 1980;24(4):153–7.

109. Morris MJ, Golovsky D, Guinness MD, et al. The value of prophylactic antibiotics in transurethral prostatic resection: a controlled trial, with observations on the origin of postoperative infection. Br J Urol 1976;48(6):479–84. https://doi.org/10.1111/j.1464-410x.1976.tb06686.x.

110. Plorde JJ, Kennedy RP, Bourne HH, et al. Course and prognosis of prostatectomy: with a note on the incidence of bacteremia and effectiveness of chemoprophylaxis. N Engl J Med 1965;272:269–77. https://doi.org/10.1056/NEJM196502112720601.

111. Marshall A. Prophylactic antimicrobial therapy in retropubic prostatectomy. Br J Urol 1959;31:431–8. https://doi.org/10.1111/j.1464-410x.1959.tb09444.x.

112. OSIUS TG, TAVEL FR, HINMAN F. Tetracycline used prophylactically in transurethral procedures. Md State Med J 1965;14:37–41.

113. Kudinoff Z, Finegold SM, Kalmanson GM, et al. Use of kanamycin or urinary acidification for prophylactic chemotherapy in transurethral prostatectomy. Am J Med Sci 1966;251(1):70–4. https://doi.org/10.1097/00000441-196601000-00012.

114. Gibbons RP, Stark RA, Correa RJ, et al. The prophylactic use–or misuse–of antibiotics in transurethral prostatectomy. J Urol 1978;119(3):381–3. https://doi.org/10.1016/s0022-5347(17)57496-0.

115. Chodak GW, Plaut ME. Systemic antibiotics for prophylaxis in urologic surgery: a critical review. J Urol 1979;121(6):695–9. https://doi.org/10.1016/s0022-5347(17)56959-1.

116. Korbel EI, Maher PO. Use of prophylactic antibiotics in urethral instrumentation. J Urol 1976;116(6):744–6. https://doi.org/10.1016/s0022-5347(17)58995-8.

117. Nielsen OS, Maigaard S, Frimodt-Møller N, et al. Prophylactic antibiotics in transurethral prostatectomy. J Urol 1981;126(1):60–2. https://doi.org/10.1016/s0022-5347(17)54380-3.

118. Shah PJ, Williams G, Chaudary M. Short-term antibiotic prophylaxis and prostatectomy. Br J Urol 1981;53(4):339–43. https://doi.org/10.1111/j.1464-410x.1981.tb03193.x.

119. Prokocimer P, Quazza M, Gibert C, et al. Short-term prophylactic antibiotics in patients undergoing prostatectomy: report of a double-blind randomized trial with 2 intravenous doses of cefotaxime. J Urol 1986;135(1):60–4. https://doi.org/10.1016/s0022-5347(17)45518-2.

120. Millar MR, Inglis T, Ewing R, et al. Double-blind study comparing aztreonam with placebo for prophylaxis of infection following prostatic surgery. Br J Urol 1987;60(4):345–8. https://doi.org/10.1111/j.1464-410x.1987.tb04982.x.

121. Wolf JS, Bennett CJ, Dmochowski RR, et al. Best practice policy statement on urologic surgery antimicrobial prophylaxis. J Urol 2008;179(4):1379–90. https://doi.org/10.1016/j.juro.2008.01.068.

122. Yeung LL, Grewal S, Bullock A, et al. A comparison of chlorhexidine-alcohol versus povidone-iodine for eliminating skin flora before genitourinary prosthetic surgery: a randomized controlled trial. J Urol 2013;189(1):136–40. https://doi.org/10.1016/j.juro.2012.08.086.

123. Putnam LR, Chang CM, Rogers NB, et al. Adherence to surgical antibiotic prophylaxis remains a challenge despite multifaceted interventions. Surgery 2015;158(2):413–9. https://doi.org/10.1016/j.surg.2015.04.013.

124. Bakken JS, Borody T, Brandt LJ, et al. Treating Clostridium difficile Infection with Fecal Microbiota Transplantation. Clin Gastroenterol Hepatol 2011;9(12):1044–9. https://doi.org/10.1016/j.cgh.2011.08.014.

125. Gray K, Korn A, Zane J, et al. Preoperative Antibiotics for Dialysis Access Surgery: Are They Necessary? Ann Vasc Surg 2018;49:277–80. https://doi.org/10.1016/j.avsg.2018.02.004.

126. Gregg JR, Bhalla RG, Cook JP, et al. An Evidence-Based Protocol for Antibiotic Use Prior to Cystoscopy Decreases Antibiotic Use without Impacting Post-Procedural Symptomatic Urinary Tract Infection Rates. J Urol 2018;199(4):1004–10. https://doi.org/10.1016/j.juro.2017.10.038.

127. Herr HW. Should antibiotics be given prior to outpatient cystoscopy? A plea to urologists to practice antibiotic stewardship. Eur Urol 2014;65(4):839–42. https://doi.org/10.1016/j.eururo.2013.08.054.

128. Herr HW. The risk of urinary tract infection after flexible cystoscopy in patients with bladder tumor who did not receive prophylactic antibiotics. J Urol 2015;193(2):548–51. https://doi.org/10.1016/j.juro.2014.07.015.

129. Garcia-Perdomo HA, Jimenez-Mejias E, Lopez-Ramos H. Efficacy of antibiotic prophylaxis in cystoscopy to prevent urinary tract infection: a systematic review and meta-analysis. Int Braz J Urol 2015;41(3):412–24. https://doi.org/10.1590/S1677-5538.IBJU.2014.0198. discussion 424.

130. Mohee AR, Gascoyne-Binzi D, West R, et al. Bacteraemia during Transurethral Resection of the Prostate: What Are the Risk Factors and Is It More Common than We Think? PLoS One 2016;11(7):e0157864. https://doi.org/10.1371/journal.pone.0157864.

131. Surgical Site Infections | The Joint Commission. Available at: https://www.jointcommission.org/resources/patient-safety-topics/infection-prevention-and-control/surgical-site-infections/. [Accessed 18 March 2024].

132. Hebert KJ, Kohler TS. Penile Prosthesis Infection: Myths and Realities. World J Mens Health 2019;37(3):276–87. https://doi.org/10.5534/wjmh.180123.

133. Faller M, Kohler T. The Status of Biofilms in Penile Implants. Microorganisms 2017;5(2):19. https://doi.org/10.3390/microorganisms5020019.

134. Gross MS, Phillips EA, Carrasquillo RJ, et al. Multicenter Investigation of the Micro-Organisms Involved in Penile Prosthesis Infection: An Analysis of the Efficacy of the AUA and EAU Guidelines for Penile Prosthesis Prophylaxis. J Sex Med 2017;14(3):455–63. https://doi.org/10.1016/j.jsxm.2017.01.007.

135. Charani E, de Barra E, Rawson TM, et al. Antibiotic prescribing in general medical and surgical specialties: a prospective cohort study. Antimicrob Resist Infect Control 2019;8:151. https://doi.org/10.1186/s13756-019-0603-6.

136. Aiken AM, Wanyoro AK, Mwangi J, et al. Changing use of surgical antibiotic prophylaxis in Thika Hospital, Kenya: a quality improvement intervention with an interrupted time series design. PLoS One 2013;8(11):e78942. https://doi.org/10.1371/journal.pone.0078942.

137. GlobalSurg Collaborative. Surgical site infection after gastrointestinal surgery in high-income, middle-income, and low-income countries: a prospective, international, multicentre cohort study. Lancet Infect Dis 2018;18(5):516–25. https://doi.org/10.1016/S1473-3099(18)30101-4.

138. Berrondo C, Carone M, Katz C, et al. Adherence to Perioperative Antibiotic Prophylaxis Recommendations and Its Impact on Postoperative Surgical Site Infections. Cureus 2022;14(6):e25859. https://doi.org/10.7759/cureus.25859.

139. Gouvêa M, de Oliveira Novaes C, Pereira DMT, et al. Adherence to guidelines for surgical antibiotic prophylaxis: a review. Braz J Infect Dis 2015;19(5): 517–24. https://doi.org/10.1016/j.bjid.2015.06.004.

140. Anderson DJ, Kaye KS, Chen LF, et al. Clinical and financial outcomes due to methicillin resistant Staphylococcus aureus surgical site infection: a multi-center matched outcomes study. PLoS One 2009;4(12):e8305. https://doi.org/10.1371/journal. pone.0008305.

141. O'Brien WJ, Gupta K, Itani KMF. Association of Postoperative Infection With Risk of Long-term Infection and Mortality. JAMA Surg 2020;155(1): 61–8. https://doi.org/10.1001/jamasurg.2019.4539.

142. Jiang S, Wei Y, Ke H, et al. Building a nomogram plot based on the nanopore targeted sequencing for predicting urinary tract pathogens and differentiating from colonizing bacteria. Front Cell Infect Microbiol 2023;13:1142426. https://doi.org/10. 3389/fcimb.2023.1142426.

143. Yang M, Li Y, Huang F. A nomogram for predicting postoperative urosepsis following retrograde intrarenal surgery in upper urinary calculi patients with negative preoperative urine culture. Sci Rep 2023;13(1): 2123. https://doi.org/10.1038/s41598-023-29352-y.

144. Wang F, Wang X, Shi Y, et al. Development of a risk nomogram predicting urinary tract infection in patients with indwelling urinary catheter after radical surgery for cervical cancer. Progres En Urol J Assoc Francaise Urol Soc Francaise Urol 2023; 33(10):492–502. https://doi.org/10.1016/j.purol. 2023.08.017.

145. McFarland LV, Mulligan ME, Kwok RY, et al. Nosocomial acquisition of Clostridium difficile infection. N Engl J Med 1989;320(4):204–10. https://doi.org/ 10.1056/NEJM198901263200402.

146. Lessa FC, Mu Y, Bamberg WM, et al. Burden of Clostridium difficile infection in the United States. N Engl J Med 2015;372(9):825–34. https://doi.org/ 10.1056/NEJMoa1408913.

147. Poeran J, Mazumdar M, Rasul R, et al. Antibiotic prophylaxis and risk of Clostridium difficile infection after coronary artery bypass graft surgery. J Thorac Cardiovasc Surg 2016;151(2):589–97. e2. https://doi.org/10.1016/j.jtcvs.2015.09.090.

148. Balch A, Wendelboe AM, Vesely SK, et al. Antibiotic prophylaxis for surgical site infections as a risk factor for infection with Clostridium difficile. PLoS One 2017;12(6):e0179117. https://doi.org/ 10.1371/journal.pone.0179117.

149. Carignan A, Allard C, Pépin J, et al. Risk of Clostridium difficile infection after perioperative antibacterial prophylaxis before and during an outbreak of infection due to a hypervirulent strain. Clin Infect Dis 2008; 46(12):1838–43. https://doi.org/10.1086/588291.

150. Wren SM, Ahmed N, Jamal A, et al. Preoperative oral antibiotics in colorectal surgery increase the rate of Clostridium difficile colitis. Arch Surg Chic Ill 1960 2005;140(8):752–6. https://doi.org/10. 1001/archsurg.140.8.752.

151. Kirkwood KA, Gulack BC, Iribarne A, et al. A multi-institutional cohort study confirming the risks of Clostridium difficile infection associated with prolonged antibiotic prophylaxis. J Thorac Cardiovasc Surg 2018;155(2):670–8.e1. https://doi.org/10. 1016/j.jtcvs.2017.09.089.

152. Teng C, Reveles KR, Obodozie-Ofoegbu OO, et al. Clostridium difficile Infection Risk with Important Antibiotic Classes: An Analysis of the FDA Adverse Event Reporting System. Int J Med Sci 2019;16(5): 630–5. https://doi.org/10.7150/ijms.30739.

153. Hess A, Byerly S, Lenart E, et al. Risk factors for clostridium difficile infection in general surgery patients. Am J Surg 2023;225(1):118–21. https://doi. org/10.1016/j.amjsurg.2022.09.031.

154. Abdelsattar ZM, Krapohl G, Alrahmani L, et al. Postoperative burden of hospital-acquired Clostridium difficile infection. Infect Control Hosp Epidemiol 2015;36(1):40–6. https://doi.org/10.1017/ ice.2014.8.

155. Poylin V, Hawkins AT, Bhama AR, et al. The American Society of Colon and Rectal Surgeons Clinical Practice Guidelines for the Management of Clostridioides difficile Infection. Dis Colon Rectum 2021;64(6):650–68. https://doi.org/10.1097/DCR.0000000000002047.

156. Kociolek LK, Gerding DN, Carrico R, et al. Strategies to prevent Clostridioides difficile infections in acute-care hospitals: 2022 Update. Infect Control Hosp Epidemiol 2023;44(4):527–49. https://doi. org/10.1017/ice.2023.18.

157. Box MJ, Ortwine KN, Goicoechea M, Scripps Antimicrobial Stewardship Program (SASP). No Impact of Probiotics to Reduce Clostridium difficile Infection in Hospitalized Patients: A Real-world Experience. Open Forum Infect Dis 2018;5(12):ofy192. https://doi.org/10.1093/ofid/ofy192.

158. Ehrhardt S, Guo N, Hinz R, et al. Saccharomyces boulardii to Prevent Antibiotic-Associated Diarrhea: A Randomized, Double-Masked, Placebo-Controlled Trial. Open Forum Infect Dis 2016;3(1): ofw011. https://doi.org/10.1093/ofid/ofw011.

159. Allen SJ, Wareham K, Wang D, et al. A high-dose preparation of lactobacilli and bifidobacteria in the prevention of antibiotic-associated and Clostridium difficile diarrhoea in older people admitted to hospital: a multicentre, randomised, double-blind, placebo-controlled, parallel arm trial (PLACIDE). Health Technol Assess Winch Engl 2013; 17(57):1–140. https://doi.org/10.3310/hta17570.

160. Cai J, Zhao C, Du Y, et al. Comparative efficacy and tolerability of probiotics for antibiotic-associated diarrhea: Systematic review with network meta-analysis. United Eur Gastroenterol J 2018;6(2):169–80. https://doi.org/10.1177/2050640617736987.

161. Auclair J, Frappier M, Millette M. Lactobacillus acidophilus CL1285, Lactobacillus casei LBC80R, and Lactobacillus rhamnosus CLR2 (Bio-K+): Characterization, Manufacture, Mechanisms of Action, and Quality Control of a Specific Probiotic Combination for Primary Prevention of Clostridium difficile Infection. Clin Infect Dis 2015;60(Suppl 2): S135–43. https://doi.org/10.1093/cid/civ179.

162. Johnson S, Maziade PJ, McFarland LV, et al. Is primary prevention of Clostridium difficile infection possible with specific probiotics? Int J Infect Dis IJID 2012;16(11):e786–92. https://doi.org/10.1016/j.ijid.2012.06.005.

163. de Bruyn G, Gordon DL, Steiner T, et al. Safety, immunogenicity, and efficacy of a Clostridioides difficile toxoid vaccine candidate: a phase 3 multicentre, observer-blind, randomised, controlled trial. Lancet Infect Dis 2021;21(2):252–62. https://doi.org/10.1016/S1473-3099(20)30331-5.

164. Shenoy ES, Macy E, Rowe T, et al. Evaluation and Management of Penicillin Allergy: A Review. JAMA 2019;321(2):188–99. https://doi.org/10.1001/jama.2018.19283.

165. Sexton ME, Kuruvilla ME. Management of Penicillin Allergy in the Perioperative Setting. Antibiot Basel Switz 2024;13(2):157. https://doi.org/10.3390/antibiotics13020157.

166. Sousa-Pinto B, Blumenthal KG, Courtney L, et al. Assessment of the Frequency of Dual Allergy to Penicillins and Cefazolin: A Systematic Review and Meta-analysis. JAMA Surg 2021;156(4):e210021. https://doi.org/10.1001/jamasurg.2021.0021.

167. Maisat W, Bermudez M, Yuki K. Use of clindamycin as an alternative antibiotic prophylaxis. Perioper Care Oper Room Manag 2022;28:100278. https://doi.org/10.1016/j.pcorm.2022.100278.

168. Sivagnanam S, Deleu D. Red man syndrome. Crit Care Lond Engl 2003;7(2):119–20. https://doi.org/10.1186/cc1871.

169. Legendre DP, Muzny CA, Marshall GD, et al. Antibiotic hypersensitivity reactions and approaches to desensitization. Clin Infect Dis 2014;58(8): 1140–8. https://doi.org/10.1093/cid/cit949.

170. Maker JH, Stroup CM, Huang V, et al. Antibiotic Hypersensitivity Mechanisms. Pharm Basel Switz 2019;7(3): 122. https://doi.org/10.3390/pharmacy7030122.

Antibiotic Prophylaxis for Genitourinary Procedures in Patients with Artificial Joint Replacement and Artificial Heart Valves

Briana Goddard, MD*, Daniel Stein, MD, MHS

KEYWORDS

- Prosthetic joint infection • Prosthetic valve endocarditis • Antibiotic prophylaxis
- Genitourinary procedure

KEY POINTS

- When choosing to administer antibiotic prophylaxis, the risk of infectious complications must be carefully weighed against the risks of administering antibiotics.
- Patients with prosthetic joints should receive antibiotic prophylaxis for genitourinary procedures if the patient is within 2 years of arthroplasty, or if they are at high risk for infection based on the procedure being performed and their individual comorbidities.
- Antibiotic prophylaxis should not be given for the sole purpose of prevention of infective endocarditis, even in the setting of a high-risk cardiac patient.

BACKGROUND

Prosthetic joints infection (PJI) and prosthetic valve endocarditis (PVE) are relatively uncommon but serious infectious complications. The incidence of PJI after hip or knee arthroplasty is 1% to 2%. Approximately 1 million hip and knee arthroplasties are performed annually in the United States, leading to a significant number of cases of PJI despite a low incidence.[1–3] Treatment for PJI includes surgical debridement, removal and replacement of the joint, and a long duration of antibiotic therapy.[3] These infections increase patient morbidity, lead to longer hospital stays, can impair patients' quality of life, and incur a large economic impact. It is estimated that within 10 years costs associated with infections of prosthetic hips and knees will total 1.8 billion dollars annually.[4–6] PVE is also associated with high morbidity and mortality. Heart valve replacement is performed in over 100,000 people annually in the United States and continues to increase.[7] The incidence of prosthetic valve infection is estimated at less than 2% per person-year and accounts for about 20% to 30% of all cases of endocarditis.[8–10] Treatment includes long duration of antibiotic therapy and in some cases surgical debridement, while complications can include heart failure and thromboembolic events.[11] Given the significant morbidity and mortality of these infectious complications, prevention of them is of great interest.

PJI and PVE can be categorized based on how long after the index procedure they occur, and

Department of Urology, George Washington University Hospital, 2150 Pennsylvania Avenue Northwest Suite 3-417, Washington, DC 20037, USA
* Corresponding author.
E-mail address: brianalgoddard@gmail.com
Twitter: @GWUrology (B.G.)

Urol Clin N Am 51 (2024) 467–474
https://doi.org/10.1016/j.ucl.2024.06.002
0094-0143/24/© 2024 Elsevier Inc. All rights reserved, including those for text and data mining, AI training, and similar technologies.

these different categories are thought to happen through different mechanisms. For PJI, early infection occurs within 3 months, delayed within 3 to 24 months, and late infections occur more than 24 months after arthorplasty.[12] Early PVE occurs within 1 year of surgery, and late occurs greater than 1 year after surgery.[13] For both PJI and PVE, early infections are thought to be acquired during the index procedure, while late infections are secondary to hematogenous seeding from episodes of bacteremia.[8,12] While patients are considered at highest risk of infection within 2 years of arthroplasty and within 1 year of prosthetic valve surgery,[2,14] the target of antibiotic prophylaxis is the prevention of late infections that occur through hematogenous seeding. Given this, urologists should know the current recommendations regarding antibiotic prophylaxis in these patient populations.

Antibiotic prophylaxis is given at the time of a procedure to reduce surgical site infections, bacteremia, and other infectious complications.[15,16] Alsaywid and colleagues performed a systematic analysis in 2013 to determine if antibiotic prophylaxis is effective in preventing bacteremia specifically for endoscopic urologic procedures. In studies that compared antibiotic prophylaxis to placebo or no treatment, antibiotic prophylaxis decreased the incidence of bacteriuria (risk ratio 0.36), bacteremia (risk ratio 0.43), symptomatic urinary tract infection (risk ratio 0.38), and high-grade fevers (risk ratio 0.41).[17]

Assessment of the risks and benefits of antimicrobial prophylaxis should include consideration of the procedure being performed, possible pathogens, the patient's ability to respond to an infection, and the potential morbidity of an infection.[16] The risk of infectious complications must also be carefully weighed against the risks of administering antibiotics, including Clostridium difficile infections, antibiotic resistance, allergic reactions, and other antibiotic side effects.[12] Each patient's individual risk factors and medical history, including a history of prosthetic joint or artificial heart valve, should be considered in a physician's antibiotic selection.

DISCUSSION
Patient Risk Factors for Infectious Complications

There are several patient factors that increase the risk of a procedure-related infection. According to the American Urologic Association (AUA) best practice statement on antimicrobial prophylaxis, patients at a higher risk of surgical site infection include those with diabetes, significant cardiovascular or pulmonary comorbidities, anatomic abnormalities of the urinary tract, poor nutritional status, tobacco use, immunocompromise, chronic colonization, concomitant infection at another site, and pregnancy.[16] While frailty may be considered a risk factor for infection, not all urologic literature has found an increase in surgical infections in patients with high frailty scores.[18]

The incidence of PJI is highest in the early and delayed postoperative period.[2] The factors that increase risk of PJI are those that increase tissue ischemia, impair wound healing, or lead to increased falls. These include tobacco use, excessive alcohol use, malnutrition, high body mass index, hepatitis C infection, peripheral artery disease, and autoimmune inflammatory arthritis.[2,3]

Patients with prosthetic valves have the highest rate of infection within the first year of surgery.[19] Additional risk factors include male gender, significant cardiovascular and pulmonary comorbidities, renal insufficiency, diabetes, liver disease, and higher body mass index.[14]

Procedural Risk Factors for Infectious Complications

In addition to patient factors, procedural factors also influence the risk of bacteremia. The risk of bacteremia during a genitourinary (GU) procedure often is the result of manipulation of the urothelial mucosa and duration of the procedure. According to the 2008 AUA best practice statement, procedures that carry a high risk of bacteremia include those with stone manipulation, ureteroscopy or pyeloscopy, incision into the urinary tract, incision into bowel, transrectal prostate biopsy, and procedures in patients with indwelling tubes that may be colonized.[20] One study found no instances of bacteremia following routine office cystoscopy—a procedure that is short in duration and does not involve breaking the mucosal barrier.[21] Another study found a bacteremia rate of 7% in patients who underwent urodynamics—a procedure that involves catheterization and bladder distention, but minimal mucosal manipulation.[22] In contrast, a study found 23% of the patients undergoing transurethral resection of the prostate—a longer procedure that does break the mucosal barrier—had transient intraoperative bacteremia despite receiving antibiotic prophylaxis.[23] In a retrospective study of 147 patients who underwent cystectomy—a lengthy procedure that involves break in the urothelial mucosa and incision into the bowel—47% developed a postoperative infection, and 18.4% developed bacteremia.[24–26] These examples demonstrate how operative factors such as surgical time and the manipulation of mucosal barriers influence the risk of postoperative infection.

Evidence for Prosthetic Joint Infection and Prosthetic Valve Endocarditis After Genitourinary Procedures

Prosthetic joints

While bacteremia due to a GU procedure is a theoretic risk for causing hematogenous seeding of a prosthetic joint or valve, data are needed to assess the actual risk of PJI after urologic procedures and the role of antibiotic prophylaxis. PJI after GU procedure does not seem to be common. In 1984, a prospective trial followed patients who received prosthetic joints for 6 years to determine the rate of PJI. These patients were not advised to take specific surgical antibiotic prophylaxis. Of the 1000 patients, 24 underwent a GU procedure during the study, and of those, none developed a PJI.[27] There have not been many prospective trials for PJI following GU procedures, and this may be due to the low overall incidence of PJI, necessitating a very large sample size. However, there are case reports of PJI following GU procedure, despite the use of standard sterile technique and antibiotic prophylaxis.[28]

In 2015, Gupta and colleagues published a retrospective case control study looking to assess the risk of PJI after GU procedure. In this study, cases were patients admitted to the hospital with a prosthetic joint infection, while controls were patients with prosthetic joints admitted to the hospital for another reason. Minor urologic and gynecologic procedures within 2 years of admission were assessed. A total of 15% of cases and 16% of controls had undergone a GU procedure in the preceding 2 years. There was no increased risk for PJI in patients who had undergone a GU procedure versus those who had not, with an odds ratio of 1.0. This study concluded that GU procedures were not a risk factor for PJI. They also found that antibiotic prophylaxis at the time of GU procedure did not decrease the risk of subsequent PJI.[29]

While there are limited data assessing PJI after GU procedure, there has been substantial investigation into the role of asymptomatic bacteriuria at the time of prosthetic joint placement. In a large study of almost 2500 patients receiving a prosthetic joint, asymptomatic bacteriuria was identified in 12.1%. In this study, the overall rate of PJI was 1.7%. While the rate of PJI was higher in the group with asymptomatic bacteriuria at 4.3% versus 1.4% in the group without bacteriuria, there was no significant difference in the rate of PJI for those treated for their asymptomatic bacteriuria

versus those who were not, at 4.7% versus 3.9%, respectively. Therefore, giving antibiotics to treat asymptomatic bacteriuria prior to arthroplasty was not recommended by the authors.[30] A 2018 meta-analysis found that while hematogenous spread of bacteria harbored in the urinary tract can occur, preoperative antibiotic treatment did not show benefit and therefore could not be recommended.[31] The relationship of asymptomatic bacteriuria and a PJI may be due to other confounding patient factors such as frailty, immunocompromise, or other susceptibilities to infection thus explaining why prophylactic antibiotics may not help. As such, the causal association between bacteriuria and joint infections needs to be better elucidated. These and similar studies begin to contribute to the existing body of knowledge on the relation of pathogens in the urinary system and infection of prosthetic joints.

Artificial valves

There have been few studies assessing the risk of PVE after GU procedures. A case-control study published in 2000 analyzed community-acquired infective endocarditis not associated with intravenous drug use and compared cases with matched community residents. Cases were more likely to have kidney disease, diabetes, previous skin infection, or to have received intravenous fluids recently. Notably, no association was seen with recent GU procedures.[32] There have been rare reports of infective endocarditis in the absence of artificial valves after GU procedure,[33] and a case-control study did find an association between *Enterococcus* native valve infective endocarditis and preceding GU procedure, with an odds ratio of 8.2.[34]

A 2011 study examined the rates of antibiotic prescriptions and the incidence of infective endocarditis in the United Kingdom before and after their guidelines changed to no longer recommend antibiotic prophylaxis prior to procedures for patients with prosthetic valves. While there were significantly fewer antibiotics prescribed, there was no change in the cases of infective endocarditis.[35,36] This further supports that antibiotic prophylaxis prior to procedures is ineffective in preventing infective endocarditis.

While limited data exist to determine the risk of PVE after GU procedure, there has been extensive investigation into the risk of PVE after dental procedures. A 2013 Cochrane review and 2022 update found the evidence is not clear if antibiotic prophylaxis is effective at preventing infective endocarditis, and it cannot be determined if the benefits outweigh the risks.[37,38] It is thought that the transient bacteremia caused from everyday routine activities, such as teeth brushing, is a higher risk for infective endocarditis than dental procedures.[39] Further data are needed to better understand the role of transient bacteremia secondary to procedures and the risk of PVE.

Guidelines for Antibiotic Prophylaxis

There are several guidelines and best practice statements to aid in antibiotic prophylaxis selection in specific patient populations. In 2017, a comprehensive guide for general surgical prophylaxis was published.[15] The AUA published a best practice statement on antibiotic prophylaxis in 2008[24] and an updated version in 2019.[16] Similarly, the American Academy of Orthopedic Surgeons (AAOS) and the American Heart Association (AHA) have release best practice statements and guidelines on this topic.

Prosthetic joints

In 2003, the AUA and AAOS released a joint statement which indicated that antibiotic prophylaxis for GU procedures is not indicated for patients with pins, plates, and screws, nor is it indicated for most patients with joint replacements. According to this statement, antibiotic prophylaxis should be considered only in high-risk patients and those within 2 years of joint replacement surgery.[40] In 2009, the AAOS released an updated statement, saying that antibiotic prophylaxis should be given to patients with prosthetic joints for any GU procedure in which there is a risk of bacteremia; however, this recommendation has since been retired.[41] The AUA white paper published in 2020 states patients with hip or knee prostheses should receive antibiotic prophylaxis for GU procedures with a high risk of bacteremia, if the patient is within 2 years of their joint replacement surgery, or if they are a high-risk patient.[16] A patient should be considered high risk based upon the risk factors for surgical site infection and PJI previously described.

Artificial valves

Guidelines released from the AHA in 1997 did recommend antibiotic prophylaxis for GU procedures in patients with prosthetic valves.[42] However, there was a rise in Enterococcus strains resistant to penicillin, vancomycin, and aminoglycosides, all antibiotics previously recommended as prophylaxis. Guidelines released by the AHA in 2007 did not recommend the use of prophylactic antibiotics solely for prevention of infective endocarditis, as there are no published data that demonstrate a conclusive link between GU procedures and infective endocarditis.[43] The AUA agrees with these recommendations; their 2020 best practice statement states that "antibiotic prophylaxis should not be given for the sole purpose of prevention of infective endocarditis, even in the setting of a high-risk cardiac patient."[16] The AUA best practice statement does make note that there may be a benefit of antibiotic prophylaxis in high-risk cardiac patients who undergo concomitant GU and oral procedures, such as buccal graft urethroplasty.[16] According to the AHA, patients with a prosthetic valve would be considered high risk and should receive prophylaxis in this scenario.[39]

Pathogens

The majority of urinary infections are caused by Escherichia coli. Other common pathogens include Klebsiella species, Enterococcus species, Streptococcus agalactiae, Proteus mirabilis, Staphylococcus saprophyticus, and Pseudomonas aeruginosa, among others.[44] These same pathogens can lead to blood stream infections. E coli is identified as the causal organism in 52% of episodes of urosepsis. Gram-positive Enterococcus species are found in about 5% of urosepsis cases.[45] Enterococcus species are the most common urinary pathogen that also cause PJI and PVE. While gram-negative bacteria are very common in urinary infections, they are much less likely to cause PJI or PVE.

Prosthetic joints

In a study of 395 total hip arthroplasties and 390 total knee arthroplasties explanted for infection over 14 years, cultures showed gram-positive bacteria in 73%, gram negative in 7%, and fungal in less than 1%. A total of 21% had no pathogen identified, and 12% were polymicrobial. The most common pathogen was Staphylococcus aureus, followed by Streptococcus species and Enterococcus species.[46] It is estimated that S aureus and Staphylococcus epidermitis account for 65% of all prosthetic joint infections.[47] Enterococcus species have been found to cause up to 5% of prosthetic joint infections, and studies suggest that patients who have Enterococcus prosthetic joint infection tend to have more comorbidities and worse outcomes.[46,48,49] In a retrospective study of 302 patients with PJI, gram-negative pathogens were identified in 11.5%. The most common gram-negative pathogens isolated in this study were E coli and P aeruginosa, followed by species of Proteus, Serratia, Klebsiella, and Morganella.[50]

Artificial valves

In a study of 780 cases of PVE, the most common pathogens were alpha-hemolytic Streptococci (29%) and S aureus (22%), followed by Enterococci (14%) and coagulase-negative Staphylococci

(12%).[51] Gram-negative infections are an uncommon cause of PVE, accounting for less than 2% of cases. This is thought to be due to a low affinity for adherence to the endocardial endothelium.[52,53]

Antibiotic Selection

Prosthetic joints

In patients with prosthetic joints and indication for antibiotic prophylaxis, The AUA recommends using a single dose of an oral quinolone 1 to 2 hours prior to the procedure, or intravenous ampicillin and gentamicin, substituting vancomycin for penicillin allergic patients.[24] Similarly, the AAOS recommends an oral or intravenous quinolone 1 hour before the procedure.[41] However, studies suggest that resistance to quinolones has been increasing.[54] Each institution should review local resistance patterns for antibiotic selection, with the earlier mentioned pathogens in consideration.

Artificial valves

Patients with artificial heart valves do not require prophylaxis on the sole basis to prevent infective endocarditis, so antibiotics should be selected based upon the procedure and the patient's previous culture data. However, in patients with artificial valves with an active infection or sepsis secondary to a GU source, empiric antibiotic coverage should cover Enterococcus species. Antibiotic options are ampicillin, amoxicillin, or vancomycin for patients with a penicillin allergy.[43] For a high-risk patient undergoing concomitant GU and oral procedure, amoxicillin is the antibiotic of choice for prophylaxis, and clindamycin or first generation cephalosporins are reasonable alternatives in the case of allergies.[55]

Application in Clinical Practice

With the several different guidelines and best practice statements released over the last 2 decades, practice patterns regarding antibiotic prophylaxis for these patient populations may vary greatly. A survey study in 2022 found that urologists and orthopedists agree that GU procedures could result in PJI, and that patients should inform their doctors if they have a prosthetic joint. While orthopedists thought antibiotics were "definitely" indicated for routine urologic procedures, urologists thought that antibiotics were "probably" indicated.[56] Further studies are needed to assess the current practice patterns of urologists, and how often antibiotic prophylaxis is administered in accordance with current best practice statements.

The AUA best practice statement encourages peri-procedural antimicrobial prophylaxis for all urologic procedures that include a break in normal tissue barriers, including skin or mucosa. Exceptions include Class I/clean procedures in adults without an increased risk for urinary infections.[16] Common procedures performed by urologists that may not require antibiotic prophylaxis in all patients include office cystoscopy, urodynamics, vasectomy, and transperineal prostate biopsy, among others. For these procedures, a urologist should reconsider the decision to forgo antibiotic prophylaxis if a patient is otherwise high risk for infection or if they are within 2 years of arthroplasty. Conversely, an artificial heart valve alone should not prompt administration of antibiotic prophylaxis for these low-risk procedures.

In Class II (clean-contaminated), III (contaminated), and IV (infected) procedures, antimicrobial prophylaxis is recommended, as the reduction in surgical site or systemic infections outweighs the risk of administering antibiotics.[16] In patients with prosthetic joints or prosthetic heart valves, antibiotic selection should consider the coverage of Enterococcus species, as this is the uropathogen most commonly identified in PJI and PVE.

SUMMARY

PJI and PVE are uncommon but severe infectious complications that lead to high morbidity and mortality. There is limited evidence to assess if GU procedures lead to bacteremia and subsequent hematogenous seeding of prosthetic joints or artificial valves. Enterococcus is the uropathogen that is most commonly associated with PJI and PVE. Current best practice statements by the AUA support antibiotic prophylaxis administration in patients with prosthetic joints undergoing GU procedure particularly if they are within 2 years of arthroplasty, if the procedure carries a higher risk of bacteremia, or if their individual comorbidities place them at a higher risk for infection. While quinolone antibiotics have been recommended, local resistance patterns should be considered. Best practice statements by the AUA and AHA do not recommend administering antibiotic prophylaxis for patients with artificial valves undergoing a GU procedure for the sole purpose of preventing infectious endocarditis.

CLINICS CARE POINTS

- The decision to administer prophylactic antibiotics prior to a genitourinary procedure should take into account the procedure being performed, possible pathogens, the patient's ability to respond to an infection, the potential morbidity of an infection, as well as the risks of antibiotic administration. These risks and benefits may change in different patient populations.

- *Enterococcus* species are the uropathogens that are most associated with PJI and with PVE.
- According to the most recent AUA best practice statement, patients with prosthetic joints should receive antibiotic prophylaxis for genitourinary procedures if the patient is within 2 years of arthroplasty, or if they are at high risk for infection based on the procedure being performed and their individual comorbidities.
- For patients with prosthetic joints, the AUA and AAOS both recommend using a quinolone 1 to 2 hours prior to the procedure for antibiotic prophylaxis. However, local resistance patterns should be considered in antibiotic selection.
- Antibiotic prophylaxis should not be given for the sole purpose of prevention of infective endocarditis, even in the setting of a high-risk cardiac patient.

DISCLOSURE

The authors have nothing to disclose.

REFERENCES

1. Ong KL, Kurtz SM, Lau E, et al. Prosthetic joint infection risk after total hip arthroplasty in the medicare population. J Arthroplasty 2009;24(6 SUPPL):105–9.
2. Weinstein EJ, Stephens-Shields AJ, Newcomb CW, et al. Incidence, microbiological studies, and factors associated with prosthetic joint infection after total knee arthroplasty. JAMA Netw Open 2023;6(10):E2340457.
3. Ayoade F, Li DD, Mabrouk A, Todd JR. Periprosthetic Joint Infection. In: StatPearls [Internet]. Treasure Island (FL): StatPearls publishing; 2024.
4. Walter N, Rupp M, Baertl S, et al. Periprosthetic joint infection. Bone Jt Res 2022;11(1):8–9.
5. Wildeman P, Rolfson O, Söderquist B, et al. What are the long-term outcomes of mortality, quality of life, and hip function after prosthetic joint infection of the hip? a 10-year follow-up from Sweden. Clin Orthop Relat Res 2021;479(10):2203–13.
6. Premkumar A, Kolin DA, Farley KX, et al. Projected economic burden of periprosthetic joint infection of the hip and knee in the United States. J Arthroplasty 2021;36(5):1484–9.e3.
7. Wang A, Athan E, Pappas PA, et al. Contemporary clinical profile and outcome of prosthetic valve endocarditis. JAMA 2007;297(12):1354–61.
8. Khalil H, Soufi S. Prosthetic Valve Endocarditis. In: StatPearls [Internet]. Treasure Island (FL): StatPearls Publishing; 2024.
9. Jiang W, Wu W, Guo R, et al. Predictors of prosthetic valve endocarditis following transcatheter aortic valve replacement: A meta-analysis. Heart Surg Forum 2021;24(1):E101–7.
10. del Val D, Panagides V, Mestres CA, et al. Infective endocarditis after transcatheter aortic valve replacement: JACC state-of-the-art review. J Am Coll Cardiol 2023;81(4):394–412.
11. Khalil H, Soufi S. Prosthetic valve endocarditis. Stat. 2022. Available at: https://www.ncbi.nlm.nih.gov/books/NBK567731/%0A.
12. Zimmerli W, Trampuz A, Ochsner PE. Prosthetic-joint infections. N Engl J Med 2004;1645–54.
13. Castillo JC, Anguita MP, Torres F, et al. Long-term prognosis of early and late prosthetic valve endocarditis. Am J Cardiol 2004;93(9):1185–7.
14. Braghieri L, Kaur S, Black CK, et al. Endocarditis after transcatheter aortic valve replacement. J Clin Med 2023;12(22).
15. Berrios-Torres S, Umscheid C, Bratzler D, et al. Center for disease control and prevention guidelines for the prevention of surgical site infection, 2017. JAMA Surg 2017;152(8):784–91.
16. Lightner DJ, Wymer K, Sanchez J, et al. Best practice statement on urologic procedures and antimicrobial prophylaxis purpose : materials and methods : results : conclusions : pre- and periprocedural prophylaxis class I/Clean procedures Class II/Clean-contaminated procedures class III/Cont. J Urol 2020;203(2):351–6.
17. Alsaywid B, Smith G. Antibiotic prophylaxis for transurethral urological surgeries: Systematic review. Urol Ann 2013;5(2):61–74.
18. Bhatia VP, Aro T, Smith SM, et al. Frailty as predictor of complications in patients undergoing percutaneous nephrolithotomy (PCNL). World J Urol 2021;39(10):3971–7.
19. Glaser N, Jackson V, Holzmann MJ, et al. Prosthetic valve endocarditis after surgical aortic valve replacement. Circulation 2017;136(3):329–31.
20. Wolf JS, Bennett CJ, Dmochowski RR, et al. Best practice policy statement on urologic surgery antimicrobial prophylaxis. J Urol 2008;179(4):1379–90.
21. Turan H, Balci U, Erdinc FS, et al. Bacteriuria, pyuria and bacteremia frequency following outpatient cystoscopy. Int J Urol 2006;13(1):25–8.
22. Onur R, Özden M, Orhan I, et al. Incidence of bacteraemia after urodynamic study. J Hosp Infect 2004;57(3):241–4.
23. Mohee AR, Gascoyne-Binzi D, West R, et al. Bacteraemia during transurethral resection of the prostate: What are the risk factors and is it more common than we think? PLoS One 2016;11(7):1–12.

24. Kolwijck E, Seegers AEM, Tops SCM, et al. Incidence and microbiology of post-operative infections after radical cystectomy and ureteral stent removal; a retrospective cohort study. BMC Infect Dis 2019; 3(19):303.

25. Griffiths L, Aro T, Samson P, et al. Prospective randomized trial of antibiotic prophylaxis duration for percutaneous nephrolithotomy in low-risk patients. J Endourol 2023;37(10):1075–80.

26. Corrales M, Sierra A, Doizi S, et al. Risk of sepsis in retrograde intrarenal surgery: a systematic review of the literature. Eur Urol Open Sci 2022;44(October): 84–91.

27. Ainscow D, Denham R. The risk of haematogenous infection in total joint replacements. J Bone Jt Surg Br 1984;66(4):580–2.

28. Dabasia H, Kokkinakis M, El-Guindi M. Haematogenous infection of a resurfacing hip replacement after transurethral resection of the prostate. Bone Joint Lett J 2009;91(6):820–1.

29. Gupta A, Osmon DR, Hanssen AD, et al. Genitourinary procedures as risk factors for prosthetic hip or knee infection: a hospital-based prospective case-control study. Open Forum Infect Dis 2015; 2(3).

30. Sousa R, Muñoz-Mahamud E, Quayle J, et al. Is asymptomatic bacteriuria a risk factor for prosthetic joint infection? Clin Infect Dis 2014;59(1):41–7.

31. Wang C, Yin D, Shi W, et al. Current evidence does not support systematic antibiotherapy prior to joint arthroplasty in patients with asymptomatic bacteriuria-a meta analysis. Int Orthop 2018;42(3): 479–85.

32. Fattahi FH, Azarshab M, Sanati H. Risk factors for infective endocarditis. J Maz Univ Med Sci 2015; 25(128):29–36.

33. Colalillo G, Cardi A, D'Elia G, et al. Unusual case of infectious endocarditis in a patient subjected to transurethral resection of the prostate (TURP) without cardiovascular risk factors. Arch Esp Urol 2021; 74(9):902–9053.

34. Mohee AR, West R, Baig W, et al. A case-control study: are urological procedures risk factors for the development of infective endocarditis? BJU Int 2014;114(1):118–24.

35. Richey R, Wray D, Stokes T. Prophylaxis against infective endocarditis: Summary of NICE guidance. Br Med J 2008;336(7647):770–1. AD.

36. Thornhill MH, Dayer MJ, Forde JM, et al. Impact of the NICE guideline recommending cessation of antibiotic prophylaxis for prevention of infective endocarditis: Before and after study. Br Med J 2011; 342(7807):13–4.

37. Glenny AM, Oliver R, Roberts GJ, et al. Antibiotics for the prophylaxis of bacterial endocarditis in dentistry. Cochrane Database Syst Rev 2013; 2013(10):14651858.

38. Rutherford SJ, Glenny A, Roberts G, et al. Antibiotic prophylaxis for preventing bacterial endocarditis following dental procedures. Cochrane Database Syst Rev 2022;10(5):5.

39. Wilson WR, Gewitz M, Lockhart PB, et al. Prevention of viridans group streptococcal infective endocarditis: a scientific statement from the American Heart Association. Circulation 2021;143(20):E963–78.

40. Antibiotic prophylaxis for urological patients with total joint replacements. J Urol 2003;169(5):1796–7.

41. Mazur DJ, Fuchs DJ, Abicht TO, et al. Update on antibiotic prophylaxis for genitourinary procedures in patients with artificial joint replacement and artificial heart valves. Urol Clin North Am 2015;42(4): 441–7.

42. Dajani A, Taubert K, Wilson W, et al. Prevention of bacterial endocarditis. Recommendations by the American Heart Association. JAMA, J Am Med Assoc 1997;277(22):1794–801.

43. Wilson W, Taubert KA, Gewitz M, et al. Prevention of infective endocarditis: Guidelines from the American Heart Association. Circulation 2007;116(15): 1736–54.

44. Foxman B. The epidemiology of urinary tract infection. Nat Rev Urol 2010;7(12):653–60.

45. Dreger NM, Degener S, Ahmad-Nejad P, et al. Urosepsis - etiology, diagnosis, and treatment. Dtsch Arztebl Int 2015;112(49):837–47.

46. Bjerke-Kroll BT, Christ AB, McLawhorn AS, et al. Periprosthetic joint infections treated with two-stage revision over 14 years: An evolving microbiology profile. J Arthroplasty 2014;29(5):877–82.

47. Esposito S, Leone S. Prosthetic joint infections: microbiology, diagnosis, management and prevention. Int J Antimicrob Agents 2008;32(4):287–93.

48. Ascione T, Balato G, Mariconda M, et al. Clinical and prognostic features of prosthetic joint infections caused by Enterococcus spp. Eur Rev Med Pharmacol Sci 2019;23(2):59–64.

49. Rasouli MR, Tripathi MS, Kenyon R, et al. Low rate of infection control in enterococcal periprosthetic joint infections infection. Clin Orthop Relat Res 2012; 470(10):2708–16.

50. Zmistowski B, Fedorka CJ, Sheehan E, et al. Prosthetic joint infection caused by gram-negative organisms. J Arthroplasty 2011;26(SUPPL. 6):104–8.

51. Berisha B, Ragnarsson S, Olaison L, et al. Microbiological etiology in prosthetic valve endocarditis: a nationwide registry study. J Intern Med 2022; 292(3):428–37.

52. Habib G, Hoen B, Tornos P, et al. Guidelines on the prevention , diagnosis , and treatment of infective endocarditis (new version 2009): The Task Force on the Prevention , Diagnosis, and Treatment of Infective Endocarditis of the European Society of Cardiology (ESC) ! Email alerts A. Eur Heart J 2009;30(19):2369–413.

53. Peralta DP, Chang AY. Escherichia coli: a rare cause of prosthetic valve endocarditis. Cureus 2023;15(5): 1–6.

54. Bader MS, Loeb M, Brooks AA. An update on the management of urinary tract infections in the era of antimicrobial resistance. Postgrad Med 2017; 129(2):242–58.

55. Ramu C, Padmanabhan TV. Indications of antibiotic prophylaxis in dental practice-Review. Asian Pac J Trop Biomed 2012;2(9):749–54.

56. Kingston R, Kiely P, McElwain J. Antibiotic prophylaxis for dental or urologic procedures following hip or knee replacement. J Infect 2002; 45(4):243–5.

The Role of the Gut Microbiome in Kidney Stone Disease

Sarah Hanstock, BSc, Ben Chew, MD, Dirk Lange, PhD*

KEYWORDS

- Kidney stone disease • Intestinal microbiome • Oxalate • *Oxalobacter formigenes*
- Short-chain fatty acids • Butyrate

KEY POINTS

- The intestinal microbiome plays a significant role in maintaining overall health.
- Healthy oxalate homeostasis involves a multispecies bacterial network in addition to *Oxalobacter formigenes*, suggesting a role for metabolic pathways beyond oxalate degradation.
- Dysbiosis of the intestinal microbiome, including the reduction of butyrate-producing bacterial species, plays a significant role in an increased risk for kidney stone formation.

BACKGROUND

Kidney stone disease (KSD) is characterized by the formation of crystal deposits in the kidney. KSD is often associated with intense pain, lasting urinary tract damage, and emergency room visits for urgent management or removal of stones. These crystals can be composed of calcium oxalate, calcium phosphate, uric acid, cysteine, and/or struvite, listed from most to least common. While rates vary by country, in North America the rate of occurrence of kidney stones ranges between 7% and 13% of individuals.[1] Interviews of patients with KSD have identified significant difficulty in disease prevention as one of the most important issues in patients' health-related quality of life.[2] As such it is important for research to focus on understanding the origins of KSD and various risk factors, to be able to address these patient-oriented goals.

The gut microbiome has been proposed as a contributing risk factor, and this may help to explain the etiology of kidney stone formation (Fig. 1). The gut microbiome is the community of bacteria that reside in the intestine. Increasingly, the microbiome has been linked to human health for both its local and distal influences on a variety of disease states, as it acts as an intersection between diet, intestinal health, immunity, and whole-body health. A healthy gut microbiome acts synergistically with a host to metabolize and produce beneficial factors and in exchange is housed in the hospitable intestine. In contrast, a dysbiotic microbiome has fallen short and created an imbalance in the microbial community and the host to increase the risk for certain diseases.

An initial connection of KSD to the gut microbiome was the finding that individuals with oral antibiotic exposure, especially in early life, had a higher risk of developing kidney stones.[3] Antibiotic exposure is an extrinsic trigger for microbiome dysbiosis, solidifying a mechanistic connection between gut microbiome dysbiosis and KSD. In this review, we plan to examine the relationship between the gut microbiome and KSD.

The Stone Centre at Vancouver General Hospital, Department of Urologic Sciences, University of British Columbia, Vancouver, Canada
* Corresponding author. The Stone Centre at Vancouver General Hospital, Jack Bell Research Centre, Room 550-3, 2660 Oak Street, Vancouver, British Columbia V6H 3Z6, Canada.
E-mail address: dirk.lange@ubc.ca

Urol Clin N Am 51 (2024) 475–482
https://doi.org/10.1016/j.ucl.2024.06.003
0094-0143/24/© 2024 Elsevier Inc. All rights are reserved, including those for text and data mining, AI training, and similar technologies.

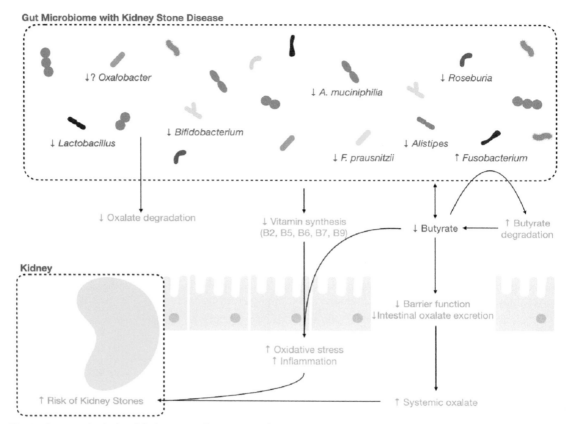

Fig. 1. Proposed relationship between the gut microbiome and KSD. The dysbiotic gut microbiome in KSD is proposed to cause a decrease in enteric oxalate degradation, decrease butyrate synthesis, and decrease vitamin synthesis.

CURRENT EVIDENCE

In order to understand microbial changes that occur in the gut of individuals with KSD, studies have compared microbial composition between individuals (both pediatric and adult) who have either active or a history of recurrent kidney stones.[4–10] In order to measure these changes, researchers have used a variety of methods designed to investigate both the microbial profile as well as factors produced by the gut microbiome. Both 16S ribosomal ribonucleic acid sequencing and shotgun metagenomic sequencing have shown utility in these studies to profile the gut microbiome, the latter method yielding a more in depth functional analysis. Metabolomic analysis has also been used in parallel with these sequencing techniques to understand changes in the intestinal environment from a biochemical perspective.[4,5,9]

Analyses of these data from microbiome sequencing can take on many forms. Most commonly, researchers will initially look at both the alpha and beta diversity, meaning the microbial diversity and the

comparative group dissimilarity, respectively. These analyses help researchers to understand trends and characterize the dysbiotic microbiome. Later, more specific analyses can be performed to look at specific species, microbial networks, and microbiome production of various metabolites to define this dysbiosis.

However, these sequencing studies do have inherent limitations. A meta-analysis examining 6 different sequencing studies identified that there are some study-specific results, with the key factors being study location, stone type, and subject age.[11] When interpreting results, we must consider these study-dependent differences, particularly in understanding why similar studies may have different results.

In parallel with these observational clinical studies, researchers have also used animal models to better understand the relevance of the gut microbiome in KSD. There is an extensive heterogeneity in the animal models selected to study KSD; however, the majority either use diet supplementation and injection of lithogenic agents or use genetic rodent models. While these studies are necessary to understand the role of the microbiome, they should all be examined with caution, as we do not yet know the role of many of these lithogenic agents on the microbiome itself. We also note that the majority of these animal models have used male mice, due to more consistency in their results. A thorough understanding of the data derived from these animal models, nonetheless, is critical to our understanding of the gut microbiome in KSD.

This section aims to characterize both the relevance of gut microbiome changes seen in KSD and their relevance to disease pathogenesis.

Oxalate Metabolism by the Gut Microbiome

Interest in the gut microbiome as a risk factor for KSD was piqued with the finding by Kaufman and colleagues[12] that individuals with recurrent calcium oxalate KSD had a lower abundance of the oxalate-degrading microbe *Oxalobacter formigenes*. Conversely, they found that there was no relationship between urinary oxalate excretion and abundance of *O formigenes*. This genus, *Oxalobacter*, was of particular interest because it can metabolize enteric oxalate. *Oxalobacter* spp use oxalate as their only carbon energy source and break it down via oxalate-degrading enzymes. Oxalate degrading function by *Oxalobacter* is facilitated by the presence of a membrane-associated oxalate antiporter (encoded by *OxlT*) for oxalate import,[13] formyl-CoA-transferase (encoded by *fcr*) for the conversion of oxalate to formate,[14] and oxalyl-CoA decarboxylase (encoded by *oxc*) for the decarboxylation of oxalyl-CoA to formyl-CoA.[15] A known risk factor for calcium oxalate KSD is oxalate consumption, and patients are recommended to reduce their oxalate consumption. Dietary oxalate is found in a variety of edible plants with especially high concentrations in spinach, rhubarb, Swiss chard, sorrel, and in lower amounts in a variety of other sources.[16] This knowledge led researchers to conclude that this may be an important metabolic pathway to enhance and to improve enteric oxalate metabolism in individuals with KSD.

Therefore, probiotic supplementation of *O formigenes* was investigated as a potential therapeutic for primary hyperoxaluria in a phase II/II clinical trial.[17] Unfortunately, there was no clinical benefit observed with probiotic supplementation; there were no significant changes in stone events, or a reduction in urine oxalate levels. While there seemed to be promise for probiotic supplementation with *O formigenes* in a clinical setting, the findings of this study suggested that targeted single-species enrichment is unlikely to be a successful strategy to treat microbiome dysbiosis in KSD.

Recent sequencing studies have not found consistent results when comparing abundance of *Oxalobacter* spp between individuals with KSD and with healthy controls. Some studies report that they see no significant differences in abundance of *Oxalobacter* between individuals with KSD and healthy controls.[5,8] Rather, shotgun metagenomic sequencing studies have found that individuals with KSD have a lower abundance of other oxalate-degrading bacteria including *Lactobacillus* and *Bifidobacterium* spp.[5,18–20] These bacteria possess the necessary proteins for oxalate metabolism, similar to *O formigenes*. These studies suggests that oxalate-degradation requires a network of bacteria to metabolically support one another and do not depend on a singular bacterial species.[11,13]

Other probiotic supplements, which include these other oxalate-degrading bacteria have also been tested. Research studies examining the effect of *Lactobacillus* and *Bifidobacterium* probiotics for KSD showed to either have a significant reduction or have a trend to reduce urinary oxalate levels.[21–24] There was a substantial individual variability in the efficacy of urinary oxalate reduction by these probiotics. It is still unclear what the clinical relevance is, as no study has demonstrated a reduction in rates of stone formation with these probiotics.

The Role of Butyrate

The underwhelming results from trials involving probiotic supplementation of *O formigenes* suggests that the relevance of gut microbiome dysbiosis to KSD may be understood through other factors. While *O formigenes* stole the spotlight from other microbiome changes, clinical studies employing sequencing of the gut microbiome of individuals with KSD have shown changes in abundance of other microbes that are not directly related to oxalate degradation. Clinical studies using shotgun metagenomic sequencing, run in parallel with metabolomics analysis, have demonstrated that there is also a reduced abundance of short-chain fatty acid (SCFA)-producing microbes in individuals with KSD.[4,5]

SCFAs are metabolites that are produced from microbial fiber fermentation. There are a variety of SCFAs including acetic acid, propionic acid, lactic acid, and isovaleric acid, but the SCFA observed to have the strongest negative correlation with KSD is butyric acid. Butyric acid, or butyrate, is produced by a variety of microbes in the gut including species from the phyla Firmicutes and Bacteroidetes.[25] Specifically in KSD, we see a decreased abundance in butyrate-producing bacteria including *Faecalibacterium prausnitzii*,[4,6,9,26] *Roseburia*,[5] *Alistipes* spp,[4] and *Akkermansia muciniphila*.[4] Furthermore, analysis has identified that a key butyrate synthesis enzyme, butyryl-coA synthetase, and resulting stool butyrate levels were significantly lower in individuals with KSD.[4,5,8]

Physiologically, this butyrate plays an important role as a primary energy source for the adjacent colonocytes.[25] At the intestine, butyrate can also influence inflammation, intestinal barrier function, ion transport, and oxidative stress pathways.[27] Butyrate can be absorbed into the systemic circulation and have distal effects.

There are a few animal studies that have investigated direct butyrate supplementation in rodent models for KSD. In one of these studies, it was found that butyrate supplementation significantly reduce renal calcium oxalate crystal deposits, in an ethylene glycol model of KSD.[28] Two additional studies that investigated sodium butyrate supplementation, either in an injectable glyoxylate mouse model[29] or with an ethylene glycol rat model,[30] consistently demonstrated that butyrate supplementation significantly reduced renal calcium oxalate deposits.

These animal models suggest that butyrate is a potent antilithogenic supplement. While the mechanism is unclear, these early studies suggest that butyrate may have this effect by influencing oxalate transport pathways and have distal antiinflammatory effects at the kidney. In the ethylene glycol mouse model, Liu and colleagues[28,31] suggest that butyrate may prevent renal crystal deposition by modulating oxalate homeostasis to favor intestinal oxalate excretion. Oxalate homeostasis at the intestine is regulated by both paracellular and transcellular absorption and excretion. Paracellular transport is determined by intestinal barrier function, particularly tight junction protein functioning. Butyrate is known to regulate expression and localization of tight junction proteins to enhance the integrity of the intestinal barrier, thus could modulate paracellular oxalate transport in the gut.[32] Transcellular transport of oxalate is regulated by a variety of solute carrier (SLC) transporter proteins, SLC26A1, SLC26A3, and SLC26A6. Butyrate has been used to increase the expression of these SLC transporters in successful treatment of congenital chloride diarrhea, a genetic condition characterized by loss-of-function mutations for the gene encoding SLC26A3.[27,33] Epigenetic and in vitro experiments have demonstrated

that butyrate may regulate the expression of SLC26A1[34–36] and SLC26A6.[12,18,19]

Aside from the local intestinal effects, butyrate may have distal effects. We know that KSD is not dependent on hyperoxaluria and requires a susceptible renal environment to begin stone formation. Tubular cell damage, often caused by oxidative stress (eg, mitochondrial dysfunction), is an important initial step in disease pathogenesis to allow for renal crystal deposition.[37,38] Animal models studying both KSD[30] and other kidney diseases[39,40] suggest that butyrate is able to reduce renal inflammation and oxidative stress. Butyrate is able to modulate renal detoxification pathways, specifically by increasing CYP2C9, which can dampen oxidative stress and inflammatory pathways.[30] Through this mechanism, butyrate may act via a 2 pronged process, both modifying the local intestinal environment to modulate oxalate homeostasis and influencing the distal renal environment to reduce cellular damage through oxidative stress pathways.

Butyrate may also have distal influence at the kidney through immunomodulation. It is known that the immune environment at the kidney is important for regulating renal inflammation and crystal clearance. In particular, the balance of M1/M2-like macrophages can dictate the rate of crystal clearance by phagocytosis.[41] Butyrate absorbed into the systemic circulation can elicit an effect to shift polarization of immune cell populations by acting on various G-protein-coupled receptors (GPRs). In a mouse model of glyoxylate-induced nephrolithiasis, Jin and colleagues[29] demonstrated that knockdown of GPR43 impaired the ability of butyrate to ameliorate renal calcium oxalate crystal deposition. They suggest that this is mediated though a shift in the immune environment of the kidney to be an antilithogenic environment.

While calcium oxalate stones have dominated research on the connection to butyrate, there are other potential connections to other stone types. Intriguingly, individuals with uric acid stones were found to have an increased abundance of *Bacteroides* and *Fusobacterium* in their gut microbiome compared to healthy controls.[42] Particularly, *Fusobacterium* is associated with degradation of SCFAs, thus limiting their bioavailability to the host. Studies investigating the microbiome of patients with gout, another condition with disruptions in uric acid homeostasis, have found that these individuals have a lower abundance of the butyrate-producing microbiome, alongside lower microbial diversity.[43] One study investigated the change in the gut microbiome with potassium sodium hydrogen citrate treatment of uric acid stones and found that through the course of treatment, the microbiome shifted toward a more healthy microbiome with decreases in the abundance of pathogenic *Fusobacterium*, increases in SCFA-producing bacteria, and increases in fecal butyrate levels posttreatment.[44] Interestingly, butyrate and uric acid share an intestinal efflux transporter ATP binding cassette subfamily G member 2 (ABCG2) suggesting a potential connection between these substrates at the subcellular level.[45] More research needs to be done to understand the connection among the gut microbiome, SCFAs, and uric acid stones.

Vitamin Metabolism

The gut microbiome is a network of bacteria, many of which produce essential metabolites for other bacteria in the community. Similar to the shift in perspective away from a single species causing disease, as seen with *O formigenes*, a shift toward understanding the complex interactions between functional pathways and various microbes is important. A review article by Chmiel and colleagues[46] proposed that a consequence of the microbiome dysbiosis seen in KSD is the lack of microbial vitamin biosynthesis. Additionally, this study suggests that individual discrepancies in response to vitamin supplementation for KSD may be due to the breakdown and limited bioavailability by some of these microbes. Sequencing studies confirm that some vitamin biosynthesis pathways are decreased in individuals with KSD.[15,47] Particularly microbial biosynthesis networks related to biosynthesis of riboflavin (vitamin B2), coenzyme A (pantothenic acid/vitamin B5 is a key precursor), pyridoxine (vitamin B6), biotin (vitamin B7), and folate (vitamin B9) were found to be absent in individuals with KSD. These vitamins have relevance in KSD as they play roles in mineral homeostasis, inflammation, and management of oxidative stress. While these few studies speculate that a dysbiotic gut microbiome in KSD interferes with vitamin biosynthesis and breakdown, we have yet to establish a mechanistic connection.

DISCUSSION

Research into the relevance of the gut microbiome suggests that we cannot simply look at KSD as a disease of the kidney, but instead as an integrative disease closely related to microbial pathways. Although the connection between the microbiome and KSD is still being established, both clinical sequencing studies and interventional animal trials suggest that there is potential for microbiome-related treatments for KSD. This

research is important because it helps to uncover the origin of KSD in populations where there is not a clear genetic or environmental cause. There are 2 clinical outcomes that should be of interest here. First is the ability for microbiome dysbiosis to serve as a biomarker for disease and second is the opportunity for microbiome interventions to be used to complement or replace current conventional treatments and be integrated into prophylactic care.

In the review article by Hinojosa-Gonalez and colleagues,[48] it is suggested that gut microbiome sequencing could act as an important biomarker for KSD. Specifically analyzing individual microbiome composition, together with metabolomics analysis, this would allow for individuals at risk for KSD to be identified. The salivary microbiome, which can be analyzed easily collectable saliva samples, may also be able to serve as a biomarker. This has also been identified to be distinct in individuals with KSD.[47] In the field of inflammatory bowel disease research, we see that the gut microbiome may be used as a biomarker to aid in early diagnosis, disease classification, and to predict response to therapy.[43] As such, research on the gut microbiome as a biomarker in KSD could assist with understanding the origin of disease, and eventually inform personalized medicine.

In regards to treatments, there are many options for the development of future microbiome interventions, each with differing efficacy. To date, the only direct microbiome interventions for KSD have been oral probiotic supplementation with underwhelming success. Since microbiome-targeted therapeutics are quite new, future research should continue to explore the options of these treatments for KSD. These options include probiotics, prebiotics, postbiotics, fecal microbiota transplantation (FMT), and antibiotic treatment. Given the current research in both animal and human studies, these treatments need to broadly target the microbial networks to either increase oxalate-degrading pathways or increase butyrate-synthesis pathways.

Probiotics

Probiotics refer to direct supplementation of a microbe, or combination of microbes. As discussed earlier, probiotic supplementation with *O formigenes* was found to be unsuccessful in preventing stone recurrence and reducing urinary oxalate levels.[17] However, other probiotic supplements, which are currently available, have been suggested to be trialed in KSD. Specifically, probiotic supplementation with *Lactobacillus* and

Bifidobacterium strains, identified in sequencing studies as having oxalate-degrading capacity,[5,18,19] could reduce urinary oxalate levels but has no impact on stone formation.[21–24]

While the majority of probiotics focus on oxalate-degrading bacteria, probiotic supplementation of SCFA-producing *Lactiplantibacillus plantarum* N-1 and J-15 has been successful in an ethylene glycol rat model of KSD.[49,50] *L plantarum* probiotic supplements were able to significantly reduce renal crystal deposits by decreasing urinary oxalate, reducing renal inflammation, and enhancing intestinal barrier function. Further exploration into probiotic supplementation of SCFA-producing bacteria for KSD should be done, so see if these results translate into a clinical population.

Prebiotics

In comparison to probiotic therapies, prebiotics aim to nourish certain microbiome communities. The majority of prebiotics is oligosaccharide carbohydrates but can also include other dietary factors.[51] By nourishing bacterial communities, prebiotics allow for a shift in the gut microbiome environment to target expansion of a certain microbial community. For example, inulin is a prebiotic, which can lead to an increase in abundance of butyrate-producing bacteria and a subsequent increase in butyrate levels.[52] While no research has tested independent prebiotic supplementation for individuals with KSD, we do, in fact, see that fiber consumption is inversely correlated with risk of KSD.[53,54]

Given the evidence for the role of butyrate, and success of supplementation in reducing renal crystal deposits in animal models,[28,29] prebiotics should be investigated in studies for both calcium-based stone and uric acid stone prophylaxis and treatment. Clinical recommendations for KSD already include various dietary recommendations, so implementation of prebiotic regimens could include changing those dietary recommendations to encourage consumption of prebiotic-rich foods. Where individuals are told to avoid certain high-oxalate foods, there should be a matched suggestion for what they should consume instead so that individuals are not limiting their fibre consumption.

Similar to probiotics, there is a high variability in individual prebiotic response since the efficacy is largely determined by the existing microbes in an individual.[52] As such, there is a good potential for synbiotics, a combination probiotic and prebiotic, to both provide and nourish oxalate-degrading and butyrate-producing communities. In vitro experiments have suggested that synbiotics may have more efficacy from an oxalate-degrading perspective.[55]

Postbiotics

One of the newest areas of microbiome interventions is the idea of supplementing microbiome-derived metabolites to see their beneficial effects without having to manipulate the microbiome directly. Given the current evidence, sodium butyrate would be a good postbiotic candidate as it has been used in animal experiments[28,29]; however, oral administration in humans is limited due to its unpleasant smell and taste. Instead, the butyrate prodrug tributyrin could be trialed to negate these limiting effects seen with sodium butyrate.[56] More research needs to be done to understand the mechanism, role, and risks of these postbiotic molecules prior to application to a clinical setting.

Fecal Microbiota Transplantation

FMT is a method whereby there is stool transplanted, typically from a healthy nondiseased individual to a diseased individual. In contrast to the use of a probiotic, this method involves the introduction of another microbiome instead of trying to make single species changes. Rodent studies have investigated FMT and found that these were able to significantly reduce urine oxalate levels, while increasing cecal expression of the oxalate transporter SLC26A6.[57,58] To date there have been no studies that investigate FMT for KSD. Prior to such trials, we would need to establish key biomarkers for an antilithogenic gut microbiome to identify healthy donors.

SUMMARY

It is evident that microbiome dysbiosis is closely related to the etiology of KSD and influences a multitude of pathways. Due to our knowledge gaps on this topic, it is still unclear if microbiome interventions can be translated to demonstrate clinical efficacy. Current evidence suggests that the enhancement of butyrate-producing pathways should be the next step for KSD research and translation into a clinical setting. There are a number of tools for accomplishing this and include probiotics, prebiotics, symbiotic, postbiotics, and FMT, each with their own advantages and risks. While we are not yet at a point where we can make clinical recommendations for KSD, there are many simple dietary or supplement-based approaches that could be applied in the future for prophylaxis or treatment of KSD.

DISCLOSURE

None.

REFERENCES

1. Sorokin I, Mamoulakis C, Miyazawa K, et al. Epidemiology of stone disease across the world. World J Urol 2017;35(9):1301–20.

2. Raja A, Wood F, Joshi HB. The impact of urinary stone disease and their treatment on patients' quality of life: a qualitative study. Urolithiasis 2020;48(3):227–34.

3. Tasian GE, Jemielita T, Goldfarb DS, et al. Oral Antibiotic Exposure and Kidney Stone Disease. J Am Soc Nephrol 2018;29(6):1731–40.

4. Choy W, Adler A, Morgan-Lang C, et al. Deficient butyrate metabolism in the intestinal microbiome is a potential risk factor for recurrent kidney stone disease. Urolithiasis 2024;52:38.

5. Denburg MR, Koepsell K, Lee JJ, et al. Perturbations of the Gut Microbiome and Metabolome in Children with Calcium Oxalate Kidney Stone Disease. J Am Soc Nephrol 2020;31(6):1358–69.

6. Ticinesi A, Milani C, Guerra A, et al. Understanding the gut-kidney axis in nephrolithiasis: an analysis of the gut microbiota composition and functionality of stone formers. Gut 2018;67(12):2097–106.

7. Zhao E, Zhang W, Geng B, et al. Intestinal dysbacteriosis leads to kidney stone disease. Mol Med Rep 2021;23(3):180.

8. Stern JM, Moazami S, Qiu Y, et al. Evidence for a distinct gut microbiome in kidney stone formers compared to non-stone formers. Urolithiasis 2016;44(5):399–407.

9. Chen F, Bao X, Liu S, et al. Gut microbiota affect the formation of calcium oxalate renal calculi caused by high daily tea consumption. Appl Microbiol Biotechnol 2021;105(2):789–802.

10. Tang R, Jiang Y, Tan A, et al. 16S rRNA gene sequencing reveals altered composition of gut microbiota in individuals with kidney stones. Urolithiasis 2018;46(6):503–14.

11. Kachroo N, Lange D, Penniston KL, et al. Meta-analysis of Clinical Microbiome Studies in Urolithiasis Reveal Age, Stone Composition, and Study Location as the Predominant Factors in Urolithiasis-Associated Microbiome Composition. mBio 2021;12(4):e0200721.

12. Kaufman DW, Kelly JP, Curhan GC, et al. Oxalobacter formigenes May Reduce the Risk of Calcium Oxalate Kidney Stones. J Am Soc Nephrol 2008;19(6):1197–203.

13. Heymann J, Sarker R, Hirai T, et al. Projection structure and molecular architecture of OxlT, a bacterial membrane transporter. EMBO J 2001;20:4408–13.

14. Khammar N, Martin G, Ferro K, et al. Use of the *frc* gene as a molecular marker to characterize oxalate-oxidizing bacterial abundance and diversity structure in soil. J Microbiol Methods 2009;76(2):120–7.

15. Suryavanshi MV, Bhute SS, Jadhav SD, et al. Hyperoxaluria leads to dysbiosis and drives selective enrichment of oxalate metabolizing bacterial species in recurrent kidney stone endures. Sci Rep 2016;6(1):34712.

16. Salgado N, Silva MA, Figueira ME, et al. Oxalate in Foods: Extraction Conditions, Analytical Methods, Occurrence, and Health Implications. Foods 2023;12(17):3201.

17. Milliner D, Hoppe B, Groothoff J. A randomised Phase II/III study to evaluate the efficacy and safety of orally administered Oxalobacter formigenes to treat primary hyperoxaluria. Urolithiasis 2018;46(4):313–23.

18. Karamad D, Khosravi-Darani K, Khaneghah AM, et al. Probiotic Oxalate-Degrading Bacteria: New Insight of Environmental Variables and Expression of the oxc and frc Genes on Oxalate Degradation Activity. Foods 2022;11(18):2876.

19. Tavasoli S, Alebouyeh M, Naji M, et al. Association of intestinal oxalate-degrading bacteria with recurrent calcium kidney stone formation and hyperoxaluria: a case–control study. BJU Int 2020;125(1):133–43.

20. Miller AW, Choy D, Penniston KL, et al. Inhibition of urinary stone disease by a multi-species bacterial network ensures healthy oxalate homeostasis. Kidney Int 2019;96(1):180–8.

21. Campieri C, Campieri M, Bertuzzi V, et al. Reduction of oxaluria after an oral course of lactic acid bacteria at high concentration. Kidney Int 2001;60(3):1097–105.

22. Lieske JC, Goldfarb DS, De Simone C, et al. Use of a probioitic to decrease enteric hyperoxaluria. Kidney Int 2005;68(3):1244–9.

23. Nogueira FRR, Marques NC, Froeder L, et al. Effects of Lactobacillus casei and Bifidobacterium breve on urinary oxalate excretion in nephrolithiasis patients. 2009. Available at: http://repositorio.unifesp.br/handle/11600/31407. [Accessed 21 March 2024].

24. Goldfarb D, Modersitzki F, Asplin J. A Randomized, Controlled Trial of Lactic Acid Bacteria for Idiopathic Hyperoxaluria. Clin J Am Soc Nephrol : CJASN 2007;2:745–9.

25. Liu H, Wang J, He T, et al. Butyrate: A Double-Edged Sword for Health? Adv Nutr 2018;9(1):21–9.

26. Kim HN, Kim JH, Chang Y, et al. Gut microbiota and the prevalence and incidence of renal stones. Sci Rep 2022;12(1):3732.

27. Canani RB, Costanzo MD, Leone L, et al. Potential beneficial effects of butyrate in intestinal and extra-intestinal diseases. World J Gastroenterol 2011;17(12):1519–28.

28. Liu Y, Jin X, Ma Y, et al. Short-Chain Fatty Acids Reduced Renal Calcium Oxalate Stones by Regulating the Expression of Intestinal Oxalate Transporter SLC26A6. mSystems 2021;6(6):e0104521.

29. Jin X, Jian Z, Chen X, et al. Short Chain Fatty Acids Prevent Glyoxylate-Induced Calcium Oxalate Stones by GPR43-Dependent Immunomodulatory Mechanism.

Front Immunol 2021;12. Available at: https://www.frontiersin.org/journals/immunology/articles/10.3389/fimmu.2021.729382. [Accessed 5 February 2024].

30. Zhou Z, Zhou X, Zhang Y, et al. Butyric acid inhibits oxidative stress and inflammation injury in calcium oxalate nephrolithiasis by targeting CYP2C9. Food Chem Toxicol 2023;178:113925.

31. Simeoli R, Mattace Raso G, Pirozzi C, et al. An orally administered butyrate-releasing derivative reduces neutrophil recruitment and inflammation in dextran sulphate sodium-induced murine colitis. Br J Pharmacol 2017;174(11):1484–96.

32. Peng L, Li ZR, Green RS, et al. Butyrate Enhances the Intestinal Barrier by Facilitating Tight Junction Assembly via Activation of AMP-Activated Protein Kinase in Caco-2 Cell Monolayers. J Nutr 2009;139(9):1619–25.

33. Canani RB, Terrin G, Cirillo P, et al. Butyrate as an effective treatment of congenital chloride diarrhea. Gastroenterology 2004;127(2):630–4.

34. Lund P, Gates L, Leboeuf M, et al. Stable isotope tracing in vivo reveals a metabolic bridge linking the microbiota to host histone acetylation. Cell Rep 2022;41:111809.

35. Canani RB, Terrin G, Elce A, et al. Genotype-dependency of butyrate efficacy in children with congenital chloride diarrhea. Orphanet J Rare Dis 2013;8:194.

36. Chernova MN, Jiang L, Friedman DJ, et al. Functional comparison of mouse slc26a6 anion exchanger with human SLC26A6 polypeptide variants: differences in anion selectivity, regulation, and electrogenicity. J Biol Chem 2005;280(9):8564–80.

37. Chaiyarit S, Thongboonkerd V. Mitochondrial Dysfunction and Kidney Stone Disease. Front Physiol 2020;11. https://doi.org/10.3389/fphys.2020.566506.

38. Ke R, He Y, Chen C. Association between oxidative balance score and kidney stone in United States adults: analysis from NHANES 2007-2018. Front Physiol 2023;14. https://doi.org/10.3389/fphys.2023.1275750.

39. Felizardo RJF, de Almeida DC, Pereira RL, et al. Gut microbial metabolite butyrate protects against proteinuric kidney disease through epigenetic- and GPR109a-mediated mechanisms. FASEB J 2019;33(11):11894–908.

40. Cheng X, Zhou T, He Y, et al. The role and mechanism of butyrate in the prevention and treatment of diabetic kidney disease. Front Microbiol 2022;13:961536.

41. Taguchi K, Okada A, Hamamoto S, et al. M1/M2-macrophage phenotypes regulate renal calcium oxalate crystal development. Sci Rep 2016;6(1):35167.

42. Cao C, Fan B, Zhu J, et al. Association of Gut Microbiota and Biochemical Features in a Chinese Population With Renal Uric Acid Stone. Front Pharmacol 2022;13:888883.

43. Guo Z, Zhang J, Wang Z, et al. Intestinal Microbiota Distinguish Gout Patients from Healthy Humans. Sci Rep 2016;6(1):20602.

44. Cao C, Li F, Ding Q, et al. Potassium sodium hydrogen citrate intervention on gut microbiota and clinical features in uric acid stone patients. Appl Microbiol Biotechnol 2024;108(1):51.

45. Xie QS, Zhang JX, Liu M, et al. Short-chain fatty acids exert opposite effects on the expression and function of p-glycoprotein and breast cancer resistance protein in rat intestine. Acta Pharmacol Sin 2021;42(3):470–81.

46. Chmiel JA, Stuivenberg GA, Al KF, et al. Vitamins as regulators of calcium-containing kidney stones — new perspectives on the role of the gut microbiome. Nat Rev Urol 2023;20(10):615–37.

47. Al KF, Joris BR, Daisley BA, et al. Multi-site microbiota alteration is a hallmark of kidney stone formation. Microbiome 2023;11(1):263.

48. Hinojosa-Gonzalez DE, Eisner BH. Biomarkers in Urolithiasis. Urol Clin North Am 2023;50(1):19–29.

49. Wei Z, Cui Y, Tian L, et al. Probiotic Lactiplantibacillus plantarum N-1 could prevent ethylene glycol-induced kidney stones by regulating gut microbiota and enhancing intestinal barrier function. Faseb J 2021;35(11):e21937.

50. Tian L, Liu Y, Xu X, et al. Lactiplantibacillus plantarum J-15 reduced calcium oxalate kidney stones by regulating intestinal microbiota, metabolism, and inflammation in rats. FASEB J 2022;36(6):e22340.

51. You S, Ma Y, Yan B, et al. The promotion mechanism of prebiotics for probiotics: A review. Front Nutr 2022;9:1000517.

52. Holmes ZC, Villa MM, Durand HK, et al. Microbiota responses to different prebiotics are conserved within individuals and associated with habitual fiber intake. Microbiome 2022;10(1):114.

53. Sorensen MD, Hsi RS, Chi T, et al. Dietary Intake of Fiber, Fruit, and Vegetables Decrease the Risk of Incident Kidney Stones in Women: A Women's Health Initiative (WHI) Report. J Urol 2014;192(6):1694–9.

54. Lin BB, Lin ME, Huang RH, et al. Dietary and lifestyle factors for primary prevention of nephrolithiasis: a systematic review and meta-analysis. BMC Nephrol 2020;21(1):267.

55. Önal Darilmaz D, Sönmez Ş, Beyatli Y. The effects of inulin as a prebiotic supplement and the synbiotic interactions of probiotics to improve oxalate degrading activity. Int J Food Sci Technol 2019;54(1):121–31.

56. Heidor R, Ortega JF, de Conti A, et al. Anticarcinogenic actions of tributyrin, a butyric acid prodrug. Curr Drug Targets 2012;13(14):1720–9.

57. Stern JM, Urban-Maldonado M, Usyk M, et al. Fecal transplant modifies urine chemistry risk factors for urinary stone disease. Physiol Rep 2019;7(4):e14012.

58. Miller AW, Oakeson KF, Dale C, et al. Microbial Community Transplant Results in Increased and Long-Term Oxalate Degradation. Microb Ecol 2016;72(2):470–8.

Best Practices in Treatment of Fungal Urinary Tract Infections

Reid A. Stubbee, MD, Joanna Orzel, MD, Chad R. Tracy, MD*

KEYWORDS

• Candiduria • Funguria • Fluconazole • Fungus ball • Amphotericin B • Urinary tract infection

KEY POINTS

- *Candida* species are the third most commonly identified pathogen in urine cultures obtained in hospitalized patients.
- Differentiation of clinically significant fungal urinary tract infections is challenging as they most often present asymptomatically.
- Treatment of candiduria is based upon the severity and location of the infection in the urinary tract with surgical intervention occasionally required for infection with upper urinary tract involvement or obstruction.
- Nephrostomy tubes, antifungal renal instillation, and endoscopic surgical management are the mainstays of treatment for fungus balls identified in the urinary system.
- *Candida auris* represents a newly identified highly resistant fungal pathogen that will require continued research and understanding as more cases are reported with its presence as a uropathogen.

INTRODUCTION

The finding of a fungal pathogen within a urine culture and as a potential cause of a urinary tract infection (UTI) can present complex management scenarios to the urologist in practice. Clinically, this condition can present with a wide range of symptoms from asymptomatic to critically ill patients. Appropriate treatment is not always straight forward and management varies based on the clinical situation, patient risk factors, and severity of illness. The following review will cover the epidemiology and risk factors associated with fungal urinary tract infections, the pathogenesis of these infections, the diagnostic studies associated with identifying these infections, and current trends in medical and surgical treatment of fungal UTIs.

EPIDEMIOLOGY AND RISK FACTORS

Fungal isolates in urine specimens are more commonly found in nosocomial settings than in the ambulatory setting. Studies have demonstrated the prevalence of fungal pathogens within clean catch urine samples varying from <1% in the outpatient setting to 5% to 10% of positive urine cultures for patients in a hospitalized setting.[1] In a large multicenter European study evaluating nosocomial UTIs, *Candida* species were the third most common uropathogen comprising about 10% of the positive urine specimens obtained.[2] In this study, about 1 in 3 admitted patients had a positive urine culture with any organism, while 1 in 32 hospitalized patients had a urine culture positive for *Candida* species.[2] This data are similar amongst patients in the intensive care unit (ICU) with an additional

Department of Urology, University of Iowa Hospitals and Clinics, University of Iowa, 200 Hawkins Drive, Iowa City, IA 52245, USA
* Corresponding author.
E-mail address: chad-tracy@uiowa.edu

Urol Clin N Am 51 (2024) 483–492
https://doi.org/10.1016/j.ucl.2024.06.006
0094-0143/24/© 2024 Elsevier Inc. All rights are reserved, including those for text and data mining, AI training, and similar technologies.

study from France noting incidence of candiduria at 27.4 per 1000 admissions.[3]

Candida albicans is the most common fungal uropathogen comprising 50% to 70% of fungal urinary isolates.[4] *Candida glabrata* and *Candida tropicalis* are found to be the second most common uropathogens usually ranging between 10% and 35% of positive samples each depending on the series and geographic location.[4] Other *Candida* species identified as uropathogens include *Candida parapsilosis* and *Candida krusei* although these are less commonly identified.[4] *Candida auris*, an emerging multidrug-resistant fungal pathogen associated with high levels of mortality, has rarely been seen in urinary isolates. This species was first identified in the United States in 2015 and has only a few case reports noted to guide identification and management.[5] Identification of non-*Candida* fungal species within urine cultures is a rare phenomenon.

Risk factors for fungal urinary tract infections are well defined, with a strong predilection for patients with certain underlying comorbid medical conditions. Demographic characteristics associated with fungal urinary tract infection include the extremes of age and female sex.[6] Underlying medical conditions, including diabetes, urinary tract abnormalities, malignancy, and malnutrition, also predispose patients to a higher risk of fungal urinary tract infections.[7] Additionally, the presence of a fungal urinary pathogen is strongly associated with any type of urinary tract instrumentation or surgical procedure. Studies have demonstrated that >80% of urine cultures with a fungal pathogen occur in patients with a current indwelling urinary drainage device at the time of the sample or within 30 days prior.[7] Interestingly, non-urologic surgical intervention can also predispose patients to fungal urinary tract infections as >50% of positive fungal cultures occur in patients having undergone a non-urologic surgical procedure within 1 month of their diagnosis.[7] Other factors predisposing patients to fungal urinary tract infections include both prior antibiotic and antifungal use which are associated with an increased risk of both *C glabrata* and systemic fungemia.[8]

Risk of mortality in patients with fungal urinary tract infection remains high in hospitalized patients and is even higher in those patients receiving ICU care. In a 2000 multicenter study in the United States, the mortality rate in patients with candiduria was 19.8% although progression to candidemia was low at 1.3%.[7] A 2007 study from France found even higher rates of mortality in ICU patients with candiduria at 31.3%.[3] A separate study in 2017 analyzed the genetic strains of *Candida* in patients with both candiduria and candidemia noting only 4/141 (2.8%) patients having the same genetic strain of *Candida* in both blood and urine.[9] Despite high rates of mortality within hospitalized patients with candiduria, it does not appear that the presence of fungal species in the urine is the main driver of mortality or progression but rather serves as a surrogate of medical complexity in patients with a high-risk acute or advanced illness.[7]

PATHOGENESIS

Fungal infections in the urine can occur from both a retrograde mechanism from the lower urinary tract and an antegrade spread from a hematogenous route into the upper urinary tract. *Candida* species have poor adherence to bladder mucosa often requiring a secondary abnormality to take hold and spread, with urinary obstruction or immunosuppression often required for these infections to propagate.[1] The creation of a biofilm from an indwelling urinary drainage device can also provide a source for infection and serves as a common etiology in fungal UTIs.[1] Vesicoureteral reflux or upper urinary tract obstruction can allow the infection to spread into the kidneys resulting in a fungal pyelonephritis. Upper urinary tract involvement can also occur through hematogenous spread into the kidneys as the pathogen invades from the bloodstream into the renal tubules.[1]

CLINICAL PRESENTATION AND DIAGNOSIS

Fungal urinary tract infections vary widely in their presentation from clinically asymptomatic to severe life-threatening illness. Fortunately, the majority of patients with funguria are asymptomatic at presentation with only 2% to 10% of patients with funguria presenting with classical symptoms commonly associated with urinary tract infection.[7,10] Symptoms of a fungal urinary tract infection are similar to those with a bacterial urinary tract infection, including urinary urgency, frequency, dysuria, suprapubic pain and tenderness, or flank pain.[10] Because of the low rate of symptomatic UTIs in patients with a fungus present on urine culture, determining appropriate treatment for these patients represents a clinical challenge.

The gold standard of diagnosis of a fungal urinary tract infection is a urine culture, however, there is little data to guide minimum values for colony counts and differentiate colonization from infection, further complicating the treatment paradigm.[11] While the presence of pyuria on microscopic urinalysis may aid in the diagnosis of fungal urinary tract infection, this finding has limited utility in diagnostic confirmation. Certain patient groups, including those patients with indwelling urinary drainage devices and elderly nursing home residents, will almost always have pyuria along with a positive urine culture.[12] Thus, the best use for microscopic urinalysis is for its negative predictive value as the absence of pyuria can aid in labeling a urine culture with positive findings of fungi as a contaminant rather than infection.[12] Similarly, colony count cutoffs for fungal urine cultures have not been established, making the use of colony forming units (CFU) unreliable to indicate the presence or absence of infection.[13] Previous studies have examined further markers to identify fungal UTIs but none are currently used in clinical practice due to limited practical utility. Fungal casts in urine specimens have been found to be diagnostic of kidney involvement and fungal pyelonephritis; however, the process to complete this test is time intensive and does not result in an expedient diagnosis.[13] Even results from urine cultures alone do not always lead to an expedient diagnosis as certain species including *Candida glabrata* can take up to 48 hours to appear using standard urine culture plating techniques.[13] To minimize the contamination effects of indwelling catheters or clean catch samples, a repeat urine sample with a new catheterized specimen or repeat culture after removal of an old indwelling urinary drainage device can serve as an additional potential tool to determine colonization versus contamination from a fungal UTI.[4]

Use of diagnostic imaging for patients with funguria is limited to patients with significant symptomatic infection and can be used to help identify an upper or lower urinary tract presence of infection. Renal and bladder ultrasound, which is able to identify clinical features of pyelonephritis, abscess, fungus balls, and obstructive uropathy, is often the first-line option for diagnostic imaging. This modality is cost effective, does not require contrast or radiation, and is easily available at most facilities.[14] On ultrasound, fungal pyelonephritis may be identified by layered wall thickening in the calyces and renal pelvis along with increased vascularity within the kidney on color Doppler.[14] Loss of corticomedullary differentiation can also be present although this finding is non-specific and variably present.[14] Fungus balls are identified by the presence of echogenic debris or mass within the collecting system without evidence of blood flow on color Doppler.[14] Ultrasound can also identify hydronephrosis, which may prompt further investigation into a source of obstruction leading to urinary stasis.

CT Urogram, a triphasic study with a non-contrasted, contrasted, and excretory phase, can also be pursued based on the clinical situation as it has improved sensitivity in identification of pyelonephritis, abscess, emphysematous infection, and obstructive pathology in comparison to ultrasound.[13] Contrasted MRI and renal cortical scintigraphy with Tc-99m dimercaptosuccinic acid (DMSA) may be used in select cases based on renal function or when trying to avoid radiation exposure. Ultimately, complex cases may require a multidisciplinary team to determine prudent imaging selection for each clinical scenario.

Medical and Pharmacologic Management

Clinical practice guidelines for the treatment of candidiasis have been released by the Infectious Disease Society of America (IDSA) and were most recently updated in 2016. The guidelines include a section discussing treatment of patients with urinary tract infection from *Candida* species.[15] These guidelines stratify treatment groups based upon the severity of illness and location of infection.[15]

ASYMPTOMATIC CANDIDURIA

The general IDSA recommendation for management of asymptomatic candiduria is conservative with avoidance of antifungal treatment outside of a few select patient populations. These groups are limited to neutropenic patients, infants with birth weights lower than 1500 g, and patients who will undergo procedural or surgical urologic intervention.[15] Treatment in these cases is recommended to guard against the risk of systemic dissemination of the fungal pathogen. For all asymptomatic patients, recommendations include removal of indwelling urinary drainage instruments when possible and management of medical comorbidities such as diabetes. In patients without risk factors, these conservative measures alone may be enough to eradicate the presence of candiduria.[4] In a study of hospitalized patients with candiduria, treatment with removal of indwelling urinary catheter alone eliminated candiduria in 41/116 (35.3%) patients,[7] with antifungal treatment (with or without catheter removal) demonstrating only slightly higher rates of resolution at 130/259 (50.2%) of patients.[7] Despite a slightly higher rate of clearance immediately after treatment cessation, further studies have shown that within weeks of treatment cessation, rates of candiduria between groups receiving antifungals and those who do not are almost identical. Similarly, a placebo- controlled trial with treatment of 200 mg daily fluconazole demonstrated identical rates of candiduria 2 weeks after the end of treatment in the placebo and antifungal groups.[16] This study again found that catheter removal or exchange alone in the placebo group had a significant benefit with regards to eradication of candiduria.[16] Importantly, no patient in either group developed progression to pyelonephritis or fungemia demonstrating limited morbidity and mortality with forgoing treatment.[16] Due to these findings, treatment for candiduria should be reserved for critically ill patients or those who need short-term clearance of candiduria, such as those undergoing an invasive urologic procedure.

SPECIAL POPULATIONS—ASYMPTOMATIC CANDIDURIA

Recommendation for treatment of patients with asymptomatic candiduria is limited to 3 populations by the IDSA: neutropenic patients, very low birthweight neonates (<1500 g), and patients undergoing a urologic procedure, all of whom are at increased risk of progressing to candidemia.[15] Candiduria in neutropenic patients and very low birthweight infants more likely results from hematogenous antegrade seeding of the fungal pathogen into the kidney and should prompt more aggressive treatment and investigation due to their underlying immunocompromised status.[15] Systemic candidemia has a much greater mortality risk highlighting the importance of treatment in this population.[3] Patients undergoing urologic instrumentation, especially ureteroscopy, are at risk of hematogenous seeding through pyelovenous backflow from increased intrarenal pressure from fluid irrigation during the procedure with many case reports documenting occurrence of post-procedural fungemia.[17,18] The American Urologic Association recommends prophylactic treatment for this group with IDSA guidelines giving specific recommendations for the use of oral fluconazole 400 mg (~6 mg/kg) OR AmB Deoxycholate 0.3 to 0.6 mg/kg/day for several days before and after the procedure.[15,19]

Treatment of Symptomatic Candiduria

It is prudent to distinguish between colonization and true urinary tract infection prior to deciding whether or not to pursue treatment. IDSA guidelines for treatment of symptomatic candiduria are based primarily around the type of infectious organism. Treatment agents listed in the guidelines include anti-fungal options such as fluconazole, amphotericin B deoxycholate, and oral flucytosine, and weight-based dosing is critical to providing an appropriate treatment.[15] Different *Candida* species possess certain inherent antifungal resistance patterns which must be considered when selecting the proper treatment. Not all antifungal agents can be used for treatment of urinary tract infections as urine concentration must be adequate to inhibit fungal growth. Notably, echinocandins such as

caspofungin do not appear in the IDSA guidelines as they have poor urine penetration with treatment.[20] IDSA guideline-recommended agents for the treatment of symptomatic *Candida* cystitis are listed in **Table 1**.[15]

Alternative options for systemic antifungal treatment include bladder irrigation with amphotericin B. Trials have demonstrated benefit in clearance of candiduria in fungal cystitis, though it is generally less optimal due to its transient effect.[15] Several studies have been performed to examine the optimal protocol for use with notable high rates of candiduria clearance at the end of treatment. A 2009 metanalysis revealed that 80% to 90% of patients treated with bladder irrigation with amphotericin B had clearance of candiduria after the final day of treatment, a notably higher rate of clearance than for systemic fluconazole.[24] However, the treatment effect was short lived as 5 days after the cessation of bladder irrigation clearance rates were identical between groups treated with systemic fluconazole and amphotericin B bladder irrigation.[24] The metanalysis noted that optimal treatment was performed with continuous rather than intermittent irrigation and 5 days of treatment provided more benefit than shorter durations. Adverse effects were minimal.[24] IDSA guidelines do not formally recommend amphotericin B bladder irrigation but note that a 5 day course of continuous irrigation with 50 mg/L in sterile water for 5 days can be an option for patients with fluconazole-resistant pathogens.[15] It may also be useful in anuric patients as drug delivery of antifungal agents is reliant on excretion in the urine to maintain adequate concentration for pathogen eradication. Care must be taken in patient selection with this treatment to rule out upper tract or systemic infection before initiation.

Treatment of Candida Pyelonephritis

IDSA guidelines differentiate treatment recommendations between patients with *Candida* cystitis and *Candida* pyelonephritis.[15] Treatment recommendations are again driven by species-appropriate antifungals generally for a longer duration or higher dose course of treatment. The guidelines are careful to note that the route of pyelonephritis is important to differentiate to determine the appropriate treatment. Hematogenous spread of fungal infection into the kidneys should be treated as candidemia and is different than an ascending urinary tract infection, which will be discussed in this section.

In addition to antifungal treatment, IDSA guidelines recommend prompt intervention to resolve any possible urinary tract obstruction and, when

Table 1
Treatment of symptomatic *Candida* cystitis[15,20–23]

Medication	Species Treated and Resistances	Mechanism	Dose	Side Effects	Contraindications	Renal Function Correction
Fluconazole	All fluconazole-susceptible species (*C albicans*, *C tropicalis*, *C parapsilosis*), *C glabrata* with some resistance, *C krusei* with complete resistance	Inhibits synthesis of ergosterol increasing fungal cellular membrane permeability	2 wk duration 200 mg/day PO 800 mg/day PO for susceptible *C glabrata*	Gastrointestinal symptoms, hepatotoxicity, QT prolongation, torsades de pointes, skin rash, severe skin reactions, dizziness, seizures	Coadministration with other QT prolonging drugs, coadministration with drugs metabolized by CYP3A4	CrCL <50 mL/min reduce dose by 50% Dialysis patients—administer full dose 3 × weekly after dialysis
AmB Deoxycholate	*C krusei*, Fluconazole-resistant *C glabrata*	Binds to ergosterol increasing fungal cell membrane permeability through pore channels	1–7 d duration 0.3–0.6 mg/kg/day IV Used with or without flucytosine for *C glabrata*	Binds to cholesterol in human cell membranes leading to toxicity, electrolyte abnormalities, fevers, nephrotoxicity, encephalopathy, bone marrow suppression, neutropenia	Anaphylaxis or acute infusion reactions Lipid formation does not have adequate urine concentration	No dosage adjustment required
Flucytosine	Fluconazole-resistant *C glabrata*; *C krusei* is resistant	Impairs fungal cell DNA, RNA, and protein synthesis	2 wk duration 25 mg/kg 4 times daily Can be used for *C glabrata*	Gastrointestinal symptoms, skin rash, hepatitis, nephrotoxicity, bone marrow suppression, pancytopenia, agranulocytosis, inflammatory bowel diseases	Neutropenic patients or patients with liver disease	CrCl 21–40 mL/min—25 mg/kg BID CrCl 10–20 mL/min—25 mg/kg daily CrCl <10 mL/min—25 mg/kg Q48 h Dialysis Patients—25–50 mg/kg/dose every 48–72 h after dialysis

feasible, remove or replace ureteral stents or nephrostomy tubes in patients with these interventions in place.[15] While no studies have compared rates of clearance of fungal pyelonephritis with or without ureteral stent or percutaneous nephrostomy tubes (PCN) exchange during antifungal treatment, it may be posited that this could aid in clearance based upon studies demonstrating the utility of indwelling catheter exchange or removal during treatment.[16]

IDSA guidelines do not include the use of echinocandins (caspofungin) for treatment of symptomatic ascending *Candida* pyelonephritis due to the low urinary concentration of the medication achieved with systemic administration. However, there are case reports in demonstrating successful treatment with these agents.[20] Proposed benefits of this treatment include achieving high concentration in the renal tissues preventing further invasion and spread from the upper urinary tract.[20] Though urine concentration of this drug is low, a small portion of the active drug does pass into the urine and can be used as an option for fluconazole-resistant species such as *Candida* glabrata as a less toxic agent than amphotericin B.[20] **Table 2** lists antifungal agents used for ascending symptomatic *Candida* pyelonephritis.

Interventional Treatment for Fungal Urinary Tract Infections

Fungus balls, an aggregation of necrotic renal epithelial and urothelial cells from infection mixed with fungal cells, represent a challenging complication of fungal UTIs and may be present with or without concomitant urinary tract obstruction (lower or upper urinary tract).[1] IDSA guidelines recommend 3 main principles of treatment for the presence of fungus balls: surgical intervention, antifungal treatment for cystitis or pyelonephritis as discussed in previous sections, and irrigation of AmB deoxycholate through nephrostomy tubes if present.[15] A stepwise approach to treatment is prudent in these conditions as there is no current algorithm in place to determine when each of these recommendations is required. Surgical intervention through nephrostomy tube placement, percutaneous nephroscopy, or ureteroscopy may not always be in the best interest of the patient as fungus balls are uncommon in patients without significant perioperative risk factors for an anesthetic complication. While the resolution of fungal balls with antifungals alone is not well reported in the adult population, limited case reports in

Table 2
Treatment of symptomatic ascending *Candida* pyelonephritis[15,20–23]

Medication	Species Treated and Resistances	Dose	Renal Function Correction
Fluconazole	All fluconazole-susceptible species (C albicans, C tropicalis, C parapsilosis). C glabrata with some resistance, C krusei with complete resistance	2 wk duration 200–400 mg/day PO 800 mg/day PO for susceptible C glabrata	CrCL <50 mL/min reduce dose by 50% Dialysis patients—administer full dose 3 × weekly after dialysis
AmB Deoxycholate	C krusei, Fluconazole-resistant C glabrata	1–7 d duration 0.3–0.6 mg/kg/day IV Used with or without flucytosine for C glabrata	No dosage adjustment required
Flucytosine	Fluconazole-resistant C glabrata, C krusei is resistant	2 wk duration 25 mg/kg 4 times daily Can be used as monotherapy for C glabrata	CrCl 21–40 mL/min— 25 mg/kg BID CrCl 10–20 mL/min— 25 mg/kg daily CrCl <10 mL/min— 25 mg/kg Q 48 h Dialysis Patients— 25–50 mg/kg/dose every 48–72 h after dialysis
Caspofungin	All Candida species. Non-Infectious Disease Society of America (IDSA) guideline use for fluconazole-resistant species	2–3 wk 70 mg IV day 1 then 50 mg daily thereafter	No dosage adjustment required

the neonatal population have shown successful resolution with antifungal agents (fluconazole or amphotericin B).[25]

Antifungal Renal Irrigation

As in all settings of obstruction with concomitant infection, prompt drainage and resolution of obstruction in hydronephrotic kidneys is paramount. In the upper urinary tract, PCNs are placed for maximal drainage as they can also provide a method for irrigation and instillation of treatment antifungals. IDSA guidelines recommend the use of AmB deoxycholate at a dose of 25 to 50 mg in 200 to 500 mL of sterile water to instill into the kidney through a nephrostomy tube as treatment for fungus balls.[15] Case studies have demonstrated patient tolerance of a rate of 30 mL/h with treatment duration variable from 5 days or until resolution.[26,27] Importantly, it is critical to not increase intrarenal pressures during irrigation. As such, patients who undergo renal irrigation should have a concomitant stent placed or another mechanism for countercurrent flow such as an additional nephrostomy tube.[26] In all cases, irrigation should be started with normal saline to determine any symptoms prior to initiation of antifungal treatment and treatment should always be done under gravity rather than through an automated pump. IDSA guidelines recommend the use of sterile water as the diluent as amphotericin B is not known to be compatible with normal saline.[15,28] The exact duration of this treatment has not been well studied.

Fluconazole irrigation has also been used in case reports though this agent is not within IDSA guidelines. Similar care should be taken in the use of this agent to prevent an increase in intrarenal pressure and ensure countercurrent flow. Successful eradication of renal fungus balls has been documented with instillation of 300 mg fluconazole diluted in 500 mL of normal saline at 62.5 mL/h for 8 hours per day for 1 week as well as instillation of the same mixture at 40 mL/hr for 12 hours per day for 1 week in different patients. No adverse effects were noted in either case report.[27,29] Instillation of streptokinase via nephrostomy tube was also identified in a case report of a neonate with a fungus ball as a successful salvage therapy after failure of antifungal instillation. Instillation of a 5 mL dose of 3000 units/mL streptokinase twice daily for 3 days was found to aid in breaking apart the fungal material with the use of antifungal therapy in 2 neonatal patients.[30]

Urologic Surgical Interventions

If non-operative management fails to resolve a fungus ball despite use of antifungal renal instillation and systemic antifungal therapy, more invasive surgical intervention may be warranted. Various techniques have been reported in the literature, including transurethral resection within the bladder or distal ureter, percutaneous nephroscopy, or ureteroscopy with placement of ureteral access sheath for irrigation and basket removal of the fungus balls.[31–33] Nephroscopy with percutaneous access may be more efficacious in removal of a large volume of material than ureteroscopy as seen in the treatment of kidney stones though it is associated with greater surgical risk than ureteroscopy. Multiple procedures may be required if ureteroscopic access for fungus ball removal is selected due to challenges in endoscopic removal of material with this method.[32] In rare cases, the fungal collection can present as a renal abscess rather than within the collecting system. This has not been reported extensively but a case report in the literature describes a case of C tropicalis fungemia and subsequent renal abscess, which was treated with percutaneous drainage.[34] As a last resort, nephrectomy can be considered with failure of all antifungal therapy and minimally invasive intervention.

EMERGING PATHOGENS AND FUTURE DIRECTIONS

Candida auris is a fungal pathogen that was first isolated in Japan in 2009 and has since been identified in a multitude of countries across the globe. C auris poses a unique threat due to its ability to persistently colonize human skin and surfaces in health care environments, leading to outbreaks in the health care setting. Furthermore, several strains of this pathogen have been identified as pan-resistant, making treatment of this pathogen challenging.[35] In addition to the resistance patterns, this pathogen is incredibly resilient and carries a high mortality with any infection. Identification of C auris may be difficult, such that matrix-assisted laser desorption/ionization-time of flight (MALDI-TOF) and molecular-based systems (eg, real-time polymerase chain reaction [PCR]) should be used for correct identification.[36] In a review of 11 patient case reports with C auris, all strains were fluconazole resistant.[5] The authors proposed a systematic approach to treatment of C auris UTIs, which starts with infection control, isolation measures, and source control. Treatment pathways are then identified depending on patient characteristics and clinical history.[5] Asymptomatic patients without critical illness or comorbidities such as recent surgery, invasive lines, or diabetes were recommended to be monitored rather than to undergo anti-fungal therapy.[5] If the patient is symptomatic or has any of these comorbid conditions, then identification of resistance patterns is recommended to identify treatment. Options for treatment include either systemic amphotericin B deoxycholate with concomitant bladder irrigation along with systemic flucytosine or therapy with echinocandins. Discontinuation of therapy and infection control measures were recommended 14 days after a negative culture and resolution of infectious symptoms are obtained.[5] Due to the characteristics of persistence, resistance, and mortality, *C auris* is a fungus being closely monitored by the Centers for Disease Control and Prevention (CDC).

Future directions of research in fungal UTIs should include the discussion of the utility of prophylaxis, which the IDSA guidelines address only in the setting of prevention of invasive candidiasis in the ICU. However, because the kidneys are the most common organs involved with systemic candidiasis, it remains clinically relevant for the urologist to consider.[37] Research should also be undertaken to develop treatment algorithms that are easily accessible due to increasing resistance patterns. A study by Albahar and colleagues aimed to assess the impact of antifungal stewardship on clinical and performance measures.[38] They included 41 studies in their analysis and found that interventions for antifungal stewardship measures ranged from audits and feedback to developing guidelines for administration and use of antifungals. Twenty-two of the 41 studies reported mortality as an outcome measure, whereas 13 of the 22 studies stated significant differences in mortality between the intervention and nonintervention groups along with decreased use of antifungal agents.[38] Many institutions already have antimicrobial stewardship teams in place; these teams could potentially expand to encompass antifungal stewardship models using the same principles to identify which patients will and will not benefit from antifungal treatment.

SUMMARY

Fungal UTIs are an increasingly common problem for current and future urologists. Current challenges lie in identification of exactly which patients warrant treatment and determination of gold standard treatments for complex scenarios where invasive management strategies are required. Identification often requires a heightened clinical acumen, with attention to patients at particular risk. Appropriate treatment often requires a multimodal approach using diligent clinical evaluation, species-appropriate antifungal treatment, removal or replacement of urinary devices, improved urinary drainage, and, when necessary, minimally invasive surgical intervention.

CLINICS CARE POINTS

- The gold standard of diagnosis of a fungal urinary tract infection is a urine culture; however there are few diagnostic tools alone that can determine whether or not the finding requires treatment.
- Diagnostic imaging is reserved for patients with significant symptomatic infection or known anatomic abnormalities. Renal and bladder ultrasound is typically the first-line modality though it has less sensitivity for identification of important findings than a CT Urogram.
- Asymptomatic infections do not typically require antifungal treatment and can be managed alone with conservative measures such as catheter exchange or removal except for a select few patient populations which include neutropenic patients, infants with birthweights less than 1500 g, and patients undergoing procedural or surgical urologic intervention
- Antifungal therapy is reserved for symptomatic patients with agent choice dependent on the fungal species and location of infection.
- Procedural or surgical intervention is considered for patients with urinary tract obstruction or the presence of fungus balls within the urinary tract.

DISCLOSURES

These authors have nothing to disclose.

REFERENCES

1. Fisher JF. Candida urinary tract infections–epidemiology, pathogenesis, diagnosis, and treatment: executive summary. Clin Infect Dis 2011;52(Suppl 6): S429–32. https://doi.org/10.1093/cid/cir108.
2. Bouza E, San Juan R, Muñoz P, et al. A European perspective on nosocomial urinary tract infections I. Report on the microbiology workload, etiology and antimicrobial susceptibility (ESGNI-003 study). European Study Group on Nosocomial Infections. Clin Microbiol Infect 2001;7(10):523–31. https://doi.org/10.1046/j.1198-743x.2001.00326.x.
3. Bougnoux ME, Kac G, Aegerter P, et al. Candidemia and candiduria in critically ill patients admitted to

intensive care units in France: incidence, molecular diversity, management and outcome. Intensive Care Med 2008;34(2):292–9. https://doi.org/10.1007/s00134-007-0865-y.

4. Kauffman CA. Diagnosis and management of fungal urinary tract infection. Infect Dis Clin North Am 2014;28(1):61–74. https://doi.org/10.1016/j.idc.2013.09.004.

5. Griffith N, Danziger L. Candida auris Urinary Tract Infections and Possible Treatment. Antibiotics (Basel) 2020;9(12). https://doi.org/10.3390/antibiotics9120898.

6. Dias V. Candida species in the urinary tract: is it a fungal infection or not? Future Microbiol 2020;15:81–3. https://doi.org/10.2217/fmb-2019-0262.

7. Kauffman CA, Vazquez JA, Sobel JD, et al. Prospective multicenter surveillance study of funguria in hospitalized patients. The National Institute for Allergy and Infectious Diseases (NIAID) Mycoses Study Group. Clin Infect Dis 2000;30(1):14–8. https://doi.org/10.1086/313583.

8. Harris AD, Castro J, Sheppard DC, et al. Risk factors for nosocomial candiduria due to Candida glabrata and Candida albicans. Clin Infect Dis 1999;29(4):926–8. https://doi.org/10.1086/520460.

9. Drogari-Apiranthitou M, Anyfantis I, Galani I, et al. Association Between Candiduria and Candidemia: A Clinical and Molecular Analysis of Cases. Mycopathologia 2017;182(11–12):1045–52. https://doi.org/10.1007/s11046-017-0180-2.

10. Storfer SP, Medoff G, Fraser VJ, et al. Candiduria: Retrospective Review in Hospitalized Patients. Infect Dis Clin Pract 1994;3(1):23–9.

11. Kauffman CA. Candiduria. Clin Infect Dis 2005;41(Supplement_6):S371–6. https://doi.org/10.1086/430918.

12. Nicolle LE. A practical guide to antimicrobial management of complicated urinary tract infection. Drugs Aging 2001;18(4):243–54. https://doi.org/10.2165/00002512-200118040-00002.

13. Kauffman CA, Fisher JF, Sobel JD, et al. Candida urinary tract infections–diagnosis. Clin Infect Dis 2011;52(Suppl 6):S452–6. https://doi.org/10.1093/cid/cir111.

14. Sadegi BJ, Patel BK, Wilbur AC, et al. Primary Renal Candidiasis. J Ultrasound Med 2009;28(4):507–14.

15. Pappas PG, Kauffman CA, Andes DR, et al. Clinical Practice Guideline for the Management of Candidiasis: 2016 Update by the Infectious Diseases Society of America. Clin Infect Dis 2015;62(4):e1–50. https://doi.org/10.1093/cid/civ933.

16. Sobel JD, Kauffman CA, McKinsey D, et al. Candiduria: A Randomized, Double-Blind Study of Treatment with Fluconazole and Placebo. Clin Infect Dis 2000;30(1):19–24. https://doi.org/10.1086/313580.

17. Tokas T, Herrmann TRW, Skolarikos A, et al. Pressure matters: intrarenal pressures during normal and pathological conditions, and impact of increased values to renal physiology. World J Urol 2019;37(1):125–31. https://doi.org/10.1007/s00345-018-2378-4.

18. Beck SM, Finley DS, Deane LA. Fungal urosepsis after ureteroscopy in cirrhotic patients: a word of caution. Urology 2008;72(2):291–3. https://doi.org/10.1016/j.urology.2008.01.005.

19. Lightner DJ, Wymer K, Sanchez J, et al. Best Practice Statement on Urologic Procedures and Antimicrobial Prophylaxis. J Urol 2020;203(2):351–6. https://doi.org/10.1097/ju.0000000000000509.

20. Sobel JD, Bradshaw SK, Lipka CJ, et al. Caspofungin in the treatment of symptomatic candiduria. Clin Infect Dis 2007;44(5):e46–9. https://doi.org/10.1086/510432.

21. Noor A, Preuss C. Amphotericin B. StatPearls. 2023. Available at: https://www.ncbi.nlm.nih.gov/books/NBK482327/.

22. Padda IS, Parmar M. Flucytosine. StatPearls. 2023. Available at: https://www.ncbi.nlm.nih.gov/books/NBK557607/.

23. Govindarajan A, Bistas KG, Ingold CJ, et al. Fluconazole. StatPearls. 2023. Available at: https://www.ncbi.nlm.nih.gov/books/NBK537158/.

24. Tuon FF, Amato VS, Penteado Filho SR. Bladder irrigation with amphotericin B and fungal urinary tract infection–systematic review with meta-analysis. Int J Infect Dis 2009;13(6):701–6. https://doi.org/10.1016/j.ijid.2008.10.012.

25. Vázquez-Tsuji O, Campos-Rivera T, Ahumada-Mendoza H, et al. Renal ultrasonography and detection of pseudomycelium in urine as means of diagnosis of renal fungus balls in neonates. Mycopathologia 2005;159(3):331–7. https://doi.org/10.1007/s11046-004-3713-4.

26. Tan WP, Turba UC, Deane LA. Renal fungus ball: a challenging clinical problem. Urologia 2017;84(2):113–5. https://doi.org/10.5301/uro.5000201.

27. Abdeljaleel OA, Alnadhari I, Mahmoud S, et al. Treatment of Renal Fungal Ball with Fluconazole Instillation Through a Nephrostomy Tube: Case Report and Literature Review. Am J Case Rep 2018;19:1179–83. https://doi.org/10.12659/ajcr.911113.

28. Díaz Giraldo J, Valencia Quintero AF, Botero Aguirre JP. Letter to editor regarding "Renal fungus ball: a challenging clinical problem". Urologia 2019;86(3):126. https://doi.org/10.1177/0391560319827445.

29. Chacko AZ, Misra S. Successful treatment of ureteral-stent-related fungal ball using fluconazole instillation through a nephrostomy tube. Urol Case Rep 2023;50:102522. https://doi.org/10.1016/j.eucr.2023.102522.

30. Bisht V, Voort JV. Clinical practice: Obstructive renal candidiasis in infancy. Eur J Pediatr 2011;170(10):1227–35. https://doi.org/10.1007/s00431-011-1514-6.

31. Davis NF, Smyth LG, Mulcahy E, et al. Ureteric obstruction due to fungus-ball in a chronically

immunosuppressed patient. Can Urol Assoc J 2013; 7(5–6):E355–8. https://doi.org/10.5489/cuaj.1214.

32. Abuelnaga M, Khoshzaban S, Reda Badr M, et al. Successful Endoscopic Management of a Renal Fungal Ball using Flexible Ureterorenoscopy. Case Rep Urol 2019;2019:9241928. https://doi.org/10. 1155/2019/9241928.

33. Zhang X, Liu J, Xia Q, et al. Endoscopic removal of giant fungus balls growing in the renal pelvis and urinary bladder due to long-term retention of ureteral stent: A case report. Urol Case Rep 2023; 48:102393. https://doi.org/10.1016/j.eucr.2023.10 2393.

34. Simhadri PK, Vaitla P, Sriperumbuduri S, et al. Sodium-glucose Co-transporter-2 Inhibitors Causing Candida tropicalis Fungemia and Renal Abscess.

JCEM Case Rep 2024;2(2):luae010. https://doi.org/ 10.1210/jcemcr/luae010.

35. Chowdhary A, Jain K, Chauhan N. Candida auris Genetics and Emergence. Annu Rev Microbiol 2023;77:583–602. https://doi.org/10.1146/annurev-micro-032521-015858.

36. Centers for Disease Control and Prevention. Candida auris. Available at: https://www.cdc.gov/fungal/candida-auris/index.html.

37. Lehner T. Systemic candidiasis and renal involvement. Lancet 1964;2(7348):1414–6. https://doi.org/ 10.1016/s0140-6736(64)91984-1.

38. Albahar F, Alhamad H, Abu Assab M, et al. The Impact of Antifungal Stewardship on Clinical and Performance Measures: A Global Systematic Review. Trop Med Infect Dis 2023;9(1). https://doi.org/ 10.3390/tropicalmed9010008.

Clinical Microbiome Testing for Urology

Glenn T. Werneburg, MD, PhD[a], Michael H. Hsieh, MD, PhD[b],*

KEYWORDS

- Microbiome • Microbiota • Next-generation sequencing • Urinary tract infection • Bacteria
- Culture • Antibiotic • Prophylaxis

KEY POINTS

- The urine culture is imperfect, and a series of alternative approaches is in development to assist in diagnosis, treatment, and prevention of urinary tract infection (UTI).
- Culture-independent approaches generally do not distinguish between viable and nonviable bacteria, and their clinical implementation may result in a higher degree of overtreatment of asymptomatic bacteriuria.
- Culture-independent approaches for microbiota testing may play important future roles in cases wherein asymptomatic bacteriuria treatment is warranted: prior to endourologic surgery and during pregnancy.
- Fecal microbiota transplant, probiotic therapy, and bacteriophage therapy are promising opportunities for future investigation regarding their potential to intentionally modulate the microbiome in order to reduce UTI risk.

INTRODUCTION

Thirty-eight trillion bacteria are present in an average human.[1] This corresponds to more than 1 bacterium per human cell. With the advent of more sensitive modalities for microbial detection, it is unsurprising that the healthy urinary tract contains bacteria, and many studies have demonstrated a complex urinary microbiome.[2,3] The microbiota in other urologic tissue niches including the prostate,[4] bladder,[5] and kidney,[6] have also been characterized.

Data regarding associations of urologic microbiota with different functional[7] and oncologic conditions[8] are accruing rapidly. Given detectable differences between healthy control patients and those with such urologic conditions, there is a strong interest in the clinical implementation of microbiota testing. To that end, there are many examples of direct-to-consumer marketing of microbiota detection tests and other products claiming to guide clinical treatment of infection. While there are robust efforts to understand the clinical utility of microbiome testing in urologic oncology, stones, infertility, and other subspecialties, we have confined the scope of our review to urinary tract infection (UTI). Here we discuss the evidence for and against the implementation of microbiome testing for UTI. We discuss the available evidence, current state of the field, and future directions. We first describe the different modalities of testing for urinary microbiota. We then focus on the utility of clinical microbiome testing to guide UTI treatment, prophylactic therapy, and prevention.

DISCUSSION

Herein we will discuss the general testing approaches to detection of microbiota. Then, we

Funding: No external funding was associated with this article.

[a] Department of Urology, Glickman Urological and Kidney Institute, Cleveland Clinic Foundation, 9500 Euclid Avenue, Cleveland, OH 44195, USA; [b] Division of Urology, Children's National Hospital, 111 Michigan Avenue Northwest, Washington, DC 20010, USA

* Corresponding author.

E-mail address: mhsieh@childrensnational.org

Urol Clin N Am 51 (2024) 493–504

https://doi.org/10.1016/j.ucl.2024.06.007

organize our discussion based on how clinical microbiome testing may guide the treatment, prophylaxis, and prevention of UTI. For each, we will discuss the clinical evidence and knowledge gaps regarding the clinical utility of microbiome testing. In **Table 1**, we provide strengths and limitations of each of these approaches.

Techniques for Microbiota Testing

Urine culture

The urine culture has been used clinically since the 1950's when Kass and colleagues proposed a quantitative cutoff of 10^5 CFU per mL to diagnose those with upper tract UTI. This cutpoint was

Table 1
Strengths and limitations of culture-dependent and culture-independent laboratory assays for urinary tract infection diagnosis

Approach	Strength	Limitations
Standard urine culture	• Captures only viable microbiota • Allows for organism quantification • Accurately captures sensitivity and resistance profiles	• Requires up to 3 d for final results • Empiric therapy during the waiting period may provide inappropriate coverage in 30% of cases • No consensus on threshold for positivity (10,000 CFU/mL vs 100,000 CFU/mL vs other) • Only optimized to detect typical uropathogens
Expanded quantitative urine culture (EQUC)	• May detect fastidious, slow growing, and other atypical microbiota • Allows for organism quantification	• Limited clinical data • No difference in UTI outcome when treated based on standard vs EQUC culture • Increased time from sample collection to final result • Increased cost • Increased sensitivity could lead to higher rates of treatment of asymptomatic bacteriuria and reduced antibiotic stewardship
Next-generation sequencing	• Highly sensitive for detection of microbiota • Rapid turnaround time	• Inability to distinguish between viable and nonviable bacteria, and DNA fragments • Antibiotic resistance gene detection may not correlate well with antibiotic resistance phenotype given diverse mechanisms of gene regulation • Antibiotic resistance genes detected may be from nonviable organism or other noninfecting bacteria • High sensitivity for uropathogenic and non-uropathogenic organisms and nonviable organisms may lead to higher rates of inappropriate treatment of asymptomatic bacteriuria and reduced antibiotic stewardship • Lack of clinical data limit interpretability

(continued on next page)

Table 1 *(continued)*		
Approach	**Strength**	**Limitations**
Next-generation sequencing with viability modifications (eg, propidium monoazide-based PCR assay)	• May distinguish between viable and nonviable bacteria • Rapid turnaround time	• Increased sensitivity may lead to higher rates of inappropriate treatment of asymptomatic bacteriuria (even if only viable commensals detected) and reduced antibiotic stewardship • Lack of clinical data limit interpretability

based on the finding that 95% of patients with pyelonephritis met this culture criterion.[9–11] Based on this small cohort of patients with upper tract infection, the testing cutoff was generalized to simple cystitis as well. However, a series of investigations and resultant guidelines have subsequently supported that a cutpoint of less than 10^5 CFU per mL may be associated with UTI and be a more appropriate threshold for a UTI diagnosis.[12–17] The urine culture is limited by the lack of consensus regarding the threshold for its positivity. This test is also imperfect for other reasons. For example, a large proportion of individuals harbors bacteria even in the absence of symptoms.[18] This phenomenon, termed "asymptomatic bacteriuria", generally does not warrant treatment. However, it is known that many individuals with asymptomatic bacteriuria receive treatment. In a 2020 study, 54% of patients who had culture-proven bacteriuria in the absence of symptoms were treated with antibiotics.[19]

Sensitivity and resistance testing is frequently coupled with the urine culture. The time-to-result for antibiotic sensitivities may be up to 72 hours. During this waiting period, empiric antibiotics are often prescribed. However, it has been shown that the empiric coverage is inappropriate in up to 30% of cases.[20] Further, there is a high incidence of urine culture contamination.[21,22] Urine culture also lacks sensitivity in the context of clinically relevant scenarios including recent antibiotic administration. For example, cultures lose sensitivity as early as 90 minutes following a single empiric antibiotic dose.[23] It also lacks sensitivity for infection diagnosis in the context of an obstructing ureteral stone.[24]

Enhanced urine culture for atypical organisms

Due to the limitations of standard urine culture, there has been considerable interest in other approaches to detect clinically-relevant urinary microbiota. While the traditional urine culture selects for common aerobic uropathogens, in some cases, there may be a high clinical suspicion for an atypical organism. For example, in an immunocompromised or neutropenic host *Candida albicans* may be suspected.[25] Importantly, such individuals with candiduria are at increased risk of associated mortality.[26,27] While fungi may be isolated from standard urine culture, other media may be necessary for acceptable cultivation. For example, Sabouraud dextrose agar is not typically a standard culture medium used for urine, but is optimized for fungal growth, and may more sensitively detect *Candida spp*. In one study that analyzed urine specimens wherein microscopy demonstrated fungi, there was *C. albicans* growth on standard culture in 37% of specimens, whereas there was growth in 98% of cases on Sabouraud dextrose agar.[27]

In other cases, clinical or laboratory evidence may be suggestive of genitourinary tuberculosis. The gold standard test for the diagnosis of genitourinary tuberculosis is the augmented urine culture using Lowenstein-Jensen medium. This medium is not typically used for urine culture, but should be considered when there is a high index of suspicion. *Mycobacteria* exhibit slow growth kinetics, and can take up to 6 weeks for isolation on culture.[28] In addition, false positives may be seen in the context of the non-pathogenic species such as *Mycobacterium smegmatis* in the urine.[28]

Fastidious bacteria such as the facultative anaerobes *Ureaplasma spp* and *Mycoplasma hominis* may be associated with UTI, but are both notoriously difficult and time-consuming to isolate on standard culture.[25] Further, to differentiate *Ureaplasma* from *Mycoplasma*, inoculation in a differential culture medium termed A7 agar may be required.[25] Given these difficulties, culture has generally been replaced with polymerase chain reaction (PCR)-based approaches and next-generation sequencing for the detection of these organisms. Further, it is controversial whether these microbes are associated with infection or lower urinary tract symptoms, and recent evidence shows that they are present in similar frequencies in the urine of those with and without symptoms.[29]

Expanded quantitative urine culture

The expanded quantitative urine culture (EQUC) is arguably an improvement upon conventional urine culture in some cohorts. It utilizes a modified approach in order to cultivate a broader proportion of live microbiota than is achievable via standard culturing approaches.[30] This test was developed in part to bridge the gap between culture-independent approaches, which cannot differentiate between alive and dead bacteria, and the standard culture, which is optimized to grow only a subset of bacteria. The EQUC generally includes a larger sample volume, more growth media, longer incubation times, and different atmospheric conditions than the standard culture.[25,30,31] Specifically, specimens are plated on blood agar, chocolate agar, and Columbia Nalidixic Acid Agar (CNA) plates. Both aerobic and anaerobic environments are used, as well as 30°C and 35°C incubation temperatures, and plates are incubated for up to 5 days. A streamlined EQUC protocol has also been reported: plating 100 μL on blood, MacConkey, and CNA agars in a 5% carbon dioxide incubator for 48 hours.[31,32] EQUC detected bacteria in 80% of urine samples in those without UTI. 92% of these specimens had no reported growth using standard laboratory culture.[30] In another study, 79% of urine specimens grew bacteria by EQUC, but 90% of these had no growth on conventional urine culture.[33] While EQUC has significant future potential for the diagnosis and management of UTI, its utility remains to established clinically. In a randomized clinical trial, individuals who were treated based on EQUC results had no difference in symptom resolution versus those treated based on standard culture results.[34] The majority (66%) of patients who did not receive antibiotics due to culture negative or non-uropathogen predominance also reported symptom resolution. The authors note that the high proportion of *Escherichia coli* UTI in their cohort may have masked a group that would benefit from EQUC-guided therapy. However, follow-up studies are needed to test this hypothesis, and to determine whether and to what extent any subgroup would benefit from EQUC-guided relative to standard culture-guided treatment. Antibiotic prescription rate was similar between the standard culture (51%) and EQUC groups (54%). While antibiotic treatment rates were similar in this cohort, it is possible that the inherent increased sensitivity of EQUC could lead to higher rates of inappropriate treatment of asymptomatic bacteriuria, and further investigation will be needed to rigorously assess this possibility.

Next generation sequencing

Next generation sequencing (NGS) is a culture-independent approach for microbial detection. Initially developed by microbial ecologists, it generally uses a PCR-based approach for the amplification of 16s rRNA genes in their hypervariable regions.[32] The 16s rRNA is highly conserved amongst bacteria, but its hypervariable regions serve as a unique "fingerprint". Through sequencing of these regions and comparison to reference databases, even closely-related microbial species can be detected and differentiated based on NGS results.

16s NGS techniques generate results faster than standard culture. Further, they are more sensitive in the detection of bacteria in urine specimens.[35] In fact, NGS-based approaches were used to first define the urinary microbiome and help shift the understanding from the urine being a sterile liquid to one harboring microbiota even in the healthy state.[36] While the application of NGS techniques to the clinical diagnosis and management of urologic infection is alluring, these potential benefits come at the cost of lower specificity and other limitations. For example, such techniques will detect bacteria even in the urine from healthy individuals with no signs or symptoms of urologic infection. In this review, we focus on the use of NGS techniques in UTI. We examine the current literature, and discuss the future opportunities surrounding this technology as it relates to diagnosis, treatment, and prevention. We provide a summary of future research opportunities for validation of existing approaches and development of novel approaches in **Table 2**.

Clinical Microbiome Testing to Guide Urinary Tract Infection Diagnosis and Treatment

As discussed earlier in this review, urine culture takes up to 3 days to result and antibiotics empirically prescribed during this period do not provide appropriate coverage of the infecting organism(s) in up to 30% of cases,.[20] Thus, this setting is one of the most pertinent opportunities for the implementation of microbiome testing via NGS or other culture-independent techniques, which can produce results within hours (**Table 3**).

Culture-independent molecular techniques such as NGS for UTI diagnosis have potential to improve antibiotic stewardship through the rapid identification of an infecting organism and its antibiotic resistance genes, but there are confounding factors that must be considered. NGS-based approaches are very sensitive for urinary microbiota and have been shown to be noninferior to standard culture in uropathogen detection in urine.[37] However,

Table 2
Future research opportunities for clinical microbiome testing

Research Area	Details
Clinical validation	• All enhanced culture and culture independent methods require further clinical validation in the form of clinical trials to establish their utility, or lack thereof, across patient cohorts • Studies must compare rates of UTI cure between standard culture-driven therapy and alternative assay-driven therapy • Studies must also consider rates of antibiotic treatment between cohorts • When interpreting study results, investigators and readers should weigh the risks and benefits of increasingly sensitive assays. These include the risk of increasing rates of treatment of asymptomatic bacteriuria, risk of treatment of nonviable or other non-infecting organisms, and the possibility of reduced antibiotic stewardship at the population level. The risks of collateral damage of antibiotics should also be considered including the rise of subsequent resistance, the risk of Clostridioides difficile colitis, bacterial vaginosis, and others.
Identification and study of improved culture-independent assays	• The ideal culture independent assay will distinguish viable from nonviable organisms • The ideal culture independent assay will assess antibiotic resistance both by genotype and phenotype, given that the presence of resistance genes does not necessarily correlate with resistance of an infecting organism • The ideal culture independent assay will provide results rapidly in order to reduce the time to final results associated with standard culture • The ideal culture independent assay will be easily interpretable by clinicians, and caution the interpreter regarding its limitations
Improved understanding of the gut-urine-UTI axis, the vagina-urine-UTI axis, and their potential for modulation	• Research should further characterize the physiologic gut, vaginal, and urine microbiomes in diverse patient cohorts • Research should address how gut and/or vaginal dysbiosis may affect urinary microbiota dysbiosis and its association with urinary tract infection • Whether and how diet, probiotics, antibiotics, and other environmental factors may protect or adversely affect the microbial communities of the gut, vagina, and urine is a viable area for research • The ability to modulate the gut, vaginal, and urinary microbiomes in order to maintain or restore healthy microbial communities is an open and promising area for investigation. Potential opportunities to do so may include targeted probiotics, fecal transplantation therapy, dietary modifications, vaccination, bacteriophage therapy, or targeting of microbial quorum-sensing.

culture-independent detection is independent of microbial viability. In one study, there was no difference in the NGS-positivity of urine specimens from individuals with symptomatic recurrent UTI versus asymptomatic controls.[38] Specifically, 74% of individuals with recurrent UTI had microbiota detected on NGS, compared to 71% of asymptomatic controls ($P = .64$). In another study, patients were randomized to treatment either based on culture or NGS results.[39] While the NGS group had greater improvement in symptoms, it is important to note that 100% of patients with lower urinary tract symptoms and 95% of healthy controls had NGS-positive urine specimens.[39] There are several additional instances wherein culture-negative urinary specimens are positive using molecular techniques. For example, in a study of 582 elderly patients with symptoms of UTI, PCR was positive while standard urine culture was negative in 22% of cases.[37] Because culture-independent techniques detect live and dead bacteria, as well as DNA fragments and commensal microbiota, clinical implementation of such assays may risk overtreatment with antibiotics, the converse of the goal of the approach. Modifications to culture-independent PCR technology are currently under investigation to selectively amplify and detect only viable microbiota.[40,41] For example, a propidium

Table 3
Future potential applications for culture-independent clinical microbiome testing for urinary tract infection diagnosis and management

Future Application	Mechanism
UTI diagnosis	Detection of uropathogenic microbe(s) in the context of symptoms could improve time to diagnosis relative to use of standard culture, which can take up to 3 d to result
UTI treatment	Early UTI treatment guided by culture-independent assay result
Asymptomatic bacteriuria treatment	Antibiotic chosen based on urinary microbiota composition (eg, during pregnancy or prior to endourologic intervention)
UTI prevention	Gut, vaginal, and urinary microbiome testing and modulation (eg, through probiotics, fecal transplant therapy, etc.) to correct dysbiosis

monoazide-based PCR assay employs the propidium monoazide dye that can penetrate nonviable cells and covalently bond to the DNA preventing its accessibility for PCR amplification.[40] This technology may play a role in the future diagnosis of UTI and may combine the strengths of both culture-dependent and culture-independent technology, while minimizing their respective limitations.

Although there may be differences in microbial diversity between those with infection relative to healthy controls,[42] the "normal" urinary microbiome requires further characterization. Without a thorough understanding of the composition of the normal microbial community in the urinary bladder (and their differences by age, sex, and other patient factors), it is not possible to accurately identify abnormalities that would benefit from treatment.

A number of UTI diagnostic products based on culture-independent approaches are commercially available,[43] some of which engage in direct-to-consumer marketing. While such assays may be implemented in the home setting without a clinical visit, they may risk amplification of contamination during collection.[43] A further bottleneck of implementation of these products is the need for clinician interpretation in order to expedite treatment. For example, even if a culture-independent assay's results return within hours of collection, interpretation by a clinician in real time would be needed in order to implement timely and appropriate treatment. It has also been argued that, given insurance coverage for many of these tests, clinicians may falsely assume that the tests have been clinically validated, which is not always the case. To date, none of the culture-independent diagnostic tests is Food and Drug Administration approved for UTI diagnosis. Of note, the American Urologic Association guidelines for recurrent UTI in

women notes that, while molecular testing technologies may provide accurate and rapid information and hold promise for the future, more evidence is needed before their incorporation in the guideline as there is concern that adoption may lead to antibiotic overtreatment.[44]

An additional potential opportunity for culture-independent methods to guide UTI treatment is the detection of antibiotic resistance genes through PCR. It has been demonstrated that PCR-based approaches can accurately detect resistance genes present in clinical urine specimens.[45] However, the correlation between genotype and phenotype is often not clear, and there is insufficient evidence to infer antibiotic resistance phenotypes from whole genome sequencing.[46] Further, phenomena including inducible resistance, regulation of gene expression, and post-translational modification are not captured through genotyping and may contribute to antibiotic resistance.[47] Also, it is possible that a resistance gene may originate from a commensal or non-viable microbe, or a DNA fragment. Thus, culture-independent antibiotic susceptibility testing is not yet optimized to guide clinical decision-making. Integration of transcriptomics and proteomics may allow for the accurate prediction of resistance phenotype based on resistance genes,[48] and requires further study.

Clinical Microbiome Testing to Guide Treatment of Asymptomatic Bacteriuria in Select Cases

In general, asymptomatic bacteriuria does not warrant treatment. Despite this, many individuals with bacteriuria but without symptoms still receive antibiotics.[49,50] This is one of the concerns of employing increasingly sensitive testing – that greater numbers of patients will be inappropriately treated with antibiotics based on the detection of bacteria by culture-independent assays. There are 2 scenarios in which antibiotic treatment of asymptomatic bacteriuria is warranted: prior to a urologic procedure (wherein breach of urinary mucosa or upper tract manipulation is anticipated) and pregnancy.[51] Here we discuss the evidence regarding culture-independent testing in these scenarios, and the potential role for targeted antibiotic prophylaxis based on these results (see **Table 3**).

Prior to urologic procedures

Antibiotic administration for individuals with asymptomatic bacteriuria is warranted for individuals who have planned upcoming endourologic procedures.[51] Specifically, procedures wherein there is likely to be breach of the urinary tract mucosa (eg, transurethral resection of the prostate, transurethral resection of bladder tumor) or upper tract manipulation (eg, laser lithotripsy of ureteral or kidney stone). Culture-independent testing may play a significant future role in this cohort, wherein there is a high UTI risk, and an indication for administration of perioperative antibiotics despite the absence of symptoms. While preoperative treatment guided by culture-independent versus culture-based approaches have not been compared, one study has examined perioperative antibiotic prophylaxis based on NGS results. In this study, consisting of 240 individuals who were to undergo endoscopic urologic surgery and had negative urine cultures, antibiotic prophylaxis based on NGS results resulted in a reduction of postsurgical urinary tract infection by 7.1% relative to the control group that did not undergo NGS testing-based antibiotic administration.[42] The intervention group also has a lower proportion of cases wherein cefazolin prophylaxis was used, and was administered a wider variety of antibiotics. While these results are promising, future studies will be needed to determine generalizability to other surgical interventions (eg, percutaneous nephrolithotomy) and whether efficacy of preoperative treatment (before 24 hour perioperative antibiotic dosing) can be improved based on culture-independent testing results. This is a pressing open question in endoscopic urologic surgery, wherein postoperative infection can exceed 40%.[52]

During pregnancy

Asymptomatic bacteriuria occurs in 2% to 15% of all pregnancies.[53,54] The diagnostic gold standard for asymptomatic bacteriuria in pregnancy is the urine culture[54] given that rapid tests such as nitrites and the Gram-stain do not have sufficient sensitivity for the detection of urine bacteria.[55] Screening for, and treating, asymptomatic bacteriuria in pregnancy is an obstetric standard-of-care. Treatment of asymptomatic bacteriuria may reduce the risk of pyelonephritis, preterm birth, and low birth rate.[54] In a Cochrane review, treatment of asymptomatic bacteriuria was associated with a risk of pyelonephritis of 48 per 1000 individuals, as compared to 199 per 1000 of untreated individuals.[54] To date, there has been no rigorous investigation regarding the relative efficacy of screening for asymptomatic bacteriuria using culture-independent molecular diagnostic approaches. This is an important area for future investigation given that the incidence of pyelonephritis in pregnancy remains about 1%.[56]

Clinical Microbiome Testing and Modulation for the Prevention of Urinary Tract Infection

Gut microbiota

It is suspected that the etiology of many UTIs is related to the gut microbiota. Gut *Enterococcus* abundance has been shown to be associated with *Enterococcus* UTIs.[57] Similarly, gut *Escherichia* was shown to be associated with *Escherichia* UTIs.[58] In a longitudinal study, it was shown that a 1% relative gut abundance of *Escherichia* is an independent risk factor for *Escherichia* bacteriuria, and that a 1% relative gut abundance of *Enterococcus* is an independent risk factor for *Enterococcus* bacteriuria.[59] In the same study, strain analysis showed close alignment between strains in the gut and the urine, supporting a gut-urine-UTI axis. The authors suggest that modulation of the gut microbiota may be an opportunity to prevent UTI. In another study, the investigators used a multi-omics approach in a longitudinal cohort of women with and without recurrent UTI.[60] Those with recurrent UTI had gut microbiomes depleted in microbial richness and butyrate-producing bacteria relative to controls. Others have shown that *E coli* gut "blooms" may precede UTI.[61,62] The findings of these studies have important implications for the development of alternatives to traditional antibiotics that do not contribute to gut-urine axis dysbiosis, and possibly repair the dysbiotic state (see **Tables 2** and **3**).[63]

One opportunity to modulate the gut microbiome to reduce UTI risk is through fecal microbiota transplantation. Recent data support further investigation of this approach[64] Specifically, in a study wherein patients received fecal microbiota transplantation for *Clostridioides difficile* infection, there was reduced UTI frequency following the transplant.[65] The transplants also improved the antibiotic susceptibility profile of uropathogens. Case reports have also shown a reduction in UTI following fecal microbiota transplants.[66–69] One of the reports showed a reduction of the proportion of gut *Enterobacteriaceae* (the family that includes *Escherichia*, *Klebsiella*, and other uropathogenic genera) from 74% before transplant to 0.07% after transplant.[68] This presents a possible mechanism for recurrent UTI risk reduction for future study. Clinical trials and mechanistic studies are warranted to further investigate the efficacy and optimal route of administration of fecal microbiota transplantation for UTI and recurrent UTI prevention. Future research may also lead to a better understanding of the most relevant microbiota involved, and thus, a targeted cocktail may be designed including only the necessary non-pathogenic microbial isolates based on the microbial composition of individual patients.

Vaginal microbiota

The vaginal microbiota may contain uropathogenic bacteria. Specifically, the vagina may harbor *E. coli*, and individuals with a history of recurrent UTI have greater predominance of vaginal *E. coli* than healthy controls.[64,70,71] Further, in a mouse model, it has been shown that *E. coli* isolates can adhere to and invade vaginal cells.[72] It was then demonstrated that the isolates could subsequently seed the urinary bladder. *Lactobacillus spp* have been shown to be present in lower levels in the vagina in those with vaginal *E. coli* than those without vaginal *E. coli* colonization.[73] *L. spp* have also been demonstrated to inhibit *E. coli* growth,[74,75] perhaps due to a combination of maintenance of low vaginal pH, production of antimicrobial products, competition for nutrients, or other mechanisms. Hormones may modulate the vaginal microbiome. Specifically, estrogen loss during menopause may reduce the relative colonization of *L. spp*, subsequently leading to increased UTI risk and recurrent infection.[64,76] Other phenomena such as antimicrobial therapy and some contraceptives may also alter protective *Lactobacillus* populations in the vagina.[76–78] Topical estrogen administration reduces UTI risk.,[79] and its mechanism may be through the modulation of *Lactobacillus* and other vaginal microbiota.[80] In the future, targeted vaginal microbiota modulation in those with recurrent UTIs might lead to an efficient restoration of a healthy microbiota environment, and could reduce risk of recurrence (see **Table 2**). Modulation could be achieved through the administration of a cocktail of *L. spp* or its derivative surface-acting molecules,[81] or other microbiota. Such a precision cocktail could be tailored for each patient through microbiota testing and comparison of the affected individual's microbiome to those without recurrent UTI.

Urine microbiota

The urinary composition of microbiota in those with and without a history of recurrent UTI may differ.[38] A less diverse urinary microbiome may predispose an individual to UTI.[82] Knowledge of the composition of the physiologic urinary microbiome is continuing to accrue.[83] In order to develop precision therapy to modulate the urinary microbiota to reduce UTI risk, further studies are needed to characterize the healthy urinary tract microbiota, and how this differs from that of those with recurrent UTI (see **Table 2**). One promising opportunity for urinary microbiome alteration to reduce infection risk is bacteriophage therapy, or "phage" therapy. Phages are intracellular viruses that infect specific bacteria. They are currently under investigation as a possible alternative or adjunct to traditional antibiotics for UTI.[84,85] They have been shown to have good lytic activity against common uropathogens.[86] A randomized-controlled clinical trial showed that phage therapy was noninferior to antibiotics, but also not superior to placebo.[87,88] Phage selection is critical to its efficacy. There are a number of different strategies for phage selection[89]: some focus on depth of coverage (more than one phage targeting a microbial strain, to reduce phage resistance rates), and some focus on breadth of coverage (a cocktail of phages covering different microbial strains). Some phage cocktails in use are based on a one-size-fits-all approach, wherein a commercially-manufactured phage cocktail is designed to target potential pathogens based on a region's antibiogram or the other data.[88] Other cocktails are developed on a patient-by-patient basis based on the clinically-isolated microbe(s) in the context of infection.[90] Presently, there are efforts to optimize phage cocktail selection through the combination of machine learning, bacterial genomics, and the phage activity data to optimally select a phage cocktail to target an infection while minimizing phage resistance.[91] Whether and how phage therapy can be employed to shift a dysbiotic urinary microbiome to a healthy state to reduce UTI and recurrent UTI risk is an important area of future research (see **Table 2**).

SUMMARY

The urine culture is imperfect, and thus, a number of alternative approaches are in development to assist in the diagnosis, treatment, and prevention of UTI. Culture-independent approaches to UTI diagnosis generally do not distinguish between viable bacteria, non-viable bacteria, and nucleotide fragments. Interpretation of these sensitive, but often nonspecific results, could lead to overtreatment with antibiotics. Thus culture-independent approaches are generally not included in current clinical guidelines. Novel approaches such as EQUC and next-generation sequencing may play important future roles in targeting antibiotic treatment of asymptomatic bacteriuria prior to endourologic surgery or in pregnancy. Future studies are needed to determine whether and how modulation of the gut, vaginal, or urinary microbiomes could reduce the risk of UTI and recurrent UTI.

CLINICS CARE POINTS

- The urine culture is imperfect and may take up to 3 days to result. From the time the culture is collected to its final result, empiric therapy is often initiated when there is suspicion for UTI. However, empiric antibiotic therapy provides inappropriate microbial coverage in up to 30% of cases.

- Given the limitations of urine culture, a series of other techniques have been developed for UTI diagnosis. One of the most common techniques is next-generation sequencing. This test is very sensitive, and cannot differentiate between viable and nonviable bacteria. Thus, while it may result more rapidly than urine culture, it also may be associated with a higher degree of overtreatment with antibiotics. Thus, it generally is not included in current clinical guidelines for UTI diagnosis.

- Next-generation sequencing and other culture-independent techniques may play an important future role in cases wherein treatment of asymptomatic bacteriuria is warranted: prior to endourologic intervention and in pregnancy.

- Whether and how modulation of the gut, vaginal, and urinary microbiomes may reduce the risk of infection in those with recurrent UTI is a promising area for future research. Possible means of modulation may include fecal microbiota transplantation, application of topical vaginal estrogen and or probiotics, and bacteriophage therapy.

DISCLOSURES

GW consultant: Atterx Biotherapeutics, Light Line Medical. MH. Hsieh: none.

Clinical trial registration: This manuscript is not a clinical trial and thus does not warrant registration as such.

Ethics of approval and patient consent: n/a.

REFERENCES

1. Sender R, Fuchs S, Milo R. Revised estimates for the number of human and bacteria cells in the body. PLoS Biol 2016;14(8):e1002533.

2. Lewis DA, Brown R, Williams J, et al. The human urinary microbiome; bacterial DNA in voided urine of asymptomatic adults. Front Cell Infect Microbiol 2013;3:41.

3. Wolfe AJ, Brubaker L. Urobiome updates: advances in urinary microbiome research. Nat Rev Urol 2019; 16(2):73–4.

4. Werneburg GT, Adler A, Zhang A, et al. Transperineal prostate biopsy is associated with lower tissue core pathogen burden relative to transrectal biopsy: mechanistic underpinnings for lower infection risk in the transperineal approach. Urology 2022;165:1–8.

5. Wolfe AJ, Rademacher DJ, Mores CR, et al. Detection of bacteria in bladder mucosa of adult females. J Urol 2023;209(5):937–49.

6. Heidler S, Lusuardi L, Madersbacher S, et al. The microbiome in benign renal tissue and in renal cell carcinoma. Urol Int 2020;104(3–4):247–52.

7. Antunes-Lopes T, Vale L, Coelho AM, et al. The role of urinary microbiota in lower urinary tract dysfunction: a systematic review. European urology focus 2020;6(2):361–9.

8. Markowski MC, Boorjian SA, Burton JP, et al. The microbiome and genitourinary cancer: a collaborative review. Eur Urol 2019;75(4):637–46.

9. Kass EH. Chemotherapeutic and antibiotic drugs in the management of infections of the urinary tract. Am J Med 1955;18(5):764–81.

10. Kass EH. Asymptomatic infections of the urinary tract. J Urol 2002;167(2):1016–20.

11. Kass EH. Bacteriuria and the diagnosis of infections of the urinary tract: with observations on the use of methionine as a urinary antiseptic. AMA Arch Intern Med 1957;100(5):709–14.

12. Semeniuk H, Church D. Evaluation of the leukocyte esterase and nitrite urine dipstick screening tests for detection of bacteriuria in women with suspected uncomplicated urinary tract infections. J Clin Microbiol 1999;37(9):3051–2.

13. Kunin CM, VanArsdale White L, Hua Hua T. A reassessment of the importance of low-count bacteriuria in young women with acute urinary symptoms. Ann Intern Med 1993;119(6):454–60.

14. Stamm WE, Running K, McKevitt M, et al. Treatment of the acute urethral syndrome. N Engl J Med 1981; 304(16):956–8.

15. Stamm WE, Counts GW, Running KR, et al. Diagnosis of coliform infection in acutely dysuric women. N Engl J Med 1982;307(8):463–8.

16. Miller JM, Binnicker MJ, Campbell S, et al. A guide to utilization of the microbiology laboratory for diagnosis of infectious diseases: 2018 update by the Infectious Diseases Society of America and the American Society for Microbiology. Clin Infect Dis 2018;67(6):e1–94.

17. Werneburg GT, Lewis KC, Vasavada SP, et al. Urinalysis exhibits excellent predictive capacity for the

absence of urinary tract infection. Urology 2023;175: 101–6.

18. Colgan R, Nicolle LE, McGlone A, et al. Asymptomatic bacteriuria in adults. Am Fam Physician 2006; 74(6):985–90.

19. Osiemo D, Schroeder DK, Klepser DG, et al. Treatment of asymptomatic bacteriuria after implementation of an inpatient urine culture algorithm in the electronic medical record. Pharmacy 2021; 9(3):138.

20. Fleming-Dutra KE, Hersh AL, Shapiro DJ, et al. Prevalence of inappropriate antibiotic prescriptions among US ambulatory care visits, 2010-2011. JAMA 2016;315(17):1864–73.

21. Hansen MA, Valentine-King M, Zoorob R, et al. Prevalence and predictors of urine culture contamination in primary care: a cross-sectional study. Int J Nurs Stud 2022;134:104325.

22. Bekeris LG, Jones BA, Walsh MK, et al. Urine culture contamination: a College of American Pathologists Q-Probes study of 127 laboratories. Arch Pathol Lab Med 2008;132(6):913–7.

23. John G, Mugnier E, Pittet E, et al. Urinary culture sensitivity after a single empirical antibiotic dose for upper or febrile urinary tract infection: a prospective multicentre observational study. Clin Microbiol Infection 2022;28(8):1099–104.

24. Mariappan P, Loong CW. Midstream urine culture and sensitivity test is a poor predictor of infected urine proximal to the obstructing ureteral stone or infected stones: a prospective clinical study. J Urol 2004;171(6 Part 1):2142–5.

25. Xu R, Deebel N, Casals R, et al. A new gold rush: a review of current and developing diagnostic tools for urinary tract infections. Diagnostics 2021;11(3):479.

26. Álvarez-Lerma F, Nolla-Salas J, León C, et al. Candiduria in critically ill patients admitted to intensive care medical units. Intensive Care Med 2003;29: 1069–76.

27. Paul N, Mathai E, Abraham O, et al. Factors associated with candiduria and related mortality. J Infect 2007;55(5):450–5.

28. Abbara A, Davidson RN. Etiology and management of genitourinary tuberculosis. Nat Rev Urol 2011; 8(12):678–88.

29. Souders CP, Scott VC, Ackerman JE, et al. Mycoplasma and Ureaplasma molecular testing does not correlate with irritative or painful lower urinary tract symptoms. J Urol 2021;206(2):390–8.

30. Hilt EE, McKinley K, Pearce MM, et al. Urine is not sterile: use of enhanced urine culture techniques to detect resident bacterial flora in the adult female bladder. J Clin Microbiol 2014;52(3):871–6.

31. Price TK, Dune T, Hilt EE, et al. The clinical urine culture: enhanced techniques improve detection of clinically relevant microorganisms. J Clin Microbiol 2016;54(5):1216–22.

32. Gasiorek M, Hsieh MH, Forster CS. Utility of DNA next-generation sequencing and expanded quantitative urine culture in diagnosis and management of chronic or persistent lower urinary tract symptoms. J Clin Microbiol 2019;58(1). e00204-19.

33. Pearce MM, Hilt EE, Rosenfeld AB, et al. The female urinary microbiome: a comparison of women with and without urgency urinary incontinence. mBio 2014;5(4). e01283-14.

34. Barnes HC, Wolff B, Abdul-Rahim O, et al. A randomized clinical trial of standard versus expanded cultures to diagnose urinary tract infections in women. J Urol 2021;206(5):1212–21.

35. Szlachta-McGinn A, Douglass KM, Chung UYR, et al. Molecular diagnostic methods versus conventional urine culture for diagnosis and treatment of urinary tract infection: a systematic review and meta-analysis. European Urology Open Science 2022;44:113–24.

36. Wolfe AJ, Toh E, Shibata N, et al. Evidence of uncultivated bacteria in the adult female bladder. J Clin Microbiol 2012;50(4):1376–83.

37. Wojno KJ, Baunoch D, Luke N, et al. Multiplex PCR based urinary tract infection (UTI) analysis compared to traditional urine culture in identifying significant pathogens in symptomatic patients. Urology 2020;136:119–26.

38. Huang L, Li X, Wei D, et al. Differential urinary microbiota composition between women with and without recurrent urinary tract infection. Front Microbiol 2022;13:888681.

39. McDonald M, Kameh D, Johnson ME, et al. A head-to-head comparative phase II study of standard urine culture and sensitivity versus DNA next-generation sequencing testing for urinary tract infections. Rev Urol 2017;19(4):213.

40. Lee AS, Lamanna OK, Ishida K, et al. A novel propidium monoazide-based PCR assay can measure viable uropathogenic E. coli in vitro and in vivo. Front Cell Infect Microbiol 2022;12:794323.

41. Dinu L-D, Al-Zaidi QJ, Matache AG, et al. Improving the efficiency of viability-qPCR with lactic acid enhancer for the selective detection of live pathogens in foods. Foods 2024;13(7):1021.

42. Liss MA, Reveles KR, Tipton CD, et al. Comparative effectiveness randomized clinical trial using next-generation microbial sequencing to direct prophylactic antibiotic choice before urologic stone lithotripsy using an interprofessional model. Eur Urol Open Sci 2023;57:74–83.

43. Hill E, Hsieh M, Prokesch B. New direct-to-consumer urinary tract infection tests: are we ready? Philadelphia (PA): Wolters Kluwer; 2022. p. 4–6.

44. Anger J, Lee U, Ackerman AL, et al. Recurrent uncomplicated urinary tract infections in women: AUA/CUA/SUFU guideline. J Urol 2019;202(2): 282–9.

45. Schmidt K, Stanley K, Hale R, et al. Evaluation of multiplex tandem PCR (MT-PCR) assays for the detection of bacterial resistance genes among Enterobacteriaceae in clinical urines. J Antimicrob Chemother 2019;74(2):349–56.

46. Ellington M, Ekelund O, Aarestrup FM, et al. The role of whole genome sequencing in antimicrobial susceptibility testing of bacteria: report from the EU-CAST Subcommittee. Clin Microbiol Infection 2017; 23(1):2–22.

47. Motro Y, Moran-Gilad J. Next-generation sequencing applications in clinical bacteriology. Biomol Detect Quantif 2017;14:1–6.

48. Ritchie MD, Holzinger ER, Li R, et al. Methods of integrating data to uncover genotype–phenotype interactions. Nat Rev Genet 2015;16(2):85–97.

49. Rotjanapan P, Dosa D, Thomas KS. Potentially inappropriate treatment of urinary tract infections in two Rhode Island nursing homes. Arch Intern Med 2011;171(5):438–43.

50. Luu T, Albarillo FS. Asymptomatic bacteriuria: prevalence, diagnosis, management, and current antimicrobial stewardship implementations. Am J Med 2022;135(8):e236–44.

51. Nicolle LE, Gupta K, Bradley SF, et al. Clinical practice guideline for the management of asymptomatic bacteriuria: 2019 update by the Infectious Diseases Society of America. Clin Infect Dis 2019;68(10): e83–110.

52. Zhou G, Zhou Y, Chen R, et al. The influencing factors of infectious complications after percutaneous nephrolithotomy: a systematic review and meta-analysis. Urolithiasis 2022;51(1):17.

53. Ipe DS, Sundac L, Benjamin Jr WH, et al. Asymptomatic bacteriuria: prevalence rates of causal microorganisms, etiology of infection in different patient populations, and recent advances in molecular detection. FEMS Microbiol Lett 2013;346(1): 1–10.

54. Smaill FM, Vazquez JC. Antibiotics for asymptomatic bacteriuria in pregnancy. Cochrane Database Syst Rev 2019;(11):CD000490.

55. Rogozińska E, Formina S, Zamora J, et al. Accuracy of onsite tests to detect asymptomatic bacteriuria in pregnancy: a systematic review and meta-analysis. Obstet Gynecol 2016;128(3):495–503.

56. Glaser AP, Schaeffer AJ. Urinary tract infection and bacteriuria in pregnancy. Urol Clin North Am 2015; 42(4):547–60.

57. Lee JR, Muthukumar T, Dadhania D, et al. Gut microbial community structure and complications after kidney transplantation: a pilot study. Transplantation 2014;98(7):697–705.

58. Paalanne N, Husso A, Salo J, et al. Intestinal microbiome as a risk factor for urinary tract infections in children. Eur J Clin Microbiol Infect Dis 2018;37: 1881–91.

59. Magruder M, Sholi AN, Gong C, et al. Gut uropathogen abundance is a risk factor for development of bacteriuria and urinary tract infection. Nat Commun 2019;10(1):5521.

60. Worby CJ, Schreiber IVHL, Straub TJ, et al. Longitudinal multi-omics analyses link gut microbiome dysbiosis with recurrent urinary tract infections in women. Nat microbiol 2022;7(5):630–9.

61. Thänert R, Reske KA, Hink T, et al. Comparative genomics of antibiotic-resistant uropathogens implicates three routes for recurrence of urinary tract infections. mBio 2019;10(4). e01977-19.

62. Worby CJ, Olson BS, Dodson KW, et al. Establishing the role of the gut microbiota in susceptibility to recurrent urinary tract infections. J Clin Investig 2022;132(5):e158497.

63. Schembri MA, Nhu NTK, Phan M-D. Gut–bladder axis in recurrent UTI. Nature Microbiology 2022; 7(5):601–2.

64. Meštrović T, Matijašić M, Perić M, et al. The role of gut, vaginal, and urinary microbiome in urinary tract infections: from bench to bedside. Diagnostics 2020;11(1):7.

65. Tariq R, Pardi DS, Tosh PK, et al. Fecal microbiota transplantation for recurrent Clostridium difficile infection reduces recurrent urinary tract infection frequency. Clin Infect Dis 2017;65(10): 1745–7.

66. Biehl LM, Cruz Aguilar R, Farowski F, et al. Fecal microbiota transplantation in a kidney transplant recipient with recurrent urinary tract infection. Infection 2018;46:871–4.

67. Grosen AK, Povlsen JV, Lemming LE, et al. Faecal microbiota transplantation eradicated extended-spectrum beta-lactamase-producing Klebsiella pneumoniae from a renal transplant recipient with recurrent urinary tract infections. Case Rep Nephrol Dial 2019;9(2):102–7.

68. Aira A, Rubio E, Vergara Gómez A, et al. rUTI resolution after FMT for Clostridioides difficile infection: a case report. Infect Dis Ther 2021;10(2): 1065–71.

69. Wang T, Kraft CS, Woodworth MH, et al. Fecal microbiota transplant for refractory clostridium difficile infection interrupts 25-year history of recurrent urinary tract infections. Open Forum Infect Dis 2018; 5(2):ofy016.

70. Lewis AL, Gilbert NM. Roles of the vagina and the vaginal microbiota in urinary tract infection: evidence from clinical correlations and experimental models. GMS Infect Dis 2020;8:Doc02.

71. Navas-Nacher EL, Dardick F, Venegas MF, et al. Relatedness of Escherichia coli colonizing women longitudinally. Mol Urol 2001;5(1):31–6.

72. Brannon JR, Dunigan TL, Beebout CJ, et al. Invasion of vaginal epithelial cells by uropathogenic Escherichia coli. Nat Commun 2020;11(1):2803.

73. Gupta K, Stapleton AE, Hooton TM, et al. Inverse association of H2O2-producing lactobacilli and vaginal Escherichia coli colonization in women with recurrent urinary tract infections. J Infect Dis 1998;178(2):446–50.

74. Hudson PL, Hung KJ, Bergerat A, et al. Effect of vaginal Lactobacillus species on Escherichia coli growth. Urogynecology 2020;26(2):146–51.

75. Vagios S, Hesham H, Mitchell C. Understanding the potential of lactobacilli in recurrent UTI prevention. Microb Pathog 2020;148:104544.

76. Stapleton AE. The vaginal microbiota and urinary tract infection. Microbiol Spectr 2016;4(6). https://doi.org/10.1128/microbiolspec.uti-0025-2016.

77. Mayer BT, Srinivasan S, Fiedler TL, et al. Rapid and profound shifts in the vaginal microbiota following antibiotic treatment for bacterial vaginosis. J Infect Dis 2015;212(5):793–802.

78. Eschenbach DA, Patton DL, Meier A, et al. Effects of oral contraceptive pill use on vaginal flora and vaginal epithelium. Contraception 2000;62(3):107–12.

79. Perrotta C, Aznar M, Mejia R, et al. Oestrogens for preventing recurrent urinary tract infection in postmenopausal women. Cochrane Database Syst Rev 2008;(2):CD005131.

80. Jung CE, Estaki M, Chopyk J, et al. Impact of vaginal estrogen on the urobiome in postmenopausal women with recurrent urinary tract infection. Urogynecology 2022;28(1):20–6.

81. Chee WJY, Chew SY, Than LTL. Vaginal microbiota and the potential of Lactobacillus derivatives in maintaining vaginal health. Microb Cell Factories 2020;19(1):203.

82. Horwitz D, McCue T, Mapes AC, et al. Decreased microbiota diversity associated with urinary tract infection in a trial of bacterial interference. J Infect 2015;71(3):358–67.

83. Morand A, Cornu F, Dufour J-C, et al. Human bacterial repertoire of the urinary tract: a potential paradigm shift. J Clin Microbiol 2019;57(3). e00675-18.

84. Leitner L, Kessler TM, Klumpp J. Bacteriophages: a panacea in neuro-urology? European urology focus 2020;6(3):518–21.

85. Uyttebroek S, Chen B, Onsea J, et al. Safety and efficacy of phage therapy in difficult-to-treat infections: a systematic review. Lancet Infect Dis 2022;22(8):e208–20.

86. Sybesma W, Zbinden R, Kutateladze M, et al. Bacteriophages as potential treatment for urinary tract infections. Front Microbiol 2016;7:183439.

87. Leitner L, Ujmajuridze A, Chanishvili N, et al. Intravesical bacteriophages for treating urinary tract infections in patients undergoing transurethral resection of the prostate: a randomised, placebo-controlled, double-blind clinical trial. Lancet Infect Dis 2021;21(3):427–36.

88. Leitner L, Sybesma W, Chanishvili N, et al. Bacteriophages for treating urinary tract infections in patients undergoing transurethral resection of the prostate: a randomized, placebo-controlled, double-blind clinical trial. BMC Urol 2017;17:1–6.

89. Abedon ST, Danis-Wlodarczyk KM, Wozniak DJ. Phage cocktail development for bacteriophage therapy: toward improving spectrum of activity breadth and depth. Pharmaceuticals 2021;14(10):1019.

90. Green SI, Clark JR, Santos HH, et al. A retrospective, observational study of 12 cases of expanded-access customized phage therapy: production, characteristics, and clinical outcomes. Clin Infect Dis 2023;77(8):1079–91.

91. Keith M, Park de la Torriente A, Chalka A, et al. Predictive phage therapy for Escherichia coli urinary tract infections: cocktail selection for therapy based on machine learning models. Proc Natl Acad Sci U S A 2024;121(12). e2313574121.

Management of Infections Associated with Penile Prostheses and Artificial Urinary Sphincters

Amandip S. Cheema, MD, MHS*, Milan K. Patel, MD,
Ahmad M. El-Arabi, MD, Christopher M. Gonzalez, MD, MBA

KEYWORDS

- Penile prosthesis • Artificial urinary sphincter • Infection

KEY POINTS

- Rates of infection for penile prostheses (PPs) and artificial urinary sphincters (AUSs) have decreased due to improved design, improved surgical approaches, and sterility, yet infection remains a feared and detrimental complication.
- The pillars for managing a prosthetic device infection include adequate culturing of the device, initiation of broad-spectrum antibiotics, device removal with aggressive antibiotic washout, and either salvage reimplantation—which has effectively become the gold standard for managing PP infections or delayed implantation of a device—for infected AUS devices.
- The culmination of surgeon experience, modernized and improved implants, and meticulous pre-operative, intra-operative, and post-operative protocols all play an important role in preventing prosthetic infections.

INTRODUCTION

The management of erectile dysfunction and male urinary incontinence often relies on prostheses. While phosphodiesterase type 5 inhibitors and intracavernosal injection therapy can be effective in improving sexual function, penile prostheses (PPs) remain the gold standard for severe or refractory erectile dysfunction. Similarly, while a wide variety of slings and bulking agents are available to men with stress urinary incontinence, an artificial urinary sphincter (AUS) is the gold standard of treatment of those with severe incontinence. Over the years, prosthetic urology has continued to evolve and technology has advanced with an effort to improve efficacy, ease of use, and patient satisfaction. Nevertheless, the rate of complications—notably, infections—continues to be significant.

The purpose of this review is to provide the practicing urologist with a primer on preventing, recognizing, and managing these infections in urologic prostheses.

PENILE PROSTHESIS: AN OVERVIEW

Epidemiologic data suggest that the incidence of erectile dysfunction (ED) is growing. By the year 2025, it is estimated that close to 322 million men will suffer from erectile dysfunction, worldwide.[1] The management of ED can be divided into a few different broad categories: lifestyle modifications, pharmacologic therapeutics, and surgical treatment options. Although most patients may initially be recommended a trial of lifestyle changes or a phosphodiesterase (PDE)-5 inhibitor, it is important to recognize that the treatment of erectile dysfunction does not need to follow a

Department of Urology, Loyola University Medical Center, 2160 South 1st Avenue, Maywood, IL 60153, USA
* Corresponding author. 2160 South 1st Avenue, Maywood, IL 60153.
E-mail address: amandip.cheema@luhs.org

Urol Clin N Am 51 (2024) 505–515
https://doi.org/10.1016/j.ucl.2024.06.008
0094-0143/24/© 2024 Elsevier Inc. All rights are reserved, including those for text and data mining, AI training, and similar technologies.

stepwise progression. PPs are not only indicated for those patients who have failed pharmacotherapy, but also for those individuals who initially present to the urologist with severe ED and cannot undergo or tolerate nonsurgical treatment, and/or simply prefer early surgical intervention.[2]

PPs have proven to be quite successful in the management of ED especially over the years. These devices come in 3 forms: the 2 piece malleable penile prosthetic (MPP), the 2 piece inflatable penile prosthetic (IPP), and the 3 piece IPP. The nuances in choosing among these 3 prostheses types are outside the scope of this study and so will instead focus on the most commonly implanted device — the 3 piece IPP. It is estimated that 15,000 IPPs are implanted in the United States alone every year.[3]

While implant malfunction is inevitable, an IPP consistently has a lifespan of 10 to 20 years.[4] Device infection has the potential to severely limit this lifespan, often requiring early device explantation. Advances in the manufacturing of PPs, operative technique, and the understanding of relevant microbiology as well as the use of antibiotics have lowered the rates of infection. Still, rates of IPP infection are between 1% and 4%.[5] Aside from explantation, an infection can lead to numerous other negative consequences for the patient, including those pertaining to the patient's psyche, future erectile function, and personal health care costs.[6] Thus, it is critical for the urologist to have the necessary familiarity and expertise required to prevent and inevitably manage this unfortunate complication.

PENILE PROSTHESIS INFECTION
Risk Factors

Various factors may predispose a patient to be at a higher risk of developing an infection of their PP. Diabetes mellitus (DM) has long been suggested as one of those risk factors. Poor vascular flow, in particular, makes DM a risk factor for postoperative complication in patients undergoing PP implantation. A major consequence of poor vascular circulation is improper wound healing and consequently infection. Studies have used preoperative glycemic control cutoffs, in the form of hemoglobin a1c (HbA1c), to suggest that patients are at a significantly increased risk for postoperative infection.[7,8] A multicenter prospective study of over 902 patients determined that an HbA1c of 8.5% or greater was associated with increased risk of postoperative IPP infection risk.[9,10] When the HbA1c value surpasses greater than 11.5, the absolute risk of infection can rise up to 31%.[8] However, other studies have suggested that preoperative HbA1c levels are not associated

with increased postoperative infection.[11,12] In the largest ever multi-institutional cohort of diabetic men undergoing PP implantation (875 men), Osman and colleagues[13] found that neither preoperative blood glucose (PBC) levels nor HbA1c was predictive of device infection, revision, or explantation. These contradictory results suggest that perhaps another measure of preoperative glycemic control should be assessed in conjunction with HbA1c levels. One such variable that is assessed in only one of these studies is PBG levels within 6 hours of surgery. Ultimately no prospective randomized controlled study comparing infection rates between uncontrolled diabetics and controlled diabetics exists and so we believe it is ultimately up to the discretion of the operating urologist to determine their own cutoff based on their experience and comfort. Prior spinal cord injury is also thought to place a patient at higher risk of IPP infection.[14] The mechanism remains unknown but potential etiologies include an increased risk of urinary tract infections, reliance on chronic or intermittent catheterization, or delayed recognition of initial erosion.[10,15] The data for other potential patient risk factors such as obesity and immunosuppression are inconclusive.[6,10,15,16] As may be assumed, a history of prior PP surgery carries a higher risk of infection. This remains true whether the prior prosthesis was removed due to device failure or infection.[17] Infection rates, following revision surgery, have been as high as 10% to 13.3% in some studies compared to 0.46% to 2% in virgin cases.[10] In one retrospective study, the rate of infection after a third, fourth, and fifth IPP insertion was found to be 33% (4 out of 12), 50% (4 out of 8), and 100% (2 out of 2), respectively.[9] It has previously been reported that the performance of an additional procedure at time of PP implantation, such as concomitant AUS insertion, may be associated with a higher risk of infection, but this has not been well established in the literature.[6] Aside from AUS insertion, circumcision is another procedure occasionally performed at time of IPP implantation and has similarly not been associated with an increased rate of postoperative infection.[10,18] Nevertheless, we caution the reader that while these additional procedures may not themselves increase the risk for infection, an overall longer operative time may do so.[18] Lastly, PP implantation by low volume surgeons has been associated with a higher rate of device infection. In a study of close to 15,000 men, patients who underwent IPP implantation by a surgeon with an annual case volume of 31 or less were 2.1 to 2.5 times more likely to require a repeat operation due to an infectious complication.[19] This reduced rate of infection seen with high volume surgeons may be explained by shorter operative times, more experienced operating room staff, and greater adherence to preoperative and perioperative protocols.[19]

Infection Types

The timing of a PP infection can be classified as an acute infection or chronic infection. Infections of the prosthesis presenting within 6 weeks are considered acute infections, whereas infections after this period are considered chronic infections.[15]

Acute Infection

The diagnosis of a PP infection can often be difficult in the immediate postoperative setting. Scrotal edema, ecchymosis, and pain are common occurrences in the first few days to weeks following implantation. These signs or symptoms are expected. In order to diagnose a true acute PP infection, the clinician must often rely on overt clinical signs of infection (eg, fevers, tachycardia, erythema, purulence, fluctuance) or laboratory findings (eg, leukocytosis, elevated procalcitonin, elevated lactate). Scrotal hematoma, in particular, is often confused with acute infection. The presence of isolated scrotal swelling or bruising without the aforementioned infectious clues favors a diagnosis of postoperative hematoma, which can often be managed expectantly.[20] If there is suspicion of a postoperative infection, it is important to then distinguish a superficial surgical-site infection (SSI) from a true infection of the prosthetic as further management can be drastically different. A superficial skin infection can often be managed nonoperatively with a course of oral antibiotics and close clinic follow-up. The management of a PP infection almost always requires surgical intervention. In general, superficial skin infections are associated with the suture line and the surrounding skin; erythema, warmth, and mild-to-moderate edema of the penile and scrotal swelling are all consistent with the diagnosis. The components of the implanted device themselves are spared. Clinically, a superficial skin infection often presents within the first few days after implantation and with minimal-to-no systemic signs of infection. In contrast, a PP infection will often present weeks to months after implantation with more obvious systemic signs of infection. With that said, these presentations can occasionally overlap and pose a great diagnostic challenge. In this situation, there are a few potential management strategies. One option is a trial of empiric oral antibiotics with close follow-up; if improvement is seen, this favors a diagnosis of a superficial skin infection. A second option is proceeding to surgical exploration and possible explantation, as would be the treatment of a true PP infection. A third option is the use of MRI. In the setting of acute infections, especially less than 6 weeks after initial implantation, MRI is seldom used, as a diagnosis is often apparent from physical examination and laboratory analyses. However, in ambiguous situations, an MRI can provide clinical utility. An MRI can help elucidate whether an infection involves the periprosthetic space. An infection that does not involve the periprosthetic space can often be managed with antibiotic therapy alone.[21]

Chronic Infections

Chronic infections of PPs can occur months to years after surgery. Among chronic IPP infections, approximately 57% occur within the first 7 months and 94% within the first year.[22] Chronic infections of an IPP can present with persistent pain that worsens with erection and patients rarely have fever, systemic symptoms, or leukocytosis.[17,21,23] A presenting symptom of chronic infections can be device extrusion.[23] Overall, the diagnosis of a chronic IPP infection is often more challenging than in the acute setting, as the presenting signs and symptoms are less obvious. Furthermore, a device infection can be easily confused for a close mimicker: device failure. Mechanical device failure is another worrisome complication after IPP implantation and, in the months to years after surgery, can be equally or perhaps even more prevalent than device infection. In fact, one study found device failure as the inciting cause of revision surgery in 65% of cases, compared to infection in 29% of cases.[21,24] Physical examination is important, and a device that does not cycle well can indicate device failure—but this is often not enough to diagnose a device failure versus chronic infection. MRI is considered the most valuable imaging modality in assessing PPs. With regard to the 3 piece IPP, the cylinders will appear T2-hyperintense due to their fluid content. The reservoir can be identified as a T2-hyperintense round or oval cystic lesion, and the scrotal pump appears as a small T2-hyperintense oval structure. MRI is often used in a PP patient with chronic pain, as it has the ability to show even the smallest amount of periprosthetic fluid collections, edema, or gas. The use of intravenous contrast also allows for enhancement of soft tissue and prosthetic component interfaces. For these reasons, MRI can aid in the diagnosis of chronic device failure versus infection in the otherwise clinically ambiguous scenario.[21]

Inflatable Penile Prosthesis Infection Versus Malleable Penile Prosthesis Infection

When comparing rates of infection between IPPs and MPPs, the data are conflicting. Bozkurt and colleagues[25] found that the rate of infection was higher in patients with an IPP (4.2%) versus those with an MPP (1.44%), although this was not statistically significant. Earle and colleagues[26] reported an infection rate of 0% in their IPP group versus a rate of 3.5% in the MPP group; however, this study was limited by small sample size and a short follow-up window. Altunkol and colleagues[27] found the incidence of infection to be comparable, with a rate of 6.3% in the IPP group and 5.6% in the MPP group. Overall, the literature does not definitively suggest a significant difference in infectious complications following insertion of an IPP or MPP.[28] Despite this, some urologists may favor placement of an MPP in high-risk patients, as it is a simpler prosthetic with less components.

MANAGEMENT OF AN INFECTED PENILE PROSTHESIS
General Management

The management of an infected PP is ultimately surgical explantation. This entails removal of all components of the device. Even if infection is thought to be limited to a small area of the device, partial removal is not recommended due to the possibility of reinfection.[17] Previously, the standard of care for infected PPs was antibiotic therapy with immediate explantation and delayed reimplantation after 6 months. This strategy was eventually found to have many pitfalls including penile shortening (up to 2 inches), corporal fibrosis, increased complexity during revision surgery, and decreased patient satisfaction.[10,29] In 1996, Mulcahy[30] described a new protocol advocating for immediate replacement of an infected PP—the Mulcahy protocol. With this new approach, the original Mulcahy salvage series of 55 patients demonstrated a success rate of 82%. Success was defined as no subsequent signs of recurrent infection or erosion, with a mean follow-up of 35 months. Other key steps of this salvage protocol included obtaining wound cultures, corporal body irrigation with antibiotic solution followed by hydrogen peroxide and then povidone–iodine (these solutions are then used in reverse), and washout of the reservoir tract.[31]

Antimicrobials

A 2016 retrospective multi-institutional study from 25 centers reviewed intraoperative cultures obtained at time of explanation of infected IPPs. They found negative cultures in 33% of cases and gram-positive and gram-negative organisms were found in 73% and 37% of positive cultures, respectively. Candida species (11.1%), anaerobes (10.5%), and methicillin-resistant Staphylococcus aureus (MRSA) (9.2%) were found in around one-third of positive cultures.[32] When performing a salvage procedure, one should adhere to the Mulcahy protocol and, based on these data, substitute the original antimicrobial washout for an antimicrobial solution of vancomycin, piperacillin–tazobactam, and amphotericin B to irrigate the wound and new implant.

Intraoperative Recommendations

Gross and colleagues[32] developed a treatment algorithm for infected PPs. First cultures should be obtained via needle aspiration, this can be done without fear of damaging an IPP, as the device is destined to be removed and should be done prior to initiation of antibiotics. Following aspiration broad-spectrum antibiotics and antifungals can be initiated to cover MRSA, oxacillin-resistant gram-positive and gram-negative bacteria, anaerobic bacteria, and Candida species. Vancomycin, piperacillin–tazobactam, and fluconazole are recommended, although it is important that providers consider their local antibiogram when selecting initial antibiotic therapy. One should then adhere to the Mulcahy protocol to wash out the tissues and PP, as described earlier. At this time, the patient should be redraped, and gowns and gloves be changed to limit contamination before proceeding with the case.

Explantation Versus Exchange

Salvage procedures have been shown to be effective and successful in up to 93% of patients, and we feel that should be the gold standard. However, data from the National Inpatient Survey show that 82.7% of PP infections are treated with explanation only.[33] Reasons for this are likely complicated and include surgeon experience, time being less with explantation alone, and other patient and provider factors. Relative contraindications to performing a salvage procedure include a patient who is floridly septic and cannot tolerate an operative procedure, an infection that is unlikely to be cleared by such a procedure (as can be seen in immunocompromised individuals), patients with tissue necrosis-making reimplantation impossible, and bilateral erosion of cylinders into the fossa navicularis.[17] When performing a salvage procedure, it is important to consider what type of prosthesis will be used to replace the infected device. A recent multicenter study opted to use an MPP as the replacement of choice for infected implants in 58 salvage procedures, quoting a 93% success rate. The authors of this study cite the benefits to be avoiding the need to place a new reservoir and pump, shortening operative time, and minimizing corporal fibrosis. Interestingly, only 31% of patients elected to convert to an IPP from the malleable device.[2] Lopategui and colleagues[33] found that patients undergoing a salvage procedure had a corporal length loss of 0.6 cm as compared to a 3.7 cm loss in patients undergoing delayed reimplantation. Gross and colleagues[32] recommend, that whenever possible, a salvage procedure is performed using a malleable device to replace an infected PP. Patients should continue on culture-directed antibiotics for 4 to 6 weeks postoperatively. If cultures are negative, it is recommended that a 4 to 6 week course of oral antibiotics with a combination of trimethoprim–sulfamethoxazole and amoxicillin–clavulanic acid be used.[32] Oral antifungal can be deferred unless cultures are positive for *Candida* species.[32]

Biofilms

Bacteria are introduced into the surgical field at the time of surgery, whether this is from the surgical team, from the patient, or from traffic in and out of the operating room. It is believed that every implant procedure is inoculated with bacteria.[31] When a foreign body is implanted during surgery, blood covers the foreign body and results in adsorption of proteins onto the device surface. This in turn forms a conditioning layer made of albumin, fibrinogen, and other proteins.[34,35] This conditioning layer is beneficial to allow immune cells to adhere to the device, but also to planktonic bacteria to do the same. With regard to timeline, after the conditioning layer is formed, bacteria adhere within minutes, within hours they multiply and secrete biofilm, a slimy adherent substance. Costerton dubbed this "a race for the surface," with regard to the battle between the host immune cells and the bacteria. If the microbes win, then the device becomes covered in the biofilm that hampers immune defenses.[34,36] It has been reported that over 99% of bacteria are able to persist in biofilms.[37] Electron microscopy of penile implants that have been removed for reasons other than infection showed that almost all components of these devices had biofilm and colonization with bacteria.[38] Biofilms not only make it difficult for the host's immune response to attack bacteria, but they also provide an added benefit to bacteria providing bacterial resistance to antibiotics. Only about 10% of biofilms are made up of bacteria, the remainder is a biomatrix with nutrients and water channels that support the bacteria.[39] These

bacteria are active but have reduced growth when compared to their rapid multiplication during initial adhesion to the implant. They also undergo several genetic transformations making antibiotics less effective. These changes, in addition to the physical barrier of the biofilm, allow bacteria to withstand antibiotic concentrations 10 to 1000 times higher than what is needed to kill equivalent bacteria in other parts of the body.[40] This biofilm also makes it difficult to obtain adequate wound cultures, often culturing of biofilms will return as "no growth."[34] Biofilms remain a persistent threat to the success of PPs and other types of implants.

PREVENTION OF A PENILE PROSTHESIS INFECTION
Antibacterial Coatings

Since 2003, virtually every IPP sold in the Unites States has been coated with infection-preventing substances. American Medical Systems (AMS) dubbed its coating InhibiZone, whereas Coloplast utilizes a different coating. InhibiZone is a mixture of rifampin and minocycline that is applied during the manufacturing process. The dosage used is quite low in comparison to those used in systemic infections. The antibiotics begin to work as soon as they are implanted into the patient, preventing colonization of bacteria into the implanted space.[31] In a study of 11,064 patients, antibacterial coatings resulted in significant reduction in infection rates during revision and replacement surgery demonstrating a decrease from 3.7% to 2.5%.[31,41] Coloplast utilizes a hydrophilic coating that allows for the uptake of antibiotics during soaking before implantation. This has the added benefit of tailoring the antibiotics to the sites susceptibility profile and the surgeons' discretion.[17] Serefoglu and colleagues[42] showed a significant reduction of device infection from 4.6% to 1.4% using the hydrophilic-coated devices. Eid and Wilson reported on the infection rates of 704 coated devices of both variations compared to non-coated devices and found that infection rates were significantly decreased in the coated devices compared to the non-coated devices of 2% to 5.3%, respectively. They found no statistical significant difference between the AMS and Coloplast devices, the latter only being dipped in saline with no antimicrobials.[43] Antibacterial coatings have undoubtedly been one of the most important developments in reducing the rates of infection in PPs in the current era.

Preoperative Antibiotics

There have been many methods used in attempts to lower the risks of infection of PPs. In 2008, the

American Urological Association guidelines were published describing the use of prophylactic antibiotics for several urologic procedures. At that time, it was recommended that systemic vancomycin and gentamicin be given 1 hour prior to incision and continued for up to 24 hours postoperatively. A third-generation cephalosporin may be substituted for vancomycin, particularly in cases of contraindications such as allergy (Red Man syndrome) or poor renal function.[44] Gross and colleagues published on American Urologic Association (AUA) and EAU guidelines based preoperative antibiotic recommendations only covering prosthesis culture isolates 62% to 86% of the time.[10,32] The AUA updated their recommendation in 2019, with the release of their Best Practice Statement on Urologic Procedures and Antibiotic Prophylaxis. These current PP antibiotic guidelines recommend the use of an aminoglycoside and either a first-generation or second-generation cephalosporin or vancomycin. Interestingly, a recent multicenter, retrospective study has found that gentamicin and vancomycin were associated with a 2.7 times higher risk of infection in virgin IPP placements, when compared to other regimens.[45] This same study also found that the addition of antifungals was associated with a 92% reduction in infection rate, despite only 2.1% of cultures being positive for fungal organisms.[45] Further investigation into the current AUA preoperative antibiotic guidelines is needed.

Postoperative Antibiotics

The use of prophylactic postoperative antibiotics after IPP insertion, beyond 24 hours, is controversial. In other specialties such as facial and plastic reconstructive surgery, a short course of postoperative antibiotics has shown a definitive protective role in preventing SSIs.[46] However, a similar benefit has not yet been established in the field of penile reconstruction. A recent study demonstrated no difference in infection rates following IPP surgery with the addition of postoperative antibiotics in both low and high risk patients.[47] This debate is ongoing and often the use of postoperative antibiotics will be determined by each individual urologist and their anecdotal experience with such practices.

Preoperative Urine Culture

The 2 manufacturers of IPP devices (Coloplast and Boston Scientific) state that placement of their device is contraindicated in patients with an active urogenital infection. For this reason, many urologists choose to obtain a preoperative urine culture and attempt to sterilize the urine before any IPP

placement is performed.[10] A 2018 retrospective review of AUS placement and IPP placement found that 41% of patients did not have any preoperative urine culture, despite this there was no difference in infection rates compared to those that did have a preoperative urine culture.[48] There is, however, level 5 evidence (expert opinion) to support obtaining a preoperative urine culture for patients undergoing genitourinary prosthetic surgery.[10]

Operative Scrub

The literature demonstrates that when infected IPPs are explanted, the majority of them are colonized with gram-positive organism. As discussed earlier, it is believed that at the time of IPP implantation, the device becomes inoculated with bacteria, which often originates from the patients' own skin microflora. A povidone–iodine-based scrub has historically been used in patients undergoing genitourinary prosthesis placement. A 2013 randomized control trial of 100 patients placed 50 patients in chlorhexidine arm and 50 patients in a povidone–iodine arm. Pre-scrub and post-scrub skin cultures were obtained. The povidone–iodine group was found to have more positive post-scrub cultures compared to chlorhexidine (32% vs 8%; $P = .0091$).[49] Furthermore, several other randomized control trials have shown the actual rate of postoperative infections to be lower with chlorhexidine preparation. It is now recommended that alcohol-based skin prep be used for genitourinary prosthesis placement with a drying time of at least 3 minutes.[17]

Staphylococcus aureus Nasal Carriage

Cultures from infected PPs often demonstrate MRSA. It is reasonable to consider testing for nasal carriage of S aureus in patients undergoing PP placement. It has been well demonstrated in the orthopedic surgery literature that nasal carriage of S aureus is a positive risk factor for developing an S aureus SSI.[10,50] A randomized control trial has found a decreased rates of SSI with S aureus among nasal carriers with the use of preoperative showering with chlorhexidine soap and the application of nasal mupirocin for 5 days versus placebo (3.4% vs 7.7%).[10,17,51]

ARTIFICIAL URINARY SPHINCTERS: AN OVERVIEW

AUSs were introduced in 1983 and are considered the gold standard for the treatment of severe urinary incontinence with a patient satisfaction rate of over 90%.[17] In men, they are often used for incontinence following radical prostatectomy. AUS infections are difficult to characterize and rates of infection range from 0.5% to 10.6%. Oftentimes, AUS erosion and infection are grouped together as one complication in the literature. AUS infection, without erosion, is often clear-cut. A patient presents shortly in the postoperative period with incisional erythema, edema, possible purulence, fever, and leukocytosis. Ziegelmann and colleagues[52] reported on their cohort of patients who underwent primary AUS placement with over 90% of infections occurring within the first 6 months.

On the contrary, it is not clear whether erosion occurs and then leads to an infected AUS, or whether an infection precedes device erosion. Regardless, either an infected and/or eroded AUS requires explantation.

Risk Factors for Artificial Urinary Sphincter Infection

Risk factors for AUS infection are similar to those for a PP infection, such as DM and poor glucose control. Pelvic radiation is also a notable risk factor for AUS infection-erosion. Radiation damages basement membranes of blood vessels leading to occlusion and thrombosis, neovascularization leads to fibroblast proliferation, and subsequent scar formation ultimately compromising blood supply.[53] Similarly, previous urethral reconstruction is associated with AUS infection-erosion especially when the bulbourethral arteries are transected; of note, non-transecting approaches were not associated with higher rates of infection-erosion.[54] Prolonged indwelling catheter or intermittent catheterization is also associated with higher rates of AUS complications.[53] Interestingly, there is conflicting information on whether prior AUS surgery is associated with infection and erosion.[54–56]

MANAGEMENT OF AN ARTIFICIAL URINARY SPHINCTER INFECTION

As discussed earlier, AUS infections can occur at any time, although the majority occur within 1 year. As seen with PPs, superficial infections of AUS devices can present with erythema, edema, pump fixation, and/or purulence. These superficial infections occur in a similar manner to PP infections with inoculation of bacteria at the suture line at the time of surgery. Oftentimes this can be managed with antibiotics and routine follow-up.[53] Infections involving the actual AUS device should be managed similarly to true PP infections—with surgical intervention. Management will often begin with systemic antibiotics and cystoscopy and/or imaging to further assess the anatomy/device.

Once an infection is confirmed or highly suspected, the next step is subsequent removal of the AUS and all of its components. Traditional teaching is that AUS infection-erosion should be managed with urinary diversion with an indwelling urethral catheter or suprapubic cystotomy in conjunction with a prolonged course of antibiotics. This allows for urethral and periurethral tissue healing. AUS reimplantation can then be considered 4 to 6 months following removal. Prior to proceeding with replacing the device, a cystoscopy should be performed to assess for any development of a urethral stricture.[17,56] Like an infected PP, where salvage is achievable, immediate replacement of an infected AUS device has been described; however, it should be approached with great caution.[17,56] Immediate replacement of an infected AUS predisposes to early cuff erosion. If erosion is already present, immediately replacing an AUS device does not allow for urethral regeneration and the risk of infection is much higher.[17] More recently, there have been reports of AUS removal due to infection-erosion with immediate urethral reconstruction. The touted benefit of this approach is preventing the development of a bulbar urethral stricture, which would make future AUS placement less difficult.[57] An infected-eroded AUS could then be treated with (1) removal of the old infected device; (2) urethroplasty at time of infected device removal; and (3) delayed placement of a new AUS device during a subsequent procedure.[56] Reports are conflicting as some data suggest that the type of repair (indwelling Foley catheter, urethroplasty, suprapubic cystotomy, etc.) at the time of infection-erosion did not alter future urethral stricture events.[58] Further studies are needed to demonstrate a benefit of urethroplasty at time of infected-eroded AUS removal. When replacing an AUS, it is important to note that success rates are 60% to 70%.[59,60] Several approaches can be taken to increase the likelihood of a successful repeat AUS device including using alternate cuff sites, using a transcorporal (TC) approach, or downsizing of cuff size.[56] Location of a new cuff will be determined by intraoperative findings and tissue viability. Often the subsequent cuff can be placed more proximally (at the perineal body or more proximal) or distally (especially if a TC approach is used).[56] If urethral atrophy is noted, or the patient is at high risk for repeat erosion, a TC cuff placement is warranted.[17] An advantage of the TC approach is that a flap of tunica albuginea allows for the dorsal urethra to be separated from the cuff making posterior urethral injury less likely and acting as a bolster to allow for sufficient closing pressure of the cuff, while dispersing the pressure of the cuff.[17,56] It also allows for the minimal mobilization of the urethra off of the corpora cavernosa at the implantation site, with a lower chance of compromised blood supply.[17] It is important to note that the tunica albuginea has limited compressibility and so cuff sizing becomes even more important than in a traditional periurethral approach. It should be noted that there is a higher rate of urinary retention following a TC approach. There have also been some very limited reports of erectile dysfunction following the TC approach.[17]

Microbiology of Artificial Urinary Sphincter Infection-Erosion

Historically, the predominant bacteria associated with infected-eroded AUS devices were coagulase-negative staphylococcus. Since the manufacturing of antibiotic-coated devices, there has been a transition to other bacteria. Leong and colleagues[61] cultured AUS devices in their patients at time of explantation (for mechanical failure or overt infection). Cultures were positive in 87% of cases. Coagulase-negative staphylococci were the predominant bacteria, followed by commensal skin flora. Cultures from eroded-infected devices revealed more virulent organisms such as *Escherichia coli* as well as fungal species such as *Candida albicans*. Werneburg and colleagues[62] examined explanted AUS devices for any reason and found biofilms to be associated with 100% of devices, even those not removed for infection. Antibiotic resistance genes were commonly detected on these biofilms, including *rpoB* mutations that confer rifampin resistance. It is hypothesized that device-associated infections are not caused by a single organism and biofilm, but rather multiple organisms and their metabolites in biofilm that result in a dysbiotic shift allowing for the transition from a colonized asymptomatic AUS to an infected AUS requiring explantation.

PREVENTING AN ARTIFICIAL URINARY SPHINCTER INFECTION

Many of the same principles, for preventing a PP infection, also apply to preventing an AUS infection. The use of meticulous sterile technique, preoperative antibiotics, aggressive washout (especially in settings of AUS explant), and the use of antibiotic-coated devices are all used in an effort to prevent AUS-associated infection-erosions. As is seen in PP explants, AUS explants also suffer from the detrimental effects of biofilm formation. Unlike PPs, antibiotic-coated AUS devices have not shown any significant reduction in infections or explantation rates.[63] The use of postoperative oral

antibiotics also does not reduce the risk of AUS explantation, and this practice should be reconsidered in the setting of increasing antibiotic resistance.[61] As discussed with PPs, the utility of a preoperative urine culture is also controversial. Preoperative urine culture is correlated poorly with the bacteriology of infected-eroded devices.[48] In addition, there has been no difference in infection rates between patients with negative urine culture and those with asymptomatic positive cultures that were not treated.[48] As was the case with PPs, we advocate for the use of a preoperative urine culture in patients undergoing AUS placement.

COMBINED ARTIFICIAL URINARY SPHINCTER AND INFLATABLE PENILE PROSTHETIC PLACEMENT

The majority of surgeons will prefer to stage the placement of an AUS and an IPP. Reasons for this vary, but it has been demonstrated that combined placement of an AUS with an IPP is safe and feasible and just as effective as staged placement of either device—many patients also prefer only undergoing one procedure.[64] Dual placement does increase operative time, and therefore, some believe that infection risk may be higher.[56] There are very limited studies available that investigate adverse effects and benefits of a combined approach. Boysen and colleagues demonstrated that dual placement did not have adverse effects on perioperative complication rates or device survival when compared to placement of IPP or AUS alone.[64] We advise each urologist to consider a dual approach in select cases. Patients should be fully informed of the possible increased risk of infection. Dual placement of an AUS and IPP allows for 1 anesthetic event, decreased recovery time when compared to 2 procedures, and overall is more convenient for a patient.[56] If a staged approach is chosen, it is recommended that the AUS is placed first, as improved continence can improve sexual desire in patients considering future IPP placement.[56]

SUMMARY

The prosthetic urologist has many challenges, the largest of which is infection. Management of an infected PP or AUS can be difficult to diagnose, treat, and manage. Through advances in technology, better understanding of microbiology and biofilms, and improved surgical techniques, the rates of infection have fallen significantly. The pillars for managing a prosthetic device infection include adequate culturing of the device, initiation of broad-spectrum antibiotics, device removal with aggressive antibiotic washout, and either salvage reimplantation—which has effectively become the gold standard for managing PP infections or delayed implantation of a device—which is recommended for infected AUS devices.

CLINICS CARE POINTS

- Imaging, such as MRI, can be a useful tool when diagnosing PP infections.[21]

- A salvage procedure should be attempted in the majority of patients presenting with a PP infection as it has a reported success rate of up to 93% and reduces penile length loss.[2,33]

- An MPP should be the prosthetic of choice during salvage procedures.[2]

- Consider using vancomycin, piperacillin–tazobactam, and amphotericin B as the antibiotic washout solution of choice during the "Mulcahy protocol" for PP salvage.[32]

- Consider using agents other than just gentamicin and vancomycin as the preoperative antibiotics of choice during prosthetic cases, as these have been associated with a 2.7 times higher risk of infection after index cases.[45]

- Consider adding antifungal coverage as a preoperative agent, during index cases, to prevent PP infection.[45]

- Biofilms likely undergo a dysbiotic shift allowing for the transition from a colonized asymptomatic prosthetic to an infected prosthetic requiring explantation.[62]

- Simultaneous implantation of an AUS and IPP is safe and feasible in the appropriate patient population.[64]

DISCLOSURES

A.S. Cheema, M.K. Patel, and A.M. El-Arabi have nothing to disclose. C.M. Gonzalez: Aurasense: Investment Interest; Cook Medical: Consultant/Advisor.

REFERENCES

1. Aytaç Mckinlay. Krane. The likely worldwide increase in erectile dysfunction between 1995 and 2025 and some possible policy consequences. BJU Int 1999;84(1):50–6.
2. Gross MS, Phillips EA, Balen A, et al. The malleable implant salvage technique: infection outcomes after Mulcahy salvage procedure and replacement of infected inflatable penile prosthesis with malleable prosthesis. J Urol 2016;195(3):694–7.
3. Darouiche RO. Treatment of infections associated with surgical implants. N Engl J Med 2004;350(14):1422–9.
4. Wilson SK, Delk JR, Salem EA, et al. Long-term survival of inflatable penile prostheses: single surgical group experience with 2,384 first-time implants spanning two decades. J Sex Med 2007;4(4_Part_1):1074–9.
5. Narang GL, Figler BD, Coward RM. Preoperative counseling and expectation management for inflatable penile prosthesis implantation. Transl Androl Urol 2017;6(Suppl 5):S869.
6. Carvajal A, Benavides J, García-Perdomo HA, et al. Risk factors associated with penile prosthesis infection: systematic review and meta-analysis. Int J Impot Res 2020;32(6):587–97.
7. Habous M, Tal R, Tealab A, et al. Defining a glycated haemoglobin (HbA1c) level that predicts increased risk of penile implant infection. BJU Int 2018;121(2):293–300.
8. Bishop JR, Moul JW, Sihelnik SA, et al. Use of glycosylated hemoglobin to identify diabetics at high risk for penile periprosthetic infections. J Urol 1992;147(2):386–8.
9. Montgomery BD, Lomas DJ, Ziegelmann MJ, et al. Infection risk of undergoing multiple penile prostheses: an analysis of referred patient surgical histories. Int J Impot Res 2018;30(4):147–52.
10. Hebert KJ, Kohler TS. Penile prosthesis infection: myths and realities. World J Mens Health 2019;37(3):276–87.
11. Wilson SK, Carson CC, Cleves MA, et al. Quantifying risk of penile prosthesis infection with elevated glycosylated hemoglobin. J Urol 1998;159(5):1537–40.
12. Canguven O, Talib R, El Ansari W, et al. Is Hba1c level of diabetic patients associated with penile prosthesis implantation infections? Aging Male 2019;22(1):28–33.
13. Osman MM, Huynh LM, El-Khatib FM, et al. Immediate preoperative blood glucose and hemoglobin a1c levels are not predictive of postoperative infections in diabetic men undergoing penile prosthesis placement. Int J Impot Res 2021;33(3):296–302.
14. Li K, Brandes ER, Chang SL, et al. Trends in penile prosthesis implantation and analysis of predictive factors for removal. World J Urol 2019;37:639–46.
15. Swanton AR, Munarriz RM, Gross MS. Updates in penile prosthesis infections. Asian J Androl 2020;22(1):28.
16. Wilson SK, Delk JR. Inflatable penile implant infection: predisposing factors and treatment suggestions. J Urol 1995;153(3):659–61.
17. Hofer MD, Gonzalez CM. Current concepts in infections associated with penile prostheses and artificial sphincters. Urologic Clinics 2015;42(4):485–92.

18. Weinberg AC, Pagano MJ, Deibert CM, et al. Sub-coronal inflatable penile prosthesis placement with modified no-touch technique: a step-by-step approach with outcomes. J Sex Med 2016;13(2): 270–6.

19. Onyeji IC, Sui W, Pagano MJ, et al. Impact of surgeon case volume on reoperation rates after inflatable penile prosthesis surgery. J Urol 2017;197(1): 223–9.

20. CARSON CC, MULCAHY JJ, GOVIER FE, et al. Efficacy, safety and patient satisfaction outcomes of the AMS 700CX inflatable penile prosthesis: results of a long-term multicenter study. J Urol 2000;164(2): 376–80.

21. Ramanathan S, Bertolotto M, Shamsodini A, et al. Comprehensive multimodality imaging review of complications of penile prostheses. Am J Roentgenol 2018;1200–7.

22. Fishman IJ, Scott FB, Selim AM. Rescue procedure: an alternative to complete removal for treatment of infected penile prosthesis. J Urol 1987;137(6):202A.

23. Al-Shaiji TF, Yaiesh SM, Al-Terki AE, et al. Infected penile prosthesis: literature review highlighting the status quo of prevention and management. Aging Male 2020;23(5):447–56.

24. Henry GD, Karpman E, Brant W, et al. The who, how and what of real-world penile implantation in 2015: the PROPPER registry baseline data. J Urol 2016; 195(2):427–33.

25. Bozkurt IH, Arslan B, Yonguç T, et al. Patient and partner outcome of inflatable and semi-rigid penile prosthesis in a single institution. Int Braz J Urol 2015;41:535–41.

26. Earle CM, Watters GR, Tulloch AG, et al. Complications associated with penile implants used to treat impotence. Aust N Z J Surg 1989;59(12): 959–62.

27. Altunkol A, Erçil H, Şener NC, et al. Clinical evaluation of outcomes of penile prosthesis implantation and partner satisfaction. Correspondance; 2014.

28. Mahon J, Dornbier R, Wegrzyn G, et al. Infectious adverse events following the placement of a penile prosthesis: a systematic review. Sexual medicine reviews 2020;8(2):348–54.

29. Caire A, Boonjindasup A, Hellstrom W. Does a replacement or revision of an inflatable penile prosthesis lead to decreased patient satisfaction? Int J Impot Res 2011;23(2):39–42.

30. Mulcahy JJ. Long-term experience with salvage of infected penile implants. J Urol 2000;163(2):481–2.

31. Mulcahy JJ, Köhler TS, Wen L, et al. Penile implant infection prevention part II: device coatings have changed the game. Int J Impot Res 2021;33(8): 801–7.

32. Gross MS, Phillips EA, Carrasquillo RJ, et al. Multicenter investigation of the micro-organisms involved in penile prosthesis infection: an analysis of the efficacy

33. Lopategui DM, Balise RR, Bouzoubaa LA, et al. The impact of immediate salvage surgery on corporeal length preservation in patients presenting with penile implant infections. J Urol 2018;200(1):171–6.

34. Wilson SK, Gross MS. Biofilm and penile prosthesis infections in the era of coated implants: 2021 update. Int J Impot Res 2022;34(5):411–5.

35. Arciola CR, Campoccia D, Montanaro L. Implant infections: adhesion, biofilm formation and immune evasion. Nat Rev Microbiol 2018;16(7):397–409.

36. Costerton JW, Stewart PS, Greenberg EP. Bacterial biofilms: a common cause of persistent infections. Science 1999;284(5418):1318–22.

37. Vickery K, Hu H, Jacombs AS, et al. A review of bacterial biofilms and their role in device-associated infection. Healthc Infect 2013;18(2):61–6.

38. Henry GD, Wilson SK, Delk JR, et al. Penile prosthesis cultures during revision surgery: a multicenter study. J Urol 2004;172(1):153–6.

39. Flemming H-C, Wingender J, Szewzyk U, et al. Biofilms: an emergent form of bacterial life. Nat Rev Microbiol 2016;14(9):563–75.

40. Jefferson KK. What drives bacteria to produce a biofilm? FEMS Microbiol Lett 2004;236(2):163–73.

41. Nehra A, Carson IIICC, Chapin AK, et al. Long-term infection outcomes of 3-piece antibiotic impregnated penile prostheses used in replacement implant surgery. J Urol 2012;188(3):899–903.

42. Serefoglu EC, Mandava SH, Gokce A, et al. Long-term revision rate due to infection in hydrophilic-coated inflatable penile prostheses: 11-year follow-up. J Sex Med 2012;9(8):2182–6.

43. Eid JF, Wilson SK, Cleves M, et al. Coated implants and "no touch" surgical technique decreases risk of infection in inflatable penile prosthesis implantation to 0.46. Urology 2012;79(6):1310–6.

44. Wolf JS, Bennett CJ, Dmochowski RR, et al. Best practice policy statement on urologic surgery antimicrobial prophylaxis. J Urol 2008;179(4):1379–90.

45. Barham DW, Pyrgidis N, Gross MS, et al. AUA-recommended antibiotic prophylaxis for primary penile implantation results in a higher, not lower, risk for postoperative infection: a multicenter analysis. J Urol 2023;209(2):399–409.

46. Olds C, Spataro E, Li K, et al. Postoperative antibiotic use among patients undergoing functional facial plastic and reconstructive surgery. JAMA facial plastic surgery 2019;21(6):491–7.

47. Dropkin BM, Chisholm LP, Dallmer JD, et al. Penile prosthesis insertion in the era of antibiotic stewardship—are postoperative antibiotics necessary? J Urol 2020;203(3):611–4.

48. Kavoussi NL, Viers BR, Pagilara TJ, et al. Are urine cultures necessary prior to urologic prosthetic surgery? Sexual Medicine Reviews 2018;6(1):157–61.

of the AUA and EAU guidelines for penile prosthesis prophylaxis. J Sex Med 2017;14(3):455–63.

49. Yeung LL, Grewal S, Bullock A, et al. A comparison of chlorhexidine-alcohol versus povidone-iodine for eliminating skin flora before genitourinary prosthetic surgery: a randomized controlled trial. J Urol 2013; 189(1):136–40.

50. Berthelot P, Grattard F, Cazorla C, et al. Is nasal carriage of Staphylococcus aureus the main acquisition pathway for surgical-site infection in orthopaedic surgery? Eur J Clin Microbiol Infect Dis 2010;29(4): 373–82.

51. Bode LG, Kluytmans JA, Wertheim HF, et al. Preventing surgical-site infections in nasal carriers of Staphylococcus aureus. N Engl J Med 2010; 362(1):9–17.

52. Ziegelmann MJ, Hebert KJ, Linder BJ, et al. The "Minimal-Touch" Technique for Artificial Urinary Sphincter Placement: Description and Outcomes. Turkish Journal of Urology 2023;49(1):40.

53. Khouri RK, Ortiz NM, Dropkin BM, et al. Artificial urinary sphincter complications: risk factors, workup, and clinical approach. Curr Urol Rep 2021;22:1–12.

54. Maurer V, Marks P, Dahlem R, et al. Prospective analysis of artificial urinary sphincter AMS 800 implantation after buccal mucosa graft urethroplasty. World J Urol 2019;37:647–53.

55. Fuller TW, Ballon-Landa E, Gallo K, et al. Outcomes and risk factors of revision and replacement artificial urinary sphincter implantation in radiated and nonradiated cases. J Urol 2020;204(1):110–4.

56. Brant WO, Martins FE. Artificial urinary sphincter. Transl Androl Urol 2017;6(4):682.

57. Rozanski AT, Tausch TJ, Ramirez D, et al. Immediate urethral repair during explantation prevents stricture formation after artificial urinary sphincter cuff erosion. J Urol 2014;192(2):442–6.

58. Gross MS, Broghammer JA, Kaufman MR, et al. Urethral stricture outcomes after artificial urinary sphincter cuff erosion: results from a multicenter retrospective analysis. Urology 2017;104:198–203.

59. Linder BJ, de Cogain M, Elliott DS. Long-term device outcomes of artificial urinary sphincter reimplantation following prior explantation for erosion or infection. J Urol 2014;191(3):734–8.

60. Altarac S, Katušin D, Crnica S, et al. Fournier's gangrene: etiology and outcome analysis of 41 patients. Urol Int 2012;88(3):289–93.

61. Leong JY, Ancira J, Bulafka J, et al. Characterizing the biofilm of artificial urinary sphincters (AUS). Transl Androl Urol 2023;12(5):866.

62. Werneburg GT, Hettel D, Adler A, et al. Biofilms on indwelling artificial urinary sphincter devices harbor complex microbe–metabolite interaction networks and reconstitute differentially in vitro by material type. Biomedicines 2023;11(1):215.

63. Hüsch T, Kretschmer A, Thomsen F, et al. Antibiotic coating of the artificial urinary sphincter (AMS 800): is it worthwhile? Urology 2017;103:179–84.

64. Boysen WR, Cohen AJ, Kuchta K, et al. Combined placement of artificial urinary sphincter and inflatable penile prosthesis does not increase risk of perioperative complications or impact long-term device survival. Urology 2019;124:264–70.

Sexually Transmitted Infections in Transgender and Gender-Diverse Individuals
Review of Screening and Treatment Recommendations

Kristy Borawski, MD[a],*, Sherry S. Ross, MD[b]

KEYWORDS

- Transgender • Gender diverse • Sexually transmitted infections • Guidelines

KEY POINTS

- Transgender and gender-diverse individuals, especially transgender women, experience disproportionately high rates of sexually transmitted infections (STIs).
- Transgender and gender-diverse individuals continue to face barriers within the health care system. It is imperative that we as clinicians ensure that we are creating a safe, welcoming, inclusive environment in which transgender and gender-diverse individuals will feel comfortable seeking and receiving care.
- Screening for STIs should be based on the individual's anatomy and sexual practices.
- Pre-exposure and postexposure prophylaxis are important tools that should be routinely discussed in patients at risk for STIs.

INTRODUCTION

In a 2023 Gallup survey, 7.6% of US adults now identify as lesbian, gay, bisexual, transgender, queer, or some other sexual orientation (LGBTQ+), up from 5.6% 4 years prior.[1] Approximately 1 in 8 LGBTQ + adults identify as transgender with an increased incidence seen among "generation Z" individuals (those born between 1997 and 2003).[1,2] Coinciding with an increasing number of people who identify as transgender or gender diverse (TGD) is the continued barriers that TGD people face in accessing essential health care services.[3,4] Some of these barriers are denial of health services, mistreatment by clinicians and health providers' discomfort or inexperience with treating TGD individuals.[4] Nearly one-third of TGD individuals reported experiencing negative behaviors from clinicians including harassment or being denied care.[5] This can lead to delayed diagnosis of many health conditions with resultant morbidity and mortality.[4]

More than 2.5 million cases of chlamydia, gonorrhea, and syphilis were reported in the United States in 2022.[6] Transgender and gender-diverse individuals experience disproportionately high rates of sexually transmitted infections (STIs).[7,8] Transgender women (TGW) have significantly higher rates of human immunodeficiency virus (HIV) and STIs compared to transgender men and other gender-diverse individuals. For example, TGW have an almost 42 fold increase in the prevalence of HIV (14%) compared to national rates (0.3%).[9] Some report HIV rates as high as 39.5%

[a] Department of Urology, University of North Carolina School of Medicine, 170 Manning Drive, Campus Box 7235, Chapel Hill, NC 27599, USA; [b] Department of Urology, University of North Carolina Chapel Hill School of Medicine, 170 Manning Drive Campus Box 7235, Chapel Hill, NC 27599, USA
* Corresponding author.
E-mail address: Kristy_borawski@med.unc.edu

Urol Clin N Am 51 (2024) 517–524
https://doi.org/10.1016/j.ucl.2024.07.015
0094-0143/24/© 2024 Elsevier Inc. All rights are reserved, including those for text and data mining, AI training, and similar technologies.

in TGW.[10] Compared to HIV, bacterial STIs such as *Chlamydia trachomatis and Neisseria gonorrhoeae* are not well studied. A 2019 study involving 6 sites from the Sexually Transmitted Disease Surveillance Network found a higher prevalence of extragenital infections (15% rectal and 7% pharyngeal chlamydia infections, 12% rectal and 9% gonorrhea infections) compared to urogenital infections (1% chlamydia and 4% gonorrhea). Despite this, transgender men and TGW received less frequent extragenital testing (48% and 62%, respectively) compared with urogenital testing (83% and 78%).[10]

SCREENING FOR SEXUALLY TRANSMITTED INFECTIONS

The Centers for Disease Control and Prevention (CDC) recommends using the "Five P's" approach to obtaining a sexual history to assist in determining the needs for STI screening. The "Five P's" include questions about *partners, practices, protection from STIs, past history of STIs, and pregnancy intentions.*[11]

STI prevention includes an assessment of both behavioral and biologic risk in a way that is inclusive to all gender identities. To do so requires referencing genitalia and providers should start by identifying which terms are preferred by the patient.[4] A good practice is to mirror the language that the patient uses to describe his/her/their identities and his/her/their body.[3] Although prior CDC STI Treatment Guidelines recommended screening transgender and gender-diverse patients based on current anatomy and sexual behaviors, the 2021 guidelines have more site-specific recommendations given the higher incidence of extragenital infections.[8,11,12] To do so, a clear understanding is needed of the patient's anatomy and sexual behaviors. The Sexual Health Clinic in Seattle, Washington, implemented a trans-inclusive questionnaire about sexual behavior, anatomy, gender-affirming surgeries, and STI symptoms. **Table 1** highlights portions of that questionnaire.[8]

The following details the CDC screening recommendations for transgender and gender-diverse individuals[11]:

- Providers should remain aware of the symptoms of common STIs and screen for asymptomatic infections on the basis of the patient's sexual practices and anatomy.
- Annual gender-based screening recommendations for *C trachomatis* and *N gonorrhoeae)* should be adapted on the basis of anatomy.
  - All sexually active female individuals aged less than 25 years.

- Transgender men and nonbinary persons with a cervix.
- HIV screening should be discussed and offered to all transgender individuals with the frequency dictated by the level of risk.
- Transgender individuals with HIV infections who have sex with cisgender men and TGW should be screened for STIs at least annually. This includes syphilis serology, hepatitis C virus testing, and urogenital and extragenital nucleic acid amplification test (NAAT) for gonorrhea and chlamydia.
- TGW who have had vaginoplasty sites should have routine STI screening for all exposed sites.
- For transgender men with a history of metoidioplasty surgery with urethral lengthening and have not had a vaginectomy, screening for genital STIs should include a cervical swab. A urine sample will not be sufficient.
- Cervical cancer screening should follow current guidelines for all transgender and gender-diverse patients with a cervix.

EXAMINATION OF THE TRANSGENDER AND GENDER-DIVERSE PATIENT

Having decided to proceed with STI testing either because of a screening recommendation as earlier and/or symptoms, the samples need to be collected. Many transgender individuals have experienced sexual violence, and it is therefore imperative that the provider should take a chaperone trauma-informed approach to any physical examination.[13] Trauma-informed examinations are performed "with" the patients to ensure that they retain control and feel safe. This includes using gender-neutral language as previously discussed and thoroughly explaining what to expect before, during, and after any examination. Patients can choose to have support persons present or they may prefer to collect samples themselves. It is recommended that health care professionals leave the room while the patient undresses and ensure that the patient's body remains covered as much as possible during the examination. Patients who decline an examination should be offered self-testing.[14]

SEXUALLY TRANSMITTED INFECTIONS ASSOCIATED WITH URETHRITIS, PROCTITIS, CERVICITIS, AND PHARYNGITIS
Gonorrhea and Chlamydia

In a 2019 study, the rates of chlamydia and gonorrhea infections were observed in 6 US cities as part of the Sexually Transmitted Disease Surveillance

Table 1 Trans-inclusive sexual health questionnaire		
Current Anatomy	So that we may best serve you today, please tell us about your current anatomy. Which of the following do you have (select all that apply)	• Vagina/front hole • Cervix • Uterus • Ovaries/adnexa • Penis/phallus • Testes/scrotum • Prostate • I prefer to discuss my anatomy with my clinician
History of Gender-affirming Genital Surgeries	Some surgical procedures impact which STDs a person can get. Have you had any of the following? (select all that apply)	• I had a hysterectomy • I had an oophorectomy • I had a vaginectomy • I had a penectomy • I had an orchiectomy • I had a vaginoplasty via penile inversion • I had a vaginoplasty via colonic graft • I had a metoidioplasty • I had a phalloplasty • I had a scrotoplasty • Not listed, please specify _____ • None
Sexual Behavior	Please note that we know individuals use various terminologies for the body parts and the type of sex they have. In order to be approachable to everyone, we are using clinical terminology. What kinds of sex have you had in the past 12 months? (select all that apply)	• Receive oral sex (partner's mouth on my genitals • Given oral sex (my mouth on partner's genitals) • Oral–anal sex (my mouth on partner's anus/butt • Anal–oral sex (partner's mouth on my anus/butt) • Receptive anal sex (partner's penis in my anus/butt • Insertive anal sex (my penis in partner's anus/butt) • Receptive vaginal/front hole sex (my partner's penis in my vagina/front hole)

Adapted from Tordoff DM, et al. Trans-Inclusive Sexual Health Questionnaire to Improve HIV/STI Care for Transgender Patients: Anatomic-site Specific STI Prevalence and Screening Rates. 2023, Clin Inf Dis 76:e736 to 743.

Network. During a 3.5 year observation period, 12.6% of TGW and 10.5% of transgender men tested positive for gonorrhea at one or more anatomic sites. Thirteen percent of TGW and 7.7% of transgender men tested positive for chlamydia. Over 80% of TGW with positive extragenital gonorrhea or chlamydial infections had a negative urogenital test. Twenty-eight percent of transgender men had a positive extragenital infection despite a negative urogenital test.[10]

Symptoms of gonorrhea and chlamydia

Typical symptoms include urethral discharge, dysuria, urethral stinging/itching, and penile tip irritation; however, urethritis is often asymptomatic.[15,16] TGW with a neovagina can present with vaginal pain and bleeding with sexual activity. For extragenital sites, symptoms can include itchy or sore throat, difficulty swallowing, increased rectal discharge, anal itching, pain with bowel movements, and rectal bleeding.[11]

Screening

When screening for urethritis, health care providers should screen based on current anatomy and sexual function as discussed earlier. Per the 2021 CDC STI Guidelines, the following are diagnostic for a diagnosis of urethritis: mucoid, mucopurulent, or purulent discharge on examination; Gram stain of urethral secretions demonstrating 2 or more WBCs per oil immersion field; positive leukocyte esterase from a first-void urine, or 10 or more WBCs per high-pass filter from a first-void urine. In most instances, however, clinicians will utilize NAATs for gonorrhea and chlamydia. Because rates of extragenital chlamydia and gonorrhea infections are higher than genital infections in transgender men and TGW, it is imperative to collect samples from all possible sites involved in sexual activity (ie, genital, anal, oropharynx)[10,11]

Gonorrhea treatment and follow-up

Treatment guidelines do not differ for transgender patients. The CDC recommends treating gonococcal infections with ceftriaxone 500 mg intramuscular (IM) in a single dose for persons weighing less than 150 kg (1000 mg IM if >150 kg). If ceftriaxone is not available, alternative regimens are gentamicin 240 mg IM in a single dose, *PLUS* azithromycin 2 g orally in a single dose, *or* cefixime 800 mg orally in a single dose. If chlamydia has not been ruled out, doxycycline 100 mg twice daily for 7 days should be added.[11] Failure rates of non-ceftriaxone regiments for extragenital infections can be substantial, and as such, in the absence of an IgE-mediated penicillin allergy (ie, anaphylaxis or urticaria) within the preceding 10 years, CDC guidelines state that the use of third-generation and fourth-generation cephalosporins is safe.[11,16]

Individuals who test positive for gonorrhea should abstain from sexual activity for 7 days and notify all partners within the preceding 60 days. All individuals who have tested positive for gonorrhea regardless of the site should undergo routine STI screening including chlamydia, syphilis, and HIV. Genital gonorrhea infections do not require a test of cure, but all extragenital infections should have a test of cure done following treatment. All individuals should have a retest in 3 months due to high rates of recurrence.[11]

Chlamydia treatment and follow-up

As with gonorrhea, treatment guidelines do not differ for transgender patients. The recommended treatment is doxycycline 100 mg orally twice daily for 7 days. Alternative regimens include azithromycin 1 g orally in a single dose *or* azithromycin 500 mg orally in a single dose followed by 250 mg orally daily for 4 days. Concurrent treatment of gonorrhea should be considered. All patients who test positive for chlamydia should receive complete STI screening including testing for gonorrhea, syphilis, and HIV. All individuals with a chlamydial STI should refrain from sexual activity for 7 days and notify any partner from the preceding 60 days. A 3 month follow-up test is recommended although, unlike gonorrhea, a test of cure for extragenital chlamydial STIs is not recommended.[11]

Mycoplasma genitalium

Mycoplasma genitalium can cause symptomatic and asymptomatic urethritis, cervicitis and proctitis. It accounts for approximately 40% of recurrent urethritis cases. Although pharyngeal infections have been documented, currently there are no documented symptomatic oropharyngeal cases attributed to an *M genitalium* infection.[17] *M genitalium* is thought to facilitate HIV transmission through mucosal disruption, recruitment of HIV susceptible cells to the mucosal service, and direct enhancement of HIV replication.[17] Currently, there is a Food and Drug Administration (FDA)-approved NAAT for *M genitalium* although it is not recommended for use in routine STI screening. Consideration should be given to *M genitalium* screening for cases of recurrent urethritis, cervicitis, or proctitis.[11,18]

Treatment of *M genitalium* is similar to chlamydia; doxycycline 100 mg orally twice daily for 7 days. Alternative regimens include azithromycin 1 g orally in a single dose *or* azithromycin 500 mg orally in a single dose followed by 250 mg orally daily for 4 days.[11,16] Given resistance patterns, especially in Europe, the European guidelines recommend screening for macrolide resistance in those with a positive test for *M genitalium*.[19] All patients who test positive for *M genitalium* should be screened for other STIs, refrain from sexual activity until symptoms resolve, and notify all partners within the preceding 60 days.[11]

Trichomoniasis

Although trichomoniasis is the most common nonviral STI worldwide, very little is known about its prevalence in transgender and gender-diverse individuals.[7] Trichomoniasis is associated with a 1.5 fold increased risk of acquiring HIV, and as such, detection and treatment are important.[11] There is no testing available for the diagnosis of extragenital trichomoniasis nor is rectal or oral testing recommended. Current guidelines recommend testing with either NAAT or wet prep (NAAT is preferred) in cisgender women with vaginal discharge or as a screening tool in those with a high risk for infection. Given this, it could be extrapolated that the same recommendation applies to transgender men with a cervix and either symptoms or are at a high risk for infection. Current treatment recommendations are one dose of metronidazole 2 g orally or a single dose of tinidazole 2 g orally.[11]

Syphilis

Syphilis is a systemic disease caused by *Treponema pallidum,* a coiled spiral spirochete bacterium, and is classified as acquired or congenital.[16] The CDC 2022 Sexually Transmitted Infections Surveillance Report highlighted an 80% increase in syphilis cases in the past 5 years. Cases of primary and secondary syphilis increased 10% in 2022; a particularly alarming trend given that these are the most contagious stages of syphilis. Congenital syphilis cases have risen 937% in the past decade with resultant 282 stillbirths attributed to congenital syphilis in 2022.[20] Racial, ethnic, sexual, and gender minorities continue to be disproportionately impacted.[2,20] In a systematic review of the prevalence of STIs in transgender persons, the prevalence of syphilis in TGW ranged from 1.4% to 50.4% and 0% to 4.2% in transgender men.[7] In a recent longitudinal study of young sexual and gender minority adults assigned male at birth, transgender participants had higher lifetime syphilis prevalence (45.3%) than cisgender participants (24.4%).[21]

Symptoms of syphilis

Primary syphilis is hallmarked by the development of a chancre, usually painless, single, and indurated ulcer with a clean base discharging clear serum. Without intervention, this typically resolves within 3 to 8 weeks. *Secondary syphilis* is characterized by a maculopapular rash involving the palms of the hands, soles of the feet, and mucous membrane lesions involving the vagina or anus. *Latent syphilis* (divided into early and late) is defined by the lack of symptoms. *Tertiary syphilis* develops in approximately 35% of those with latent syphilis and is characterized by neurologic, cardiologic, and gummous syphilis.[11,16]

Screening for syphilis

All patients with symptoms or those who have a positive screening indication should be tested for syphilis. Although cultures for *T pallidum* are available, they are cumbersome and not widely used. A diagnosis of syphilis requires the use of 2 tests: a nontreponemal test (NTT) and a treponemal test (TT). All patients with a reactive NTT (most commonly venereal disease research laboratory [VDRL] or rapid plasma reagin) must have a confirmatory TT performed.[11,16,22] TTs detect treponemal antibiotics via various methods (FTA-ABS, TP-PA, EIAs). Although false-positive TTs are rare, they can occur in patients with collagen disease, lupus, and other infections.[11,16,23] Notably, however, once positive, a TT will likely remain positive lifelong.[11]

As with other STIs, all patients testing positive for primary and secondary syphilis should be screened for other STIs. Given the significantly increased risk of HIV in patients with syphilis, all those patients who have tested negative for HIV should be offered HIV pre-exposure prophylaxis (PrEP).[11,24]

Syphilis treatment and follow-up

Guidelines for syphilis treatment do not differ for TGD individuals. Treatment recommendation for primary, secondary, and early latent syphilis is benzathine penicillin G 2.4 million units given in one IM dose. Late latent syphilis should be treated with 2.4 million units of benzathine penicillin G intramuscularly weekly for 3 consecutive weeks.[11,25] Due to increased demand, there was a significant drug shortage starting in 2023. Per the most recent CDC update, the supply of Benzathine penicillin G is improving and was hoped to be readily available by June 2024.[26] In follow-up, clinical and laboratory testing should be done at 6 and 12 months and, for those with latent syphilis, at 24 months.[11]

HUMAN IMMUNODEFICIENCY VIRUS

Transgender individuals accounted for 2% (671) of the 36,801 new HIV diagnoses in the United States in 2019[6] Race and gender-based differences in HIV prevalence have been widely reported.[27] Ninety-three percent of those transgender individuals diagnosed with HIV in 2019 were TGW. Of those 625 cases among TGW, 46% were in Black/African Americans, 35% in Hispanic/Latino, and 13% in White TGW.[6] In a recent HIV and Transgender Communities Issue Brief, the CDC reported that data from a meta-analysis of studies from 2006 to 2017 that demonstrated laboratory-confirmed HIV prevalence were 14.1% for TGW and 3.2% for transgender men.[28] In a 2021 report of the National HIV Behavioral Surveillance, 40% of TGW had HIV with continued significant racial and ethnic differences (86% of Black TGW had HIV compared to 35% of Hispanic/Latina TGW and 17% of White TGW).[29] Given this epidemic in transgender patients, the CDC is actively partnering with public, federal, and community agencies to address the HIV epidemic in transgender individuals with a focus on HIV testing, linkage to care, and prevention services.[28]

Symptoms with Human Immunodeficiency Virus

HIV is often asymptomatic in its early stages (1–2) and typically only manifests as one progresses to stage 3 (acquired immune deficiency syndrome [AIDS]) that is diagnosed when the CD4 count is less than 200 cells/mm^3 or if the patient acquires an AIDS-defining condition.[11] HIV/AIDS can manifest in any organ system, the details of which are beyond the scope of this review.

Screening for Human Immunodeficiency Virus

As mentioned in a previous section, HIV screening should be discussed and offered to all transgender individuals with the frequency dictated by the level of risk. Individuals who test positive for another STI should have HIV testing offered. Additionally, transgender individuals with HIV infections who have sex with cisgender men and TGW should be screened for STIs at least annually.[11] The CDC recommends that HIV testing begins with a laboratory-based HIV-1/HIV-2 Ag/Ab combination assay, and if positive, it is followed by a laboratory-based assay with a supplemental HIV-1/HIV-2 antibody differentiation assay. Point-of-care HIV testing is available with results in less than 20 minutes but they may give a false negative in those with an acute HIV (ie, early) infection.[11]

Treatment Recommendations for Human Immunodeficiency Virus in Transgender Individuals

Treatment recommendations and considerations for transgender individuals are summarized in **Box 1**[30]

PREVENTION OF SEXUALLY TRANSMITTED INFECTIONS
Pre-exposure Prophylaxis

Human immunodeficiency virus
PrEP is one of the most effective ways of HIV prevention.[31] PrEP should be discussed with all sexually active adults and adolescents and strongly encouraged in those with sexual behaviors that place them at increased risk including the diagnosis of an STI within the preceding 6 months. PrEP should be offered to TGW who have sex with men and who report sexual behaviors that place them at ongoing risk for HIV exposure.[11,32] Some studies have reported decreased adherence to PrEP recommendations compared to the MSM population given the unfounded belief that there may be negative interactions between PrEP and hormone treatment.[31] However, a recent review of PrEP prescriptions among United States commercially insured transgender men and TGW demonstrated a substantial increase in PrEP prescriptions from 2014 to 2021.[27]

Two oral options for adults and adolescents weighing greater than 35 kg include[11,33]

- Emtricitabine (F) 200 mg in combination with tenofovir disoproxil fumarate (TDF) 300 mg (F/TDF)
- Emtricitabine (F) 200 mg in combination with tenofovir alafenamide (TAF) 25 mg (F/TAF). *Note that F/TAF is not approved for those at increased risk of acquiring HIV through receptive vaginal sex.*

Recently, a randomized control trial compared emtricitabine (F) 200 mg in combination with TDF 300 mg (F/TDF) versus IM cabotegravir (CAB-LA)

Box 1
Recommendations for human immunodeficiency virus treatment of transgender patients

Panel's recommendations regarding transgender people with HIV

Panel's recommendations

- Antiretroviral therapy (ART) is recommended for all transgender people with HIV to improve their health and to reduce the risk of HIV transmission to sexual partners (AI).
- HIV care services should be provided within a gender-affirmative care model to reduce potential barriers to ART adherence and to maximize the likelihood of achieving sustained viral suppression (AII).
- Prior to ART initiation, a pregnancy test should be performed for transgender individuals of childbearing potential (AIII).
- Some antiretroviral drugs may have pharmacokinetic interactions with gender-affirming hormone therapy. Clinical effects and hormone levels should be routinely monitored with appropriate titrations of estradiol, testosterone, or androgen blockers, as needed (AIII).
- Gender-affirming hormone therapies are associated with hyperlipidemia, elevated cardiovascular risk, and osteopenia; therefore, clinicians should choose an ART regimen that will not increase the risk of these adverse effects (AIII).

Rating of recommendations: A = strong; B = moderate; C = weak

Rating of evidence: I = data from randomized controlled trials; II = data from well-designed nonrandomized trials or observational cohort studies with long-term clinical outcomes; III = expert opinion

(Box from U.S. Department of Health and Human Services Guidelines for the Use of Antiretrovirals in Adults and Adolescents with HIV. 2022.)

---

600 mg IM every 8 weeks in cisgender men who have sex with men and TGW. The authors noted that CAB was superior to emtricitabine in combination with TDF with a 66% reduction in new HIV diagnoses.[34] Routine HIV testing every 3 months is recommended for those taking oral PrEP and every 4 months for those on IM CAB.[11]

Postexposure Prophylaxis

Human immunodeficiency virus
The current guidelines recommend postexposure prophylaxis (PEP) within 72 hours after a potential

nonoccupational HIV exposure that has an increased risk of HIV transmission. nPEP involves a 4 week course of TDF 300 mg with emtricitabine 200 mg daily plus raltegravir 400 mg twice daily *or* dolutegravir 50 mg daily. HIV testing is recommended at 6 weeks, 3 months, and again at 6 months after exposure.[35]

Bacterial Sexually Transmitted Infections

Two separate large trials examined the utility of postexposure doxycycline in those with a bacterial STI in the preceding year. In the Intervention Preventive de l'Exposition aux Risques avec et pour les Gays, a 47% reduction in STI incidence was reported (70% relative reduction for syphilis and chlamydia but no reduction for gonorrhea).[36]

In a more recent study, TGW and men who have sex with men who were either on HIV PrEP or living with HIV who had a bacterial STI within the past year were randomized to either 30 mg delayed release doxycycline hyclate (Doxy-PEP) taken within 72 hours (ideally <24 hours) after any condomless anogenital, vaginal, or oral sex versus no intervention. Doxy-PEP taken decreased the incidence of gonorrhea, chlamydia, and early syphilis by two-thirds.[37]

SUMMARY

Transgender and gender-diverse individuals are at an increased risk for the development of an STI and it is of the utmost importance that screening and prevention strategies are used to combat this. To do so, we as clinicians need to ensure that we are creating a safe, welcoming, inclusive environment in which transgender and gender-diverse individuals will feel comfortable seeking and receiving care.

DISCLOSURES

The authors do not have any disclosures.

REFERENCES

1. Jones J. LGBTQ+ Identification in U.S. Now at 7.6. 2024. Available at: https://news.gallup.com/poll/611864/lgbtq-identification.aspx. [Accessed 29 June 2024].
2. Badash A, Grennan D, Albrecht J. Sexually transmitted disease and HIV in transgender patients. Clin in Derm 2024;42:180–91.
3. Ard KL, MacDonald-Ly A, Demidont AC. Sexual Health Care for Transgender and Gender Diverse People. Med Clin N Am 2024;108:393–402.
4. Wascher J, Hazra A, Fisher AR. Sexual Health for Transgender and Gender Diverse Individuals: Routine Examination, Sexually Transmitted Infection Screening and Prevention. Obstet Gynecol Clin N Am 2024;51:405–24.
5. Garcia AD, Lopez X. How Cisgender Clinicians Can Help Prevent Harm During Encounters with Transgender Patients. AMA J Ethics 2022;24:E573–761.
6. Centers for Disease Control and Prevention. Fast Facts: HIV and Transgender People. 2022. Available at: https://www.cdc.gov/hiv/data-research/facts-stats/transgender-people.html. [Accessed 29 June 2024].
7. Van Gerwen OT, Jani A, Long DM, et al. Prevalence of sexually transmitted infections and human immunodeficiency virus in transgendered persons: a systematic review. Transgender Heal 2020;5:90–103.
8. Tordoff DM, Dombrowski JC, Ramchandani MS, et al. Trans-Inclusive Sexual Health Questionnaire to Improve Human Immunodeficiency Virus/Sexually Transmitted Infection (STI) Care for Transgender Patients: Anatomic Site-Specific STI Prevalence and Screening. Clin Infect Dis 2023;76:736–43.
9. Brown EE, Patel EU, Poteat TC, et al. Prevalence of Sexually Transmitted Infections Among Transgender Women with and without HIC in the Eastern and Southern United States. J Infect Dis 2024;229:1614–27.
10. Pitasi MA, Kerani RP, Kohn R, et al. Chlamydia, Gonorrhea and Human Immunodeficiency virus infection amongst transgender women and transgender men attending clinics that provides sexually transmitted disease services in six U.S. cities: Results from the sexually transmitted disease surveillance network. Sex Transm Dis 2019;46:112–7.
11. Workowski KA, Bachmann LH, Chan PA, et al. Centers for Disease Control and Prevention: Sexually Transmitted Infections Treatment Guidelines, 2021. MMWR Rep 2021;74:1–192.
12. Workowski KA, Bolan GA. Centers for Disease Control and Prevention: Sexually transmitted diseases treatment guidelines, 2015. MMWR Recomm Rep (Morb Mortal Wkly Rep) 2015;64(RR–03):1–137.
13. Poteat T. Transgender people and sexually transmitted infections (STIs). Available at: https://transcare.ucsf.edu/guidelines/stis. [Accessed 30 June 2024].
14. Gorfinkel MD, Perlow E, Macdonald S. The trauma-informed genital and gynecologic examination. Can Med J 2021;193:E1090.
15. Moi H, Blee K, Horner PJ. Management of nongonococcal urethritis. BMC Infect Dis 2015;15:294.
16. Borawski KM. Sexually Transmitted Infections. In: Partin AW, Dmochowski RR, Kavoussi LR, editors. et al Campbell-Walsh-Wein Urology. 12th edition. Elsevier; 2020. p p1251–72.
17. Crowell TA, Lawlor J, Lombardi K, et al. Anorectal and Urogenital *Mycoplasma Genitalium* in Nigerian Men who have Sex with Men and Transgender Women: Prevalence, Incidence and Association with HIV. Sex Trans Dis 2020;47:202–6.

18. Centers for Disease Control and Prevention: Mycoplasma genitalis. 2021. Available at: https://www.cdc.gov/std/treatment-guidelines/mycoplasmagenitalium.html. [Accessed 30 June 2024].

19. Jensen JS, Cusini M, Gomberg M, et al. 2021 European guideline on *Mycoplasma genitalium* infections. J Eur Acad Dermatol Venereol 2022;36:641–50.

20. Centers for Disease Control and Prevention. Sexually transmitted infections surveillance 2024. Available at Sexually Transmitted Infections Surveillance, 2022 (cdc.gov). . [Accessed 27 June 2024].

21. Xavier Hall CD, Ryan D, Hayford C. Syphilis Prevention, Incidence and Demographic Differences in a Longitidinal Study of Young Sexual and Gender Minority Adults Assigned Male at Birth. J Infect Dis 2024;229:232–6.

22. Janier M, Hegyi V, Dupin N, et al. European guideline on the management of syphilis, 2014. J Eur Acad Dermatol Venereol 2014;28:1581–93.

23. Hart G. Syphilis tests in diagnostic and therapeutic decision making. Ann Intern Med 1986;104:368–76.

24. Chesson HW, Heffelfinger JD, Voigt RF, et al. Estimates of primary and secondary syphilis rates in persons with HIV in the United States. Sex Transm Dis 2005;32:265–9.

25. Tuddenham S, Hamill MM, Ghanem KG. Diagnosis and Treatment of Sexually Transmitted Infections: A Review. JAMA 2022;327:161–72.

26. Centers for Disease Control and Prevention. FDA announcement on the Availability of Extencilline. 2024. Available at: https://www.cdc.gov/sti/php/from-the-director/2024-01-16-bachmann-extencilline.html. [Accessed 30 June 2024].

27. Huang YL, Radix A, Zhu W, et al. HIV Testing and Pre-exposure Prophylaxis Prescriptions Among U.S. Commercially Insured Transgender Men and Women, 2014 to 2021. Ann Intern Med 2024;177:12–8.

28. Centers for Disease Control and Prevention. Issue Brief: HIV and Transgender Communities: Strengthening Prevention and Care. 2024. Available at: https://www.cdc.gov/hiv/policies/data/transgender-issue-brief.html. [Accessed 29 June 2024].

29. Centers for Disease Control and Prevention. HIV Prevention, Risk Prevention and Testing Behaviors Among Transgender Women – National HIV Behavioral Surveillance, 7 U.S. Cities 2019-2020, 2021, HIV Surveillance Special report. Available at: https://stacks.cdc.gov/view/cdc/105223. [Accessed 15 June 2024].

30. Gulick RM, Lane HC, et al. U.S. Department of Health and Human Services Guidelines for the Use of Antiretrovirals in Adults and Adolescents with HIV. 2022. Available at: https://clinicalinfo.hiv.gov/sites/default/files/guidelines/documents/adult-adolescent-arv/guidelines-adult-adolescent-arv.pdf. [Accessed 30 June 2024].

31. Kania Z, Mijas M, Grabski, et al. HIV pre-exposure prophylaxis (PrEP) for transgender and nonbinary persons. Literature review and guidelines for professionals. Psychiatr Pol 2023;27:1023–35.

32. Centers for Disease Control and Prevention. US Public Health Service: Preexposure prophylaxis for the prevention of HIV infection in the United States—2021 Update: a clinical practice guideline. 2021. Available at: https://www.cdc.gov/hiv/pdf/risk/prep/cdc-hiv-prep-guidelines-2021.pdf. [Accessed 30 June 2024].

33. Centers for Disease Control and Prevention. Clinical Guidelines for PrEP. 2024. Available at: https://www.cdc.gov/hivnexus/hcp/prep. [Accessed 29 June 2024].

34. Landovitz RJ, Donnell D, Clement ME, et al. Cabotegravir for HIV Prevention in Cisgender Men and Transgender Women. N Engl J Med 2021;385:595–608.

35. Centers for Disease Control and Prevention. Updated guidelines for antiretroviral postexposure prophylaxis after sexual, injection drug use, or other nonoccupational exposure to HIV—United States. 2016. Available at: https://www.cdc.gov/hiv/pdf/programresources/cdc-hiv-npep-guidelines.pdf. [Accessed 15 June 2024].

36. Molina JM, Charreau I, Chidiac C, et al. Post-exposure prophylaxis with doxycycline to prevent sexually transmitted infections in men who have sex with men: an open-label randomized substudy of the ANRS IPERGAY trial. Lancet Infect Dis 2018;18:308–17.

37. Luetkemeyer AF, Donnel D, Dombrowski JC, et al. Postexposure Doxycycline to Prevent Bacterial Sexually Transmitted Infections. N Engl J Med 2023;338:1296–306.

Manipulating the Gut Microbiome in Urinary Tract Infection-Prone Patients

Rahul Dutta, MD, Lynn Stothers, MD, MHSc, FRCSC,
A. Lenore Ackerman, MD, PhD*

KEYWORDS

- Fecal microbiota transplant • Probiotics • Cranberry • Short chain fatty acids
- Urinary tract infection • Gut dysbiosis • Microbiome

KEY POINTS

- Antibiotics play a crucial role in inducing gut dysbiosis; cumulative antibiotic burden may worsen both the systemic inflammatory and metabolic effects of perturbations in commensal microbial communities as well as enrich for uropathogenic bacteria bearing antimicrobial resistance genes.
- The effect of the gut microbiome on urinary tract infection (UTI) risk is likely mediated by (1) direct seeding of the urinary tract by uropathogenic bacteria and (2) an indirect effect of the complex interplay between the microbiota, their metabolic byproducts, and the host immune system, making nonantibiotic approaches to the management and prevention of UTI sorely needed.
- Although cranberry supplementation has been shown in multiple studies to be protective against UTI, evidence that this effect is mediated by the gut microbiome is limited. Additional dietary interventions to reverse gut dysbiosis have been proposed, but none have as-yet been evaluated in UTI or recurrent UTI.
- The evidence for the efficacy of gut microbiome manipulation via probiotic supplementation on UTI risk is conflicting and stronger in the pediatric literature than in the adult literature.
- While evidence is still far from conclusive, fecal microbiota transplantation appears to modify the gut microbiome, improving outcomes in UTI. While promising, this therapy warrants further investigation.

INTRODUCTION

Urinary tract infections (UTIs) are the most common outpatient infections in women; globally, over 400 million individuals experience UTIs each year.[1] While most infections are self-limited, as many as 40% of women with UTI will experience infection recurrences.[2,3] Recurrent UTIs (rUTIs), defined as 2 or more infections within a 6 month period or 3 or more infections in a 12 month period,[3] are an enormous financial burden on the health care system[4] and individually can be highly disruptive to a patient's health-related quality of life, workplace productivity, and psychosocial well-being.[5–7]

Risk factors for UTI are numerous and not fully understood, including anatomic abnormalities of the lower urinary tract, postmenopausal hormonal status, use of immunomodulatory medications, spermicide-based contraception, and vaginal intercourse.[8] Most women, however, do not have identifiable anatomic or functional risk factors for recurrent infections.[9,10] Instead, it is becoming increasingly clear that *exposure to antibiotics, often given to treat UTI itself, constitute a strong and independent risk factor for UTI recurrence.*

Division of Urogynecology and Reconstructive Pelvic Surgery, David Geffen School of Medicine at UCLA, Box 951738, Los Angeles, CA 90095-1738, USA
* Corresponding author.
E-mail address: AAckerman@mednet.ucla.edu

Urol Clin N Am 51 (2024) 525–536
https://doi.org/10.1016/j.ucl.2024.07.016

Antibiotics Remain the Gold Standard for Urinary Tract Infection Treatment

Oral antibiotic therapy is the mainstay for treatment, with the American Urological Association recommending nitrofurantoin, trimethoprim-sulfamethoxazole, or fosfomycin as first-line therapies for acute, uncomplicated UTI episodes.[11] UTI is one of the most common indications for outpatient antibiotic prescriptions, comprising approximately 20% of all antibiotic prescriptions.[12] When patients experience recurrences of these kinds of infections, numerous guidelines suggest a shift in management approach from intermittent antibiotic treatment of acute episodes to prevention approaches.[13,14] Numerous approaches are acceptable, such as postcoital antibiotics, vaginal estrogen, urinary antiseptics, or continuous, low-dose antibiotics, of which low-dose antibiotic prophylaxis is the most common approach. Each of these approaches can decrease UTI incidence[14] but can be associated with the development of antimicrobial resistance as well as other antibiotic-associated adverse events, such as *Clostridium difficile* colitis.[15] The majority of patients, however, is never transitioned to prophylactic therapy and can instead continue to receive multiple courses of antibiotics yearly and dozens of antibiotic courses over years.

The consequences of such high antibiotic burdens are not fully understood, but it is becoming more widely accepted that repeated antibiotics result in disturbances in the commensal microbial communities throughout the body, including the gut and genitourinary tract. These alterations are suspected to play a central role in UTI recurrence risk. In the time in which we have seen the rapid expansion in the use of antibiotics, particularly since the introduction of second-generation fluoroquinolones in the mid-1980s, the incidence of UTI has increased sharply, climbing more than 62%, from 252 million cases in 1990 to 404 million cases in 2019.[1,16] From 2000 to 2015, global antibiotic consumption also increased approximately 65%.[17]

Several studies have specifically noted sustained alterations in urinary microbial communities in patients after repeated antibiotic treatment of UTI that are associated with both chronic lower urinary tract symptoms and altered urinary tract inflammation.[18–20] In mice, antibiotic-mediated microbial depletion alters bladder transcriptional patterns and gross histologic structure.[21] These reports have suggested a theory that while a "healthy" commensal urinary microbiome ("urobiome") supports normal bladder homeostasis, alterations in genitourinary microbial communities that do not support normal bladder function, termed as *dysbiosis*, may disrupt lower urinary tract structure and function. Changes in the microbial communities of the urinary tract, however, do not occur in isolation. In each of these situations, the inciting event disturbing the urobiome is likely to have also had profound impacts on microbial communities throughout the body, including the gut microbiome, which comprises the largest microbial reservoir in humans.

Antibiotics Impact on the Gut Microbiome

In 1941, the Lancet detailed the case of a 6 year old boy whose UTI had progressed to sepsis who made a miraculous recovery following administration of penicillin. At the time, this miraculous drug spawned hope that researchers had discovered a "magic bullet" with the potential to end infectious causes of mortality and leave the humans it was used to treat unaltered.[22] Indeed, these first reports of antibiotic use document "no toxic effects attributable to therapeutic penicillin."[23] With the introduction of additional antibiotic classes and the recognition of their seemingly boundless potential to manage bacterial infections, we have seen an explosion of widespread use in humans, farm animals, and even crops. Only recently, however, have we begun to understand the potential consequences, both societally and at an individual level, of this overexposure to antimicrobials.

In the immediate term, antimicrobials rapidly diminish the commensal microbiome, creating space into which more pathogenic organisms can expand. Accumulating antimicrobial burden also facilitates the emergence of multidrug-resistant microorganisms (MDRO), which can necessitate the use of more potent, broad-spectrum antibiotics for acute infections. This escalating cycle of antibiotic use only further exacerbates the damage to these endogenous communities in the gut. A single course of antibiotics, particularly the more broad-spectrum agents, can rapidly alter the gut microbial composition, decreasing the overall abundance of gut bacteria by as much as 30% and reducing both the evenness and richness of these communities.[24,25] The microbiota may recover after a single course, but the initial state is often not totally recovered, with several specific taxa failing to reconstitute the gut microbiome after periods as long as 6 months.[25,26] With repeated antibiotic courses, changes can persist more than a year after repeat antibiotics and also result in logarithmic increases in gut fungal burden.[27,28]

The Impact of Gut Dysbiosis on Human Health

Antibiotic-induced, microbial alterations in the gut indirectly impact overall health in the long term.

Accumulating literature elucidates connections between such disruptions in the gut microbiome and human disease both within and beyond the gastrointestinal tract, predisposing individuals to cardiovascular and metabolic conditions, neurologic disease,[29,30] psychiatric illness,[31] and autoimmunity.[32]

In animals, transient treatment with antibiotics rapidly induces systemic dysbiosis with notable physiologic perturbations that are best described in the gut,[33] leading to altered gut morphology, motility, permeability, secretion, and innervation.[33–39] Systemic immune function is also impaired, with alterations in the composition of T and B cells, impaired maturation of lymphoid follicles, and decreased expression of Toll-like receptors, which recognize microbial components.[40–44] Increased visceral hyperalgesia and systemic pain behaviors are also commonly observed in animals following antibiotic-induced dysbiosis.[45–47]

While such prospective studies are not possible in humans, observational studies have echoed the dramatic impact of antibiotics on the gut microbiota and its impact on overall health. Gut microbiota alterations result in an increased susceptibility to infections, particularly intestinal infections, which can derive from either newly acquired pathogens or the expansion of pathobiont organisms already present in the microbiota. Gut dysbiosis can also affect immune homeostasis, leading to systemic, long-term immunologic impairments.[48] Atopic, inflammatory, and autoimmune diseases (eg, asthma, Crohn's disease) have been linked to gut microbiota dysbiosis, an association that is even stronger following early life antibiotic exposures.[49] The gut microbiome also plays a crucial role in energy homeostasis and adiposity, with phylum-level changes resulting in significantly increased risks of obesity, diabetes, cardiovascular disease, and steatohepatitis.[50] Beyond these direct effects, antibiotics also alter gene expression, protein activity, and cellular metabolism in the gut, effects that can occur much more rapidly that the changes seen in gut microbial composition.[51] Given these profound and widespread effects of antibiotics, we will focus on the evidence implicating disturbances in the gut microbiome in UTI pathophysiology and explore the potential therapeutic options that arise from understanding the gut microbiome's role in urinary diseases and UTI.

Implication of the Gut Microbiome in Urinary Tract Infection Pathogenesis

As yet, there is not a clear understanding of the early molecular events involved in the progression of UTI. Several studies[52–54] support a more direct role for gut microbes in UTI pathogenesis. A leading theory is that direct physical seeding of the periurethral space with gut bacteria is the first step in the development of UTI, followed by the ascension of these microbes into the bladder up the urethra.[55] This theory is bolstered by the presence of the same uropathogen strains in the host gut and urine at the time of UTI.[52,56]

Several observational studies support the possibility that the gut may serve as a reservoir for uropathogenic bacteria, further implicating the gut microbiota in the pathogenesis of UTI.[52,53,57] In a study of nontransplant patients, Paalanne and colleagues[53] prospectively compared the gut microbiomes of children who were hospitalized with a febrile UTI and matched healthy controls. They found that the UTI group had a significantly higher relative abundance of *Enterobacter*, a known uropathogen, and less Peptostreptococcaceae than the controls. They also found, via quantitative polymerase chain reaction, high absolute abundances of *Escherichia coli* in the hospitalized children.

Magruder and colleagues[52,58] collected urine and fecal specimens at regular intervals from 168 kidney transplant recipients for 6 months following their transplant. They found that the patients who developed bacteriuria during follow-up were more likely to have UPEC Uropathogenic E. Coli (UPEC) and *Enterococcus* species in their gut compared to those without bacteriuria. 30% of their cohort developed Enterobacteriaceae bacteriuria; they found that increased relative abundances of *Faecalibacterium* and *Romboutsia* were independently, inversely associated with having Enterobacteriaceae bacteriuria. In addition, strain analysis revealed a close strain level alignment between species found in the gut and those seen in the urine in the same subjects, supporting the possibility of cross-colonization of the urinary tract with gut bacteria.

Global Effects of Gut Dysbiosis on Infection Susceptibility

Direct physical ascension and competition of uropathogens over other commensal bacteria, however, do not entirely explain the effect of the gut microbiome on rUTI and other infectious processes. More global immunologic and metabolic effects of gut dysbiosis may also play a crucial role in rUTI susceptibility. Short-chain fatty acids (SCFA), such as butyrate and acetate, are the main metabolites produced by gut microbial digestion of otherwise indigestible plant fibers consumed by their host. SCFA concentrations in the gut can be as high as 100 mM, serving as energy sources for colonocytes, acting to regulate intestinal epithelial cell growth, and helping to maintain gut epithelial barrier function. This has been studied extensively in inflammatory bowel disease (IBD)[59] such as Crohn's disease and ulcerative colitis, where supplementation of SCFA-producing bacteria has led to in vitro improvements in gut epithelial barrier function.[60] A reduction in SCFA-producing bacteria has also been seen in pathologies beyond the gut, such as allergic airway disease,[61] rheumatoid arthritis,[62] and neuropsychiatric disorders.[63]

High SCFA concentrations in the gut are also correlated with increased resistance to infections, likely via several different mechanisms. SCFAs regulate inflammatory responses, preventing aberrant activity of the host mucosal immune system against commensal gut bacteria but also boosting host defenses. In addition, SCFAs may directly inhibit both bacterial and fungal growth.[64,65] The substances can diffuse across microbial cell membranes at low pH, changing cellular osmotic balance and intracellular pH, ultimately compromising cellular metabolism and inhibiting microbial growth.[66] SCFAs may also impact virulence gene expression, which may compromise bacterial pathogenicity and increase the recognition of these pathogens by the host immune system.[64,67]

A recent study was able to observe the synergistic effects of several of the proposed mechanisms whereby gut dysbiosis contributes to UTI recurrence. Worby and colleagues[68] recently published findings that prospectively compared the gut microbiomes of women with rUTI and age-matched controls over 12 months. As in a multitude of other inflammatory conditions, they found that women with rUTI had significantly less microbial diversity in the gut than individuals without rUTI, frequently co-occurring with the loss of multiple SCFA-producing bacteria. They also found elevated levels of eotaxin 1, a chemokine that has been associated with higher levels of intestinal inflammation in patients with IBD. Unsurprisingly, they found reductions in uropathogenic gut bacteria after antibiotic treatment, though those same urinary strains returned to the gut within weeks of finishing the antibiotic. These data are supported by a recent prospective, longitudinal study of 125 women with rUTI, in which Choi and colleagues[54] observed postantibiotic *E coli* "blooms" in the gut 7 to 14 days after treatment, often exhibiting increased antimicrobial resistance genes. These data support the concept that even appropriate antibiotic regimens fail to eliminate uropathogenic bacteria from gut reservoirs, which may go on to seed subsequent UTI.

All of this evidence suggests a model of disease for patients with rUTI in which gut dysbiosis, likely a direct consequence of repeated antibiotic exposure, results in perpetuation of these recurrent infections via multiple mechanisms. Despite resolution of the acute symptoms of infection, uropathogenic bacteria are not cleared by antimicrobials, and may even be enriched by antibiotic treatment, enhancing individual risk of UTI recurrence. This dysbiosis perturbs local intestinal inflammation, which may increase the risk of translocation of these uropathogenic organisms to the urinary tract. Further, the loss of SCFA-producing bacteria impairs host immune function, decreases antibacterial defenses, and alters energy metabolism, further weakening resistance to infection recurrences. Together, these data strongly suggest that nonantibiotic approaches to manipulating the gut microbiome may be needed both to eliminate uropathogenic strains from the bladder and gut and to reverse the global impact of gut dysbiosis on patient UTI susceptibility.

POTENTIAL INTERVENTIONS TO MANIPULATE THE GUT MICROBIOME IN URINARY TRACT INFECTION
Cranberry

Consumption of cranberries (*Vaccinium macrocarpon*), either in their whole, dried, juiced, or supplement form, has been associated with a reduction in rUTI[69] and is supported, although weakly, by multiple guidelines recommendations.[13,14] While the primary mechanism of action of cranberry is thought to be the direct inhibition of uropathogenic adherence to the urothelium,[70,71] there may be secondary effects of cranberry-containing compounds of the gut microbiome.

Cranberry consumption is supported in multiple clinical guidelines, by varying strengths of evidence, in the prevention of rUTI in women.[13,14] Research in rUTI prevention has principally utilized the berry variety *V macrocarpon*. The primary mechanism of action resulting in a reduction of rUTI episodes is believed to be the presence of proanthocyanidins (PACs) in human urine interfering with adhesion of uropathogens to the urothelium. PACs have been demonstrated to appear in human urine as early as 1 hour after consumption of juice or whole fruit peaking between 1.5 and 2.5 hours postingestion.[72,73] Cranberry is available in multiple formulations and research findings related to the gut microbiome vary depending upon the preparation used: juice, whole fruit, pure tablets (100% whole fruit powder), powder combined with other supplements or whole dried fruit.

Limited data, however, suggest that cranberry supplementation may also affect gut microbial diversity,[74,75] indicating an additional mechanism of action by which cranberry may reduce rUTI risk. Bekiares and colleagues[76] studied the effect of sweetened dried cranberries on the fecal microbiome and urinary proteome of 10 healthy women over 2 weeks. They found changes in the relative abundances of multiple gut bacterial strains associated with improved health parameters, including increased *Akkermansia* and a decreased Firmicutes:Bacteroidetes ratio. They also found a decrease in uromodulin in the urine; although its role in urinary health is unclear, some studies suggest its involvement is protective against UTI.[77]

However, a longer term study of women who supplemented their diet with a cranberry beverage for 24 months found minimal alteration in the gut microbiome, except for the reduction in one species of *Flavonifractor*.[78] Despite this lack of change, a significant reduction in rUTI burden was experienced by the cohort. In 2020, the Food and Drug Administration in the United States announced that they would not object to particular qualified health claims related to rUTI prevention in healthy women for cranberry beverages containing at least 27% juice or tablets containing at least 500 mg of 100% dried fruit powder.[79] While dried fruit was excluded in the health claims advisement, the above studies suggest dried cranberries may alter gut microbial diversity,[74,75] the impact of which on rUTI prevention is not known.

Gut microbial diversity was studied with cranberry in tablet form combined with additional components. A prospective study of a tablet supplement containing cranberry (along with pumpkin seed extract, vitamin C, and vitamin B$_2$) found a significant reduction in rUTI after 6 months but no change in microbial diversity[80] further substantiating the concept that the specific formulation of cranberry may be important when effects on the gut microbiome are desired.

Probiotics

One route for gut microbiome manipulation is via probiotics, or introduction of the microorganisms themselves. Probiotics are typically well tolerated and are typically delivered orally in pill form and include both living and deceased bacterial strains. Nonviable probiotics will not reconstitute the endogenous microbiome, but instead are thought to exert beneficial effects primarily via modulation of the immune system, regulation of intestinal barrier function, as well as direct effects of bacterial products inhibiting enteropathogens.[81] Living probiotic supplementation is thought to impose these effects as well, but may also influence metabolic pathways and neural signaling in positive ways for overall health. Persistence of exogenous probiotic strains, however, is likely both strain-specific and individual-specific, which may account for the large variability in studies examining the effects of probiotics in UTI prevention.[82]

There is conflicting evidence regarding their efficacy and challenges to their administration (eg, bypassing the highly acidic environment of the stomach for bacterial establishment within the small bowel). A Cochrane review from 2015 included 9 studies of oral probiotic supplementation in women with rUTI and found "no significant benefit was demonstrated for probiotics compared with placebo or no treatment, but a benefit cannot be ruled out as the data were few, and derived from small studies with poor methodological reporting."[83] They compared studies of probiotic versus placebo as well as probiotic versus antibiotic; interestingly, they did not find a difference in the outcomes of either analysis. A subsequent Cochrane review from 2017 specifically searched for oral probiotic effect on symptomatic UTI in patients with a neurogenic bladder but found no studies that directly addressed that question.[33]

Some of the most robust evidence for probiotic supplementation and UTI risk can be found in the pediatric urology literature. A 2017 systematic review and meta-analysis by Hosseini and colleagues[84] included 10 studies on the use of probiotics in children with UTI. Overall, they found significant heterogeneity in the included studies and no significant effect with the use of probiotics as a monotherapy. However, when compared to a control group of children given antibiotic therapy alone, they did note a reduction in the incidence of UTI when probiotics were used in combination with antibiotics.

Since the publication of that report, several additional randomized trials have documented a potential effect of probiotics on UTI recurrence. Lee and colleagues[85] randomized infants with normal urinary tracts to 6 months of a probiotic, antibiotic prophylaxis, or no intervention after their first febrile UTI. They found a significant reduction in UTI incidence with probiotics relative to the no intervention group, similar to that seen in the antibiotic-treated group. Sadeghi-bojd and colleagues[86] randomized healthy children between 4 months and 5 years of age without other pathology conferring an increased risk for rUTI to an oral probiotic (containing *Lactobacillus acidophilus*, *Lactobacillus rhamnosus*, *Bifidobacterium bifidum*, and *Bifidobacterium lactis*) or placebo for 18 months after their first febrile UTI. They found significant results favoring the probiotic group for both their primary endpoint of cure at 18 months (97 vs 83%) and time to subsequent UTI (6.5 vs 3.5 months). Importantly, they noted no adverse events in either group, echoing substantive data that probiotic supplementation is safe for most populations.[82]

Other Dietary Interventions Impacting the Gut Microbiome

In other human diseases associated with dysbiosis, dietary changes may also help to restore the gut microbiome.[87–89] Diets rich in simple sugars and low in fiber promote disruptions of the intestinal barrier, increase intestinal inflammation, and negatively influence host metabolism, an effect that appears to be mediated by dietary impacts on the gut microbiome.[90] In animals, diets high in simple starches will promote the growth of E coli in the gut. Xenobiotics, such as food additives or pharmacologic agents, are substances that are foreign to the body that can also disrupt the gut microbiome. Food preservatives, dietary emulsifiers, artificial sweeteners can promote the overgrowth of proteobacteria, exacerbating inappropriate inflammatory changes and negatively impacting metabolic processes, such as glucose metabolism.[66] Thus, changes in dietary consumption could improve outcomes in rUTI, something that is supported by observational studies noting a protective effect of healthy diet (eg, vegetarian or diets higher in fruits/vegetables) on UTI risk.[91,92]

The consumption of fermented milk products, such as sour cream, yogurt, and cheese, can also protect against UTI, an effect that is likely mediated by the probiotic Lactobacillus in these foods. Women consuming fermented milk more than 3 times a week had a significantly decreased risk (odds ratio of 0.21, 95% confidence interval: 0.06, 0.66) of developing a UTI in comparison to those ingesting such products less than once a week.[93] This effect was not seen with milk alone, only with milk products containing probiotics.

Given the implication of SCFA-producing bacteria in UTI recurrence, several approaches to increasing SCFA production may be helpful, including prebiotics, probiotics, or a combination of the two. The ingestion of a diet rich in fiber helps ameliorate the severity of bacterial infections and improves resistance to viral infections in a manner correlating with increased SCFA production.[94] Lactobacillus probiotics can also stimulate the growth of SCFA-producing gut bacteria, reducing the severity of systemic infections.[95] Since 1947, a multitude of studies have documented the efficacy of SCFAs to treat infections, such as vulvovaginitis, conjunctivitis, colitis,

necrotic enteritis, septic arthritis, and even fungal infections, such as dermatomycosis.[66] Numerous studies of infection in animal models have confirmed the mechanisms behind this inhibition, noting direct impacts on pathogen growth as well as immunomodulatory effects. None of these studies, however, have examined the impact of dietary supplementation with SCFAs on UTI recurrence risk, so this approach to UTI management remains hypothetical.

Vitamin C (ascorbic acid) supplementation has also been suggested as a dietary measure that could lower the risk of UTI. In a case–control study, dietary vitamin C appeared to protect against UTI, resulting in a decreased odds ratio for UTI in both UTI-naïve and recurrent UTI populations.[96] Previously, it was thought that vitamin C could reduce UTI risk by urinary acidification, which can itself be bacteriostatic. In a prospective trial of spinal cord injury patients, however, no significant changes in urinary pH followed oral vitamin C supplementation.[97] Vitamin C increased alpha-diversity in the colon, specifically increasing Bifidobacterium abundance and SCFA production.[98,99] Vitamin C may also have direct effects on bacteria; in vitro, it could both inhibit the growth of UPEC and reverse biofilm formation.[100] In animal models, vitamin C improved UPEC UTI outcomes, lowering bacterial colony counts and improving bladder inflammation at levels similar to those of antibiotics. Although the effects differed somewhat by strain and bacterial load, the antibacterial effect of vitamin C was not influenced by the presence of antimicrobial resistance.[100] While these findings in animals are intriguing, the evidence for the use of vitamin C in humans is equivocal. The only prospective trials have been in complicated UTI populations, such as pregnant women and spinal cord injury patients, and are difficult to interpret due to small numbers, large subject dropout, lack of randomization, and differences in dosing.[97,101]

Fecal Microbiota Transplant

Another intervention aimed at manipulating the gut microbiome is fecal microbiota transplant (FMT). It involves collection of healthy stool from a donor and direct transplantation after varying degrees of processing into the upper or lower gastrointestinal tract of a recipient. Its efficacy has been well established in treating C difficile colitis,[102] IBD,[103] and other infections.[104] It is generally considered to be safe, with most adverse events being immediate and self-limited.[105]

Antibiotics can be effective at clearing an active infection, but paradoxically worsen microbial dysbiosis. Despite successful resolution of the UTI, the likelihood of repeat infection is amplified by each episode (each antibiotic course); this progressive increase in recurrence risk can be attributed to the incremental reductions in microbial diversity proportional to the number of previous antibiotic treatments. FMT is thought to reduce UTI recurrence through several mechanisms, similar to those proposed for probiotics. FMT can restore microbial diversity and allow the resurgence of protective organisms that actively compete with those organisms for niche space and resources. FMT is also thought to modulate recipient immunity, improve gut barrier function, and directly suppress uropathogens through the production of bacteriostatic or bacteriocidal peptides.

The proposed benefits of FMT over probiotics, however, come from more consistent recolonization of the gut, which appears to also result in effective reductions in antimicrobial resistance.[106] A systematic review noted the consistent efficacy of FMT in eradicating MDRO in approximately 70% of all subjects across 20 studies.[107] This strategy was effective across a range of population, including immunologically at-risk populations, such as renal transplant recipients and allogeneic hematopoietic stem cell transplant recipients.[106,108] As most recurrent infections are preceded by colonization of the infecting organism in the gut,[109] this approach of "decolonization," defined as "removing or reducing the burden of a pathogen, either temporarily or permanently," is thought to provide an effective method for reducing subsequent infection risk.[110] In addition, as MDRO-colonized patients can serve as reservoirs for transmission to others, reducing the pathogen burden in colonized individuals may improve outcomes in the larger population.

Recently, several case reports have documented improvements in or complete resolution of rUTI following FMT for non-UTI indications, such as C difficile infection.[111,112] Wood and colleagues[113] retrospectively examined FMT recipients for C difficile infection with and without a history of rUTI. The rUTI group (n = 17) exhibited a trend toward decreased UTI frequency; however, limitations of the study methodology make it difficult to draw meaningful conclusions from this report. Two retrospective analyses by Tariq and colleagues[114,115] examined the effect of FMT for recurrent C difficile infection on rUTI occurrence. They compared the incidence of UTI between 2 groups of patients with rUTI and recurrent C difficile infection: those who received FMT and those who received standard of care antibiotics. They found a significant reduction in the incidence of UTI following FMT (median infections per year: 1

after FMT vs 4 before FMT), while yearly incidence of UTI remained unchanged in subjects treated with antibiotics alone. Additionally, the antibiotic susceptibility profiles of the causative UTI organisms was more favorable after FMT relative to before. This promising "side-effect" of FMT treatment has prompted further interest into the possibility of using FMT as direct treatment of rUTI.

Multiple case reports detail the outcomes of patients treated with FMT specifically for rUTI. A case series investigating FMT for unique indications reported the resolution of recurrent MDRO E coli UTI caused by an extended-spectrum beta-lactamase (ESBL)-producing strain. FMT eradicated the MDRO isolate in the 31 year old woman's stool, and subsequent UTIs were pansensitive.[116] Another case of a 73 year old woman with severe rUTI (~10/y) and concurrent irritable bowel syndrome showed complete resolution of rUTI after FMT over an 8 month follow-up period.[117] They observed the new establishment of 12 donor-associated bacterial species in the recipient stool at follow up.

Other case reports of FMT for rUTI have focused on renal transplant recipients, a population particularly at risk for infection secondary to a lifetime requirement of immunosuppression and typical postprocedural courses of multiple antimicrobials. As a result, this population rapidly develops gut dysbiosis, demonstrating a lack of SCFA-producing bacterial strains.[118] In one case report of a patient who had lost his renal allograft to episodes of recurrent ESBL E coli pyelonephritis,[119] continued ESBL E coli colonization in the stool, considered a contraindication for transplantation, prevented him from proceeding with a second transplant after his allograft loss. Within 2 weeks of FMT, however, stool cultures demonstrated elimination of the offending bacteria, allowing him to be placed on the transplant waiting list. Another report is of a woman with 8 ESBL E coli UTI over 2 years who experienced the complete resolution of UTI symptoms and bacteriuria throughout the 9 month follow-up after FMT.[120] Finally, a man with ESBL Klebsiella pneumoniae rUTI at risk of losing his allograft experienced only one UTI, which occurred only 3 days after the FMT itself, in the 12 months following his FMT.[121]

One pilot study by Jeney and colleagues[122] for the use of FMT in rUTI was published in 2020. Eleven women who continued to experience rUTI despite at least 6 months of antibiotic suppression received FMT and were followed for 6 months thereafter. They found a nonsignificant (P = .055) decrease in the median number of UTI per patient over the 6 months after treatment compared with prior. They also observed an increase in fecal microbial alpha diversity with a nonsignificant reduction in the proportion of women with ESBL bacteria in stool cultures following FMT. Although the results were nonsignificant, they prompt further investigation with larger studies.

SUMMARY

Future UTI management practices need to be mindful of the need for better antimicrobial stewardship and our evolved understanding of how antibiotic-induced dysbiosis can exacerbate UTI risk. New UTI treatment and prevention strategies should maximize available nonantibiotic approaches informed by this understanding to improve patient outcomes, restrict rising antimicrobial resistance, and improve outcomes in people with UTI.

CLINICS CARE POINTS

- Use urine cultures to drive antibiotic choices.
- In symptomatic patients with negative cultures review and identify mimickers of UTI such as vaginal infections and genitourinary symptoms of menopause.
- Implement and maximize nonantibiotic prevention approaches including educating patients on symptoms, urine cultures and awareness of UTI mimicking disorders.

ACKNOWLEDGMENT

NIDDK K08DK118176 and Department of Defense PRMRP W81XWH2110644.

DISCLOSURE

COI for Dr A Lenore Ackerman: receives grant funding from MicrogenDx and is an advisor for AbbVie, GlaxoSmithkline and Watershed Medical. Dr Stothers and Dr Dutta no disclosures.

REFERENCES

1. Zeng Z, Zhan J, Zhang K, et al. Global, regional, and national burden of urinary tract infections from 1990 to 2019: an analysis of the global burden of disease study 2019. World J Urol 2022;40(3):755–63.
2. Gupta K, Trautner BW. Diagnosis and management of recurrent urinary tract infections in non-pregnant women. BMJ 2013;346:f3140.
3. Geerlings SE. Clinical presentations and epidemiology of urinary tract infections. Microbiol Spectr 2016;4(5).
4. Johnson JR, Stamm WE. Diagnosis and treatment of acute urinary tract infections. Infect Dis Clin North Am 1987;1(4):773–91.
5. Naber KG, Tiran-Saucedo J, Wagenlehner FME, et al. Psychosocial burden of recurrent uncomplicated urinary tract infections. GMS Infect Dis 2022;10:Doc01.
6. Newlands AF, Kramer M, Roberts L, et al. Evaluating the quality of life impact of recurrent urinary tract infection: Validation and refinement of the Recurrent UTI Impact Questionnaire (RUTIIQ). Neurourol Urodyn 2024. https://doi.org/10.1002/nau.25426.
7. Scott VCS, Thum LW, Sadun T, et al. Fear and frustration among women with recurrent urinary tract infections: findings from patient focus groups. J Urol 2021;206(3):688–95.
8. Hooton TM, Scholes D, Hughes JP, et al. A prospective study of risk factors for symptomatic urinary tract infection in young women. N Engl J Med 1996;335(7):468–74.
9. Pagano MJ, Barbalat Y, Theofanides MC, et al. Diagnostic yield of cystoscopy in the evaluation of recurrent urinary tract infection in women. Neurourol Urodyn 2017;36(3):692–6.
10. Santoni N, Ng A, Skews R, et al. Recurrent urinary tract infections in women: what is the evidence for investigating with flexible cystoscopy, imaging and urodynamics? Urol Int 2018;101(4):373–81.
11. Anger JT, Cameron AP, Madison R, et al. Urologic Diseases in America P. Predictors of implantable pulse generator placement after sacral neuromodulation: who does better? Neuromodulation 2014;17(4):381–4 [discussion 384].
12. Dolk FCK, Pouwels KB, Smith DRM, et al. Antibiotics in primary care in England: which antibiotics are prescribed and for which conditions? J Antimicrob Chemother 2018;73(suppl_2):ii2–10.
13. Kwok M, McGeorge S, Mayer-Coverdale J, et al. Guideline of guidelines: management of recurrent urinary tract infections in women. BJU Int 2022;130(Suppl 3):11–22.
14. Anger J, Lee U, Ackerman AL, et al. Recurrent uncomplicated urinary tract infections in Women: AUA/CUA/SUFU Guideline. J Urol 2019;202(2):282–9.
15. Langford BJ, Brown KA, Diong C, et al. The benefits and harms of antibiotic prophylaxis for urinary tract infection in older adults. Clin Infect Dis 2021;73(3):e782–91.
16. Yang X, Chen H, Zheng Y, et al. Disease burden and long-term trends of urinary tract infections: A worldwide report. Front Public Health 2022;10:888205.
17. Friedrich MJ. Antibiotic Consumption Increasing Globally. JAMA 2018;319(19):1973.

18. Burnett LA, Hochstedler BR, Weldon K, et al. Recurrent urinary tract infection: Association of clinical profiles with urobiome composition in women. Neurourol Urodyn 2021;40(6):1479–89.

19. Hochstedler BR, Burnett L, Price TK, et al. Urinary microbiota of women with recurrent urinary tract infection: collection and culture methods. Int Urogynecol J 2022;33(3):563–70.

20. Vaughan MH, Mao J, Karstens LA, et al. The urinary microbiome in postmenopausal women with recurrent urinary tract infections. J Urol 2021;206(5):1222–31.

21. Roje B, Elek A, Palada V, et al. Microbiota alters urinary bladder weight and gene expression. Microorganisms 2020;8(3).

22. Roux D, Pier GB, Skurnik D. Magic bullets for the 21st century: the reemergence of immunotherapy for multi- and pan-resistant microbes. J Antimicrob Chemother 2012;67(12):2785–7.

23. Abraham EP, Chain E, Fletcher CM, et al. Further observations on penicillin. Lancet 1941/08/16/ 1941;238(6155):177–89.

24. Franzosa EA, Hsu T, Sirota-Madi A, et al. Sequencing and beyond: integrating molecular 'omics' for microbial community profiling. Nat Rev Microbiol 2015;13(6):360–72.

25. Dethlefsen L, Huse S, Sogin ML, et al. The pervasive effects of an antibiotic on the human gut microbiota, as revealed by deep 16S rRNA sequencing. PLoS Biol 2008;6(11):e280.

26. Dethlefsen L, Relman DA. Incomplete recovery and individualized responses of the human distal gut microbiota to repeated antibiotic perturbation. Proc Natl Acad Sci USA 2011;108(Suppl 1):4554–61.

27. Rashid MU, Zaura E, Buijs MJ, et al. Determining the long-term effect of antibiotic administration on the human normal intestinal microbiota using culture and pyrosequencing methods. Clin Infect Dis 2015;60(Suppl 2):S77–84.

28. Shiao SL, Kershaw KM, Limon JJ, et al. Commensal bacteria and fungi differentially regulate tumor responses to radiation therapy. Cancer Cell 2021;39(9):1202–1213 e6.

29. Cryan JF, Dinan TG. Mind-altering microorganisms: the impact of the gut microbiota on brain and behaviour. Nat Rev Neurosci 2012;13(10):701–12.

30. Cryan JF, O'Riordan KJ, Sandhu K, et al. The gut microbiome in neurological disorders. Lancet Neurol 2020;19(2):179–94.

31. Jang SH, Woo YS, Lee SY, et al. The brain-gut-microbiome axis in psychiatry. Int J Mol Sci 2020;21(19).

32. Miyauchi E, Shimokawa C, Steimle A, et al. The impact of the gut microbiome on extra-intestinal autoimmune diseases. Nat Rev Immunol 2023;23(1):9–23.

33. Kennedy EA, King KY, Baldridge MT. Mouse microbiota models: comparing germ-free mice and antibiotics treatment as tools for modifying gut bacteria. Front Physiol 2018;9:1534.

34. Grasa L, Abecia L, Forcen R, et al. Antibiotic-induced depletion of murine microbiota induces mild inflammation and changes in toll-like receptor patterns and intestinal motility. Microb Ecol 2015;70(3):835–48.

35. Reikvam DH, Erofeev A, Sandvik A, et al. Depletion of murine intestinal microbiota: effects on gut mucosa and epithelial gene expression. PLoS One 2011;6(3):e17996.

36. Corbitt N, Kimura S, Isse K, et al. Gut bacteria drive Kupffer cell expansion via MAMP-mediated ICAM-1 induction on sinusoidal endothelium and influence preservation-reperfusion injury after orthotopic liver transplantation. Am J Pathol 2013;182(1):180–91.

37. Kelly CJ, Zheng L, Campbell EL, et al. Crosstalk between microbiota-derived short-chain fatty acids and intestinal epithelial HIF augments tissue barrier function. Cell Host Microbe 2015;17(5):662–71.

38. Park JH, Kotani T, Konno T, et al. Promotion of intestinal epithelial cell turnover by commensal bacteria: role of short-chain fatty acids. PLoS One 2016;11(5):e0156334.

39. Yan J, Herzog JW, Tsang K, et al. Gut microbiota induce IGF-1 and promote bone formation and growth. Proc Natl Acad Sci USA 2016;113(47):E7554–63.

40. Josefsdottir KS, Baldridge MT, Kadmon CS, et al. Antibiotics impair murine hematopoiesis by depleting the intestinal microbiota. Blood 2017;129(6):729–39.

41. Ekmekciu I, von Klitzing E, Fiebiger U, et al. Immune responses to broad-spectrum antibiotic treatment and fecal microbiota transplantation in mice. Front Immunol 2017;8:397.

42. Hill DA, Siracusa MC, Abt MC, et al. Commensal bacteria-derived signals regulate basophil hematopoiesis and allergic inflammation. Nat Med 2012;18(4):538–46.

43. Ivanov II, Frutos Rde L, Manel N, et al. Specific microbiota direct the differentiation of IL-17-producing T-helper cells in the mucosa of the small intestine. Cell Host Microbe 2008;4(4):337–49.

44. Oh JZ, Ravindran R, Chassaing B, et al. TLR5-mediated sensing of gut microbiota is necessary for antibody responses to seasonal influenza vaccination. Immunity 2014;41(3):478–92.

45. Aguilera M, Cerda-Cuellar M, Martinez V. Antibiotic-induced dysbiosis alters host-bacterial interactions and leads to colonic sensory and motor changes in mice. Gut Microb 2015;6(1):10–23.

46. Verdu EF, Bercik P, Verma-Gandhu M, et al. Specific probiotic therapy attenuates antibiotic induced visceral hypersensitivity in mice. Gut 2006;55(2):182–90.

47. Garvey M. The association between dysbiosis and neurological conditions often manifesting with chronic pain. Biomedicines 2023;11(3).

48. Francino MP. Early development of the gut microbiota and immune health. Pathogens 2014;3(3):769–90.

49. Christovich A, Luo XM. Gut microbiota, leaky gut, and autoimmune diseases. Front Immunol 2022; 13:946248.

50. Dabke K, Hendrick G, Devkota S. The gut microbiome and metabolic syndrome. J Clin Invest 2019;129(10):4050–7.

51. Perez-Cobas AE, Gosalbes MJ, Friedrichs A, et al. Gut microbiota disturbance during antibiotic therapy: a multi-omic approach. Gut 2013;62(11):1591–601.

52. Magruder M, Sholi AN, Gong C, et al. Gut uropathogen abundance is a risk factor for development of bacteriuria and urinary tract infection. Nat Commun 2019;10(1):5521.

53. Paalanne N, Husso A, Salo J, et al. Intestinal microbiome as a risk factor for urinary tract infections in children. Eur J Clin Microbiol Infect Dis 2018;37(10):1881–91.

54. Choi J, Thanert R, Reske KA, et al. Gut microbiome correlates of recurrent urinary tract infection: a longitudinal, multi-center study. EClinicalMedicine 2024;71:102490.

55. Flores-Mireles AL, Walker JN, Caparon M, et al. Urinary tract infections: epidemiology, mechanisms of infection and treatment options. Nat Rev Microbiol 2015;13(5):269–84.

56. Jantunen ME, Saxen H, Lukinmaa S, et al. Genomic identity of pyelonephritogenic Escherichia coli isolated from blood, urine and faeces of children with urosepsis. J Med Microbiol 2001;50(7):650–2.

57. Thanert R, Reske KA, Hink T, et al. Comparative Genomics of Antibiotic-Resistant Uropathogens Implicates Three Routes for Recurrence of Urinary Tract Infections. mBio 2019;10(4).

58. Magruder M, Edusei E, Zhang L, et al. Gut commensal microbiota and decreased risk for Enterobacteriaceae bacteriuria and urinary tract infection. Gut Microb 2020;12(1):1805281.

59. Ni J, Wu GD, Albenberg L, et al. Gut microbiota and IBD: causation or correlation? Nat Rev Gastroenterol Hepatol 2017;14(10):573–84.

60. Geirnaert A, Calatayud M, Grootaert C, et al. Butyrate-producing bacteria supplemented in vitro to Crohn's disease patient microbiota increased butyrate production and enhanced intestinal epithelial barrier integrity. Sci Rep 2017;7(1):11450.

61. Trompette A, Gollwitzer ES, Yadava K, et al. Gut microbiota metabolism of dietary fiber influences allergic airway disease and hematopoiesis. Nat Med 2014;20(2):159–66.

62. Takahashi D, Hoshina N, Kabumoto Y, et al. Microbiota-derived butyrate limits the autoimmune response by promoting the differentiation of follicular regulatory T cells. EBioMedicine 2020;58:102913.

63. Nikolova VL, Smith MRB, Hall LJ, et al. Perturbations in gut microbiota composition in psychiatric disorders: a review and meta-analysis. JAMA Psychiatr 2021;78(12):1343–54.

64. Lin YH, Chen Y, Smith TC 2nd, et al. Short-chain fatty acids alter metabolic and virulence attributes of borrelia burgdorferi. Infect Immun 2018;86(9).

65. Nguyen LN, Lopes LC, Cordero RJ, et al. Sodium butyrate inhibits pathogenic yeast growth and enhances the functions of macrophages. J Antimicrob Chemother 2011;66(11):2573–80.

66. Machado MG, Sencio V, Trottein F. Short-chain fatty acids as a potential treatment for infections: a closer look at the lungs. Infect Immun 2021;89(9): e0018821.

67. Lawhon SD, Maurer R, Suyemoto M, et al. Intestinal short-chain fatty acids alter Salmonella typhimurium invasion gene expression and virulence through BarA/SirA. Mol Microbiol 2002;46(5):1451–64.

68. Worby CJ, Schreiber HLt, Straub TJ, et al. Longitudinal multi-omics analyses link gut microbiome dysbiosis with recurrent urinary tract infections in women. Nat Microbiol 2022;7(5):630–9.

69. Fu Z, Liska D, Talan D, et al. Cranberry reduces the risk of urinary tract infection recurrence in otherwise healthy women: a systematic review and meta-analysis. J Nutr 2017;147(12):2282–8.

70. Ermel G, Georgeault S, Inisan C, et al. Inhibition of adhesion of uropathogenic Escherichia coli bacteria to uroepithelial cells by extracts from cranberry. J Med Food 2012;15(2):126–34.

71. Howell AB, Vorsa N, Der Marderosian A, et al. Inhibition of the adherence of P-fimbriated Escherichia coli to uroepithelial-cell surfaces by proanthocyanidin extracts from cranberries. N Engl J Med 1998; 339(15):1085–6.

72. Brown P, Stothers L. Determination of anthocyanin metabolites in biological fluids post-consumption of cranberry juice cocktail. Planta Med 2012. https://doi.org/10.1055/s-0032-1307500.

73. Amin K, Stothers L, Liu Y, et al. Effect of whole fruit cranberry on urinary proanthocyanidin metabolites in women. Journal article; Conference proceeding. Neurourol Urodyn 2019;38:S33–4.

74. Prasain JK, Barnes S. Cranberry polyphenols-gut microbiota interactions and potential health benefits: An updated review. Food Frontiers 2020;1(4): 459–64.

75. Lessard-Lord J, Roussel C, Lupien-Meilleur J, et al. Short term supplementation with cranberry extract modulates gut microbiota in human and displays a bifidogenic effect. NPJ Biofilms Microbiomes 2024;10(1):18.

76. Bekiares N, Krueger CG, Meudt JJ, et al. effect of sweetened dried cranberry consumption on urinary proteome and fecal microbiome in healthy human subjects. OMICS 2018;22(2):145–53.

77. Schaeffer C, Devuyst O, Rampoldi L. Uromodulin: roles in health and disease. Annu Rev Physiol 2021;83:477–501.

78. Straub TJ, Chou WC, Manson AL, et al. Limited effects of long-term daily cranberry consumption on the gut microbiome in a placebo-controlled study of women with recurrent urinary tract infections. BMC Microbiol 2021;21(1):53.

79. FDA Announces Qualified Health Claim for Certain Cranberry Products and Urinary Tract Infections. Available at: https://www.fda.gov/food/cfsan-con stituent-updates/fda-announces-qualified-health-cl aim-certain-cranberry-products-and-urinary-tract-infections#:~:text=%E2%80%9CConsuming%205 00%20mg%20each%20day,scientific%20evidence %20supporting%20this%20claim.%E2%80%9D. Accessed August 20, 2024.

80. Jeitler M, Michalsen A, Schwiertz A, et al. Effects of a supplement containing a cranberry extract on recurrent urinary tract infections and intestinal microbiota: a prospective, uncontrolled exploratory study. J Integr Complement Med 2022;28(5): 399–406.

81. Pique N, Berlanga M, Minana-Galbis D. Health benefits of heat-killed (tyndallized) probiotics: an overview. Int J Mol Sci 2019;20(10).

82. Suez J, Zmora N, Segal E, et al. The pros, cons, and many unknowns of probiotics. Nat Med 2019; 25(5):716–29.

83. Schwenger EM, Tejani AM, Loewen PS. Probiotics for preventing urinary tract infections in adults and children. Cochrane Database Syst Rev 2015;(12):CD008772.

84. Hosseini M, Yousefifard M, Ataei N, et al. The efficacy of probiotics in prevention of urinary tract infection in children: A systematic review and meta-analysis. J Pediatr Urol 2017;13(6):581–91.

85. Lee SJ, Cha J, Lee JW. Probiotics prophylaxis in pyelonephritis infants with normal urinary tracts. World J Pediatr 2016;12(4):425–9.

86. Sadeghi-Bojd S, Naghshizadian R, Mazaheri M, et al. Efficacy of probiotic prophylaxis after the first febrile urinary tract infection in children with normal urinary tracts. J Pediatric Infect Dis Soc 2020;9(3): 305–10.

87. Kohnert E, Kreutz C, Binder N, et al. Changes in gut microbiota after a four-week intervention with vegan vs. meat-rich diets in healthy participants: a randomized controlled trial. Microorganisms 2021;(4):9.

88. Shahinozzaman M, Raychaudhuri S, Fan S, et al. Kale attenuates inflammation and modulates gut microbial composition and function in C57BL/6J mice with diet-induced obesity. Microorganisms 2021;9(2).

89. van der Merwe M, Moore D, Hill JL, et al. The impact of a dried fruit and vegetable supplement and fiber rich shake on gut and health parameters in female healthcare workers: a placebo-controlled, double-blind, randomized clinical trial. Microorganisms 2021;9(4).

90. Vrieze A, Van Nood E, Holleman F, et al. Transfer of intestinal microbiota from lean donors increases insulin sensitivity in individuals with metabolic syndrome. Gastroenterology 2012;143(4):913–916 e7.

91. Chen YC, Chang CC, Chiu THT, et al. The risk of urinary tract infection in vegetarians and non-vegetarians: a prospective study. Sci Rep 2020; 10(1):906.

92. Mititelu M, Olteanu G, Neacsu SM, et al. Incidence of urinary infections and behavioral risk factors. Nutrients 2024;(3):16.

93. Kontiokari T, Laitinen J, Jarvi L, et al. Dietary factors protecting women from urinary tract infection. Am J Clin Nutr 2003;77(3):600–4.

94. Bernard H, Desseyn JL, Gottrand F, et al. Pectin-derived acidic oligosaccharides improve the outcome of pseudomonas aeruginosa lung infection in C57BL/6 Mice. PLoS One 2015;10(11): e0139686.

95. Nagpal R, Wang S, Ahmadi S, et al. Human-origin probiotic cocktail increases short-chain fatty acid production via modulation of mice and human gut microbiome. Sci Rep 2018;8(1):12649.

96. Foxman B, Chi JW. Health behavior and urinary tract infection in college-aged women. J Clin Epidemiol 1990;43(4):329–37.

97. Castello T, Girona L, Gomez MR, et al. The possible value of ascorbic acid as a prophylactic agent for urinary tract infection. Spinal Cord 1996;34(10):592–3.

98. Pham VT, Fehlbaum S, Seifert N, et al. Effects of colon-targeted vitamins on the composition and metabolic activity of the human gut microbiome-a pilot study. Gut Microb Jan-Dec 2021;13(1):1–20.

99. Hazan S, Dave S, Papoutsis AJ, et al. Vitamin C improves gut Bifidobacteria in humans. Future Microbiol 2022. https://doi.org/10.2217/fmb-2022-0209.

100. Hassuna NA, Rabie EM, Mahd WKM, et al. Antibacterial effect of vitamin C against uropathogenic E. coli in vitro and in vivo. BMC Microbiol 2023; 23(1):112.

101. Ochoa-Brust GJ, Fernandez AR, Villanueva-Ruiz GJ, et al. Daily intake of 100 mg ascorbic acid as urinary tract infection prophylactic agent during pregnancy. Acta Obstet Gynecol Scand 2007;86(7):783–7.

102. Cammarota G, Ianiro G, Gasbarrini A. Fecal microbiota transplantation for the treatment of Clostridium difficile infection: a systematic review. J Clin Gastroenterol 2014;48(8):693–702.

103. Imdad A, Pandit NG, Zaman M, et al. Fecal transplantation for treatment of inflammatory bowel disease. Cochrane Database Syst Rev 2023;4(4): CD012774.

104. Ghani R, Mullish BH, Roberts LA, et al. The potential utility of fecal (or intestinal) microbiota transplantation in controlling infectious diseases. Gut Microb Jan-Dec 2022;14(1):2038856.

105. Baxter M, Colville A. Adverse events in faecal microbiota transplant: a review of the literature. J Hosp Infect 2016;92(2):117–27.

106. Woodworth MH, Conrad RE, Haldopoulos M, et al. Fecal microbiota transplantation promotes reduction of antimicrobial resistance by strain replacement. Sci Transl Med 2023;15(720):eabo2750.

107. Yoon YK, Suh JW, Kang EJ, et al. Efficacy and safety of fecal microbiota transplantation for decolonization of intestinal multidrug-resistant microorganism carriage: beyond Clostridioides difficile infection. Ann Med Nov-Dec 2019;51(7–8):379–89.

108. Innes AJ, Mullish BH, Ghani R, et al. Fecal microbiota transplant mitigates adverse outcomes seen in patients colonized with multidrug-resistant organisms undergoing allogeneic hematopoietic cell transplantation. Front Cell Infect Microbiol 2021;11:684659.

109. Tosh PK, McDonald LC. Infection control in the multidrug-resistant era: tending the human microbiome. Clin Infect Dis 2012;54(5):707–13.

110. Mangalea MR, Halpin AL, Haile M, et al. Decolonization and pathogen reduction approaches to prevent antimicrobial resistance and healthcare-associated infections. Emerg Infect Dis 2024; 30(6):1069–76.

111. Ramos-Martinez A, Martinez-Ruiz R, Munez-Rubio E, et al. Effect of faecal microbiota transplantation on recurrent urinary tract infection in a patient with long-term suprapubic urinary catheter. J Hosp Infect 2020;105(2):332–3.

112. Wang Y, Wiesnoski DH, Helmink BA, et al. Fecal microbiota transplantation for refractory immune checkpoint inhibitor-associated colitis. Nat Med 2018;24(12):1804–8.

113. Wood N, Propst K, Yao M, et al. Fecal microbiota transfer for clostridium difficile infection and its effects on recurrent urinary tract infection. Urogynecology (Phila) 2023;29(10):814–26.

114. Tariq R, Pardi DS, Tosh PK, et al. Fecal microbiota transplantation for recurrent clostridium difficile infection reduces recurrent urinary tract infection frequency. Clin Infect Dis 2017;65(10):1745–7.

115. Tariq R, Tosh PK, Pardi DS, et al. Reduction in urinary tract infections in patients treated with fecal microbiota transplantation for recurrent Clostridioides difficile infection. Eur J Clin Microbiol Infect Dis 2023;42(8): 1037–41.

116. Lahtinen P, Mattila E, Anttila VJ, et al. Faecal microbiota transplantation in patients with Clostridium difficile and significant comorbidities as well as in patients with new indications: A case series. World J Gastroenterol 2017;23(39):7174–84.

117. Hocquart M, Pham T, Kuete E, et al. Successful fecal microbiota transplantation in a patient suffering from irritable bowel syndrome and recurrent urinary tract infections. Open Forum Infect Dis 2019;6(10):ofz398.

118. Swarte JC, Douwes RM, Hu S, et al. Characteristics and dysbiosis of the gut microbiome in renal transplant recipients. J Clin Med 2020;9(2).

119. Singh R, van Nood E, Nieuwdorp M, et al. Donor feces infusion for eradication of Extended Spectrum beta-Lactamase producing Escherichia coli in a patient with end stage renal disease. Clin Microbiol Infection 2014;20(11):O977–8.

120. Biehl LM, Cruz Aguilar R, Farowski F, et al. Fecal microbiota transplantation in a kidney transplant recipient with recurrent urinary tract infection. Infection 2018;46(6):871–4.

121. Grosen AK, Povlsen JV, Lemming LE, et al. Faecal microbiota transplantation eradicated extended-spectrum beta-lactamase-producing klebsiella pneumoniae from a renal transplant recipient with recurrent urinary tract infections. Case Rep Nephrol Dial May-Aug 2019;9(2):102–7.

122. Jeney SES, Lane F, Oliver A, et al. Fecal microbiota transplantation for the treatment of refractory recurrent urinary tract infection. Obstet Gynecol 2020; 136(4):771–3.

Pediatric Urinary Tract Infections

Nicole A. Belko, MD[a], Hans G. Pohl, MD[a,b],*

KEYWORDS

- Urinary tract infection • Circumcision • Bladder bowel dysfunction • RBUS • Vesicoureteral reflux
- Posterior urethral valves

KEY POINTS

- Females have overall a higher risk of urinary tract infection (UTI), except in the neonate period with uncircumcised males <1 year old carrying the greatest risk.
- The signs and symptoms of UTI differ by age group, infants with nonspecific symptoms and children with more typical symptoms.
- Circumcision in infant males results in an 85% reduction in the odds of UTI compared to uncircumcised males.
- Vesicoureteral reflux has a high rate of spontaneous resolution, especially in lower grades (I–II), making standardized treatment challenging.
- Bladder and bowel dysfunction evaluation consists of voiding and bowel diaries, renal and bladder ultrasound, and uroflow, and the diaries should be used to track treatment progress.

BACKGROUND

Pediatric urinary tract infections (UTIs) are one of the most common conditions treated in the inpatient and outpatient setting with high associated health care costs. The annual economic burden associated with inpatient UTI treatment alone in the United States is 180 million dollars.[1] UTI presents a clinical spectrum reflecting its anatomic involvement, ranging from the lower urinary tract (urethritis, cystitis, and epididymo-orchitis) to the upper urinary tract (pyelitis and pyelonephritis). Clinical symptoms range from mild lower urinary tract symptoms to severe, such as fevers, chills, abdominal/flank pain, and even hypotension. This article will review pediatric UTI epidemiology, pathophysiology, initial work up and treatment, and present case studies highlighting evaluation and management of specific clinical scenarios.

EPIDEMIOLOGY

UTIs are the second most common bacterial infection in children, with an annual incidence of 3.5%.[1,2] Pediatric UTI accounts for up to 1.75 million outpatient visits and 500 K emergency department (ED) per year.[3] The highest incidence occurs in the first year of life, with uncircumcised males <1 year old carrying the greatest risk.[4] While UTIs are overall more common in females, males have a 2-fold incidence in the neonatal period. From 1 to 6 months there is an equal ratio, and by 6 to 12 months females carry a 4-fold greater incidence of UTI. After 1 year of age, the risk in males drops and remains low throughout their lifetime (**Fig. 1**).[3] Some studies have reported a lower incidence of pediatric UTIs in African American children, but the overall results of these studies remain inconsistent.[3,5]

[a] Division of Urology, Children's National Medical Center, 111 Michigan Avenue Northwest, Washington, DC 20010, USA; [b] Department of Urology and Pediatrics, George Washington University School of Medicine and Health Sciences
* Corresponding author. Children's National Hospital, 111 Michigan Avenue, Northwest, West Wing, Suite 4400, Washington DC 20010.
E-mail address: Hpohl@childrensnational.org

Urol Clin N Am 51 (2024) 537–549
https://doi.org/10.1016/j.ucl.2024.06.004
0094-0143/24/© 2024 Elsevier Inc. All rights are reserved, including those for text and data mining, AI training, and similar technologies.

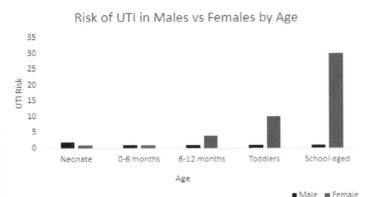

Fig. 1. Comparative risk of urinary tract infections in males versus females by age group.[3]

DIAGNOSIS & EVALUATION
History & Physical Examination

The signs and symptoms of UTI differ by age group. Infants often present with non-specific findings such as fever, irritability, poor feeding, nausea, vomiting, diarrhea, and failure to thrive.[6] Toddlers and older children have a more typical presentation; suprapubic pain, dysuria, change in voiding patterns, and flank pain (**Table 1**).

One should inquire about the severity and duration of symptoms, particularly fever, as well as risk factors, such as a prior history of UTI, bladder and bowel habits in toilet-trained children, history of abnormal imaging, and prior genitourinary (GU) or gastrointestinal surgery. Sexual history should be obtained starting in the preteen years (~12–13). Physical examination should assess abdominal distention, palpable flank mass, costovertebral angle tenderness, presence of a foreskin and phimosis, as well as inspection for perineal/vulvar, anorectal, and lumbosacral anomalies (**Table 2**).

Laboratory Work

Urine tests

The standard method for urine collection for febrile infants 2 to 24 months is suprapubic aspiration or catheterization.[7] A bagged specimen is not recommended in this population as it cannot diagnose UTI due to high rates of contamination. If a bagged specimen is positive, a repeat specimen should be obtained via catheter or aspiration. Studies comparing suprapubic aspiration to catheterization have not found either method superior in diagnosis of UTI or patient comfort.[8]

Table 1
Common signs and symptoms of urinary tract infections by age group

Infants	Toddlers	School-Aged Children
Fever	Fever	Urgency
Vomiting	Abdominal pain	Frequency
Lethargy	Vomiting	Dysuria
Irritability	Poor oral intake	Changes in continence
Poor oral intake	Irritability	Changes in voiding patterns
Failure to thrive		Abdominal pain
Less Common		
Jaundice	Hematuria	Fever
Hematuria	Lethargy	Malaise
Abdominal pain	Failure to thrive	Vomiting
Foul-smelling urine	Dysuria Foul-smelling urine	Foul-smelling urine

Table 2
Common physical examination findings in urinary tract infections

Examination Component	Examination Findings and Common Pathologies
Abdomen	Distention- *urinary retention* Suprapubic tenderness- *cystitis* Flank mass- *hydronephrosis* CVA tenderness- *upper tract infection*
GU	Phimosis Scrotal erythema, testicular tenderness- *epididymo-orchitis* Urethral irritation and discharge- *urethritis* (older children) Genital adhesions Vulvo-vaginal irritation Vaginal discharge

A mid-stream urine sample can be used for potty-trained and older children. If there is concern for contamination (multiple organisms), then a repeat catheterized specimen should be considered.

Specific urinalysis (UA) components that aid in the diagnosis of UTI are leukocyte esterase (LE), nitrates, and white blood cells (WBC) (**Table 3**). Positive LE has a sensitivity of 95% for children with symptoms, and the combination with positive nitrate has 80% to 90% sensitivity and 98% specificity for UTI diagnosis.[9] Pyuria, known as $\geq$10 WBC/high power field (HPF), has been demonstrated to be an indicator of active infection. However, recent studies suggest the presence of pyuria and bacteria on a UA has 84% positive predictive value for UTI.[9]

A urine culture (UC) is the gold standard for diagnosing a UTI in any pediatric age group and should be obtained prior to antibiotic administration.[7] A positive UC is defined as $\geq$50K colony-forming unit (CFU) of a single organism in 2 to 24-month-old children and 100K CFU of a single organism in mid-stream sample. Asymptomatic bacteriuria (ASB), which is the presence of bacteria on UC without symptoms, is important to differentiate from a "positive" culture. ASB can be seen in infants 1 to 3 months of age, older children with bladder dysfunction, neurogenic bladder (ie, Spina Bifida), and any patients with urinary devices such as catheters.[8] The inappropriate treatment of ASB in children leads to the emergence of multi-drug resistant organisms.

The American Academy of Pediatrics (AAP) guidelines recommend UA and UC in all febrile infants aged 2 to 24 months prior to administration of antibiotics.[7] Similarly, The Canadian Pediatric Society (CPS) recommends UA/UC, but the guidelines apply to all children >2 months.[10] There are no US-based guidelines for the evaluation and treatment of UTIs in older-aged children. The National Institute for Health and Care Excellence (NICE) guidelines from the United Kingdom and the European Association of Urology (EAU) recommend a positive UA only prior to the treatment of UTI in children over 3 years of age.[11,12] Furthermore, the EAU defines a positive UC as 1 to 10K CFU of a single bacterium, compared to 50K in most other definitions.[12]

Blood tests

While no specific blood tests are recommended for the initial evaluation of UTI, one shows promise as a means to identify renal parenchymal involvement among children with febrile UTI. Procalcitonin has been shown to be elevated in bacterial infections, but undetectable otherwise.[13] Meta-analyses preformed have demonstrated that an elevated procalcitonin (>0.5 ng/mL) correlates with the presence of acute pyelonephritis and predicts the evolution of renal scarring, outperforming WBC, and C-reactive protein.[14] Thus, it has been proposed as a proxy for 99m-Tc-dimercaptosuccinic acid (DMSA) scanning in the "Top-Down" Approach for the detection of vesicoureteral reflux (VUR) (see Imaging).

Imaging

Various international societies have established conflicting guidelines on standard imaging after UTI (**Table 4**).

Renal & bladder ultrasound

All guidelines recommend a Renal & bladder ultrasound (RBUS) after a febrile UTI in an infant <6 month old, but the NICE guidelines only recommend an RBUS in children >6 month old if "atypical" by guideline criteria or recurrence.[11] Additionally, the American Urologic Association (AUA) states a physician should consider RBUS in all children under <5 year old and all females regardless of age with febrile or recurrent UTIs. RBUS in this population will yield abnormal results in 15% of the time, with 1% having clinically significant abnormalities requiring continued evaluation and management.[7] A study by Nelson and colleagues demonstrated the sensitivity of RBUS for any abnormal findings on voiding cystourethrogram (VCUG) ranged from 5% to 28%, concluding RBUS to be a poor evaluation tool for GU abnormalities.[15]

Voiding cystourethrogram

A VCUG is performed by instilling contrast through a feeding tube into the bladder, and images are

Table 3
Diagnostic elements of urine analysis

UA Component	Diagnostic Information
Leukocyte Esterase	Indicates that white blood cells (WBC) are in urine *false positive*- other conditions causing inflammation in urinary tract
Nitrate	Substance produced by gram-negative bacteria *false negative*- gram-positive (Staph, Enterobacter), Pseudomonas
WBC	>10/high power field (HPF) considered indicative of infection

Table 4
Comparison of imaging recommendations between pediatric urinary tract infection guidelines

Guideline	Age	Renal & Bladder Ultrasound (RBUS)	Voiding Cystourethrogram (VCUG)	99m-Tc-Dimercaptosuccinic Acid (DMSA)
American Academy of Pediatrics[7]	2–24 mo	All children	Abnormal RBUS Complicated urinary tract infection (UTI) *Consider* in recurrence	Not recommended
CANADA[10]	>2 mo	All children <2 y	Abnormal ultra sound (US) Recurrence in children <2 y	Aid in diagnosis in the acute setting
NICE[11]	0–16 y	<6 mo: all infants >6 mo: atypical UTI or recurrence	<6 mo: atypical UTI or recurrence 6–36 mo: *consider* if atypical or recurrence + any risk factor	3 y: atypical or recurrence 3 y: recurrence
EAU[12]	0–18 y	All children with febrile UTI	<1 y: All Children >1y: Non *E coli* UTI Or Recurrent Febrite UTI *Can consider DMSA as alternative*	Alternative to VCUG (1–2 mo after infection)
ITALIAN[15]	2–36 mo	All children	Abnormal RBUS Recurrence Non-*E coli* infection	Vesicoureteral reflux (VUR) grade IV–V

obtained during filling and voiding. This allows for precise visualization of reflux and identification of potential anatomic abnormalities.[16] Thus, it is the gold standard for diagnosis of vesicoureteral reflux (VUR) and posterior urethral valves (PUVs).

The guidelines differ regarding the use of VCUG. The AAP, CPS, and Italian guidelines recommend a VCUG in response to an abnormal RBUS, while NICE and EAU stratify the need based on age and clinical characteristics, such as a non-*E coli* infection.[7,10–12,15]

99m-Tc-dimercaptosuccinic acid scan

Dimercaptosuccinic acid (DMSA) scan is performed by taking images of the kidney after injection of radioisotope to evaluate the renal uptake. This provides information regarding renal function and scarring. The AAP does not recommend DMSA in the evaluation of pediatric UTI.[7] The CPS states that DMSA can be used in the acute setting.[10] This is because it is highly sensitive and specific for the diagnosis of acute pyelonephritis with studies demonstrating sensitivity and specificity for detecting pyelonephritis 92.1%

and 93.8%, respectively.[17] DMSA can be used in clinical scenarios where this diagnosis is in question.

The EAU recommends it as an alternative to VCUG to evaluate for renal scarring. This can stratify patients who are more likely to have abnormalities on VCUG, known as the "Top-Down Approach."[12] A study retrospectively evaluating the ability for DSMA scan to predict dilating VUR during work-up for acute UTI demonstrated the sensitivities of DMSA in predicting dilating VUR were 96.15% (<6 months of age) and 100.0% (≥6 months), respectively, and negative predictive values, 97.26% and 100.0%, respectively.[18] Additionally, in patients with high-risk of renal damage and failure, DMSA scan can be considered.

The case studies presented in this article will discuss the utility of imaging in the follow-up period for children with UTIs.

TREATMENT

The initial treatment of UTIs is based on the UC results and local antibiotic resistance patterns

(**Table 5**). Trimethoprim-sulfamethoxazole has been highly prescribed in the past but has high resistance patterns.[19] Nitrofurantoin (cystitis only) or first-generation cephalosporin is commonly used for oral treatment. Intravenous (IV) antibiotic use depends on the severity of symptoms and clinical status of the patient. A duration of 7 to 10 days is typically recommended for febrile UTI, as studies have demonstrated inferior response with <7 days.[20] The American Academy of Family Physicians recommends a short course of antibiotics (2–4 days) with an afebrile UTI, but studies have not shown this to be conclusive.[21]

DISCUSSION
Case Studies

Case study #1, vesicoureteral reflux
A 2-month-old female presented to the ED with decreased oral intake, lethargy, and fever to 39 C. Aside from elevated temperature, the vital signs were normal. A physical examination was normal. Catheterized urine specimens revealed + leukocytes, + nitrates, + bacteria, >10 WBC/hpf. She was discharged on 10 days of oral antibiotic. The urine culture resulted >100K CFU/mL of *E coli*.

On follow-up, renal & bladder ultrasound (RBUS) demonstrated moderate right hydronephrosis and hydroureter, prompting a VCUG which was significant for right grade IV VUR. A DMSA renal scan performed 4 months after the febrile UTI demonstrated right upper pole renal scarring (**Fig. 2**).

VUR, the retrograde passage of urine into the ureter and kidney, is present in 30% to 40% of infants being evaluated for UTI. VUR increases the risk for pyelonephritis and renal scarring and can lead to renal disease.[22] Primary VUR is due to the lack of the passive valve mechanism of the ureterovesical junction (UVJ) and is frequently associated with laterally displaced ureteral orifice and short intramural tunnel at the UVJ.[22] Secondary VUR is a result of elevated bladder pressure during voiding. This is most seen in patients with dysfunctional voiding or neurogenic bladder.

Diagnosis The gold standard for diagnosis of VUR is VCUG.

Classification The International Reflux Study developed a 5-point grading system for VUR based on the degree of urine and amount of dilation within the upper urinary tract (**Table 6**). Grade I is the mildest with reflux into non dilated ureter, while Grade V is the most severe with reflux into the kidney accompanied by severe dilation of the collecting system and ureter.[23] Low-pressure VUR occurs during filling, while high pressure occurs during voiding.

Treatment The treatment of VUR has changed over the last several decades, with a shift from operative to non-operative management at the front-line of treatment (**Table 7**). Studies have shown that there is no uniform pathway to VUR, which has led to challenges in management of this population.[24] Overall, there is a high rate of spontaneous resolution of VUR, which is primarily influenced by the fact that most VUR is low grade (Grades 1–2). High-grade VUR (Grades 4–5) is associated with decreased resolution and increased incidence of renal disease.[25] Grade 3 VUR represents a watershed; some cases

---

Table 5
Antibiotics used in the treatment of urinary tract infection and local susceptibility patterns for commonly seen organisms

Antibiotic	Local Antibiotic Susceptibility					
	E coli	K pneumonia	P aeruginosa	P mirabilis	E cloacae	E faecalis
Oral						
Trimethoprim-sulfamethoxazole	65	73		82		
Cephalexin	69	72		71		
Nitrofurantoin	84	27				
IV						
Cefazolin	69	72		71		
Ceftriaxone	90	80	82	100	74	
Ampicillin	44	69		85		99
Gentamicin	90	90	76	99	93	
Pip-Tazo	88	79	81	100	74	

Adapted from Children's National Hospital, Washington, D.C. antibiogram.

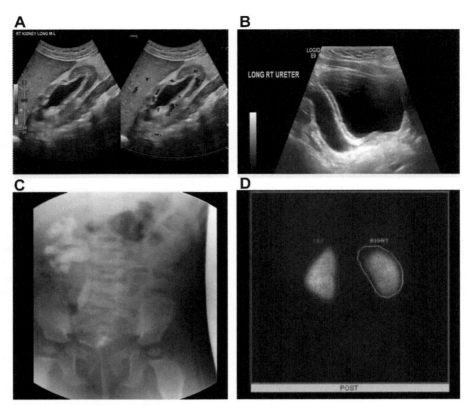

Fig. 2. (*A*) Renal & bladder ultrasound (RBUS) with moderate right hydronephrosis (*B*) Right hydroureter (*C*) Voiding cystourethrogram (VCUG) demonstrating right grade IV vesicoureteral reflux (*D*) 99m-Tc-dimercaptosuccinic acid scan with right upper pole scarring.

resolve spontaneously without recurrent UTIs and renal scarring, while others benefit from surgical management because UTI and the risk for renal scarring cannot be mitigated through preventive antibiotics.

Patient characteristics have been shown to be associated with grade of reflux. A study by Khondker and colleagues demonstrated that male sex, age <6 months, and presence of hydronephrosis are associated with high-grade reflux.[26] There are several commonly used online calculators to aid in predicting outcomes in this population utilizing patient characteristics. Age, gender, timing of VUR, presence of anomalies, grade of VUR, circumcision status, and presence of bladder and bowel dysfunction (BBD) are used to predict the child's chance of resolution or risk of breakthrough UTI (**Table 8**).

Case study #2, posterior urethral valve

A 3-month-old male presented to the ED with vomiting, diarrhea, and weight loss. In the ED, the patient was febrile 39.5 C and appeared lethargic. Patient was circumcised. Catheterized urine specimen revealed + leukocytes, + bacteria, >10 WBC/hpf. The patient was admitted for febrile UTI. RBUS obtained inpatient was positive for bilateral moderate hydronephrosis. After treatment of culture-confirmed UTI, VCUG demonstrated trabeculated bladder and a dilated posterior urethra (**Fig. 3**).

PUVsare leaflets of tissue that lead to congenital bladder outlet obstruction in males. It is the most

Table 6	
International grading system for vesicoureteral reflux[20]	
Grade	**Defining Characteristics**
I	Non-dilated ureter
II	Non-dilated ureter and renal pelvis/calyces
III	Mild-moderate dilatation/tortuosity of ureter and renal pelvis/calyces Sharp or minimally blunted fornices
IV	Blunting of forniceal angle Papillary impressions still appreciated
V	Grossly dilated collecting system with severe tortuosity Loss of papillary impressions

Table 7
Indications for surgical correction of vesicoureteral reflux

Indications	Relative Indications
• Breakthrough febrile UTI	• Parental preference
• Persistent febrile UTIs after bladder and bowel dysfunction (BBD) management	• Grade IV–V in a young child after a year of conservative management
• Failure of renal growth	• Failure to spontaneously resolve after period of watchful waiting
• Progressive renal injury	• Nephropathy at diagnosis in pubertal child
• Intolerance or non-compliance with antibiotic prophylaxis	

common cause of end-stage renal disease (ESRD) in pediatric males, with between 20% and 50% of patients progressing to ESRD in their lifetime.[27] In utero, the obstruction leads to oligohydramnios or anhydramnios, which can result in uropathy-associated pulmonary hypoplasia due to lack of amniotic fluid during lung development.

Physiologically, the outlet obstruction initially leads to an increase in voiding pressure, which results in detrusor muscle hypertrophy and increased collagen deposition. These changes to the bladder alter its storage and emptying ability. High pressures from the bladder transmit into the upper tract, causing impairment in renal function. Inability to concentrate urine results in polyuria, which leads to increased urine flow in a hostile bladder, a cycle termd as the "valve bladder cycle."[28]

Diagnosis Up to 50% of PUVs are diagnosed prenatally on RBUS with the diagnostic findings of distended thick-walled bladder and dilated posterior urethra, "the keyhole sign."[29] Postnatally, the diagnosis is typically made after a patient presents with UTIs or lower urinary tract symptoms. PUV is categorized into 3 types (**Table 9**), with Type 1 being the most common.[30]

Imaging VCUG is the standard imaging test used to diagnose PUV postnatally. Common findings include dilated posterior urethra to the level of the valves, trabeculated bladder with diverticula, hydroureteronephrosis, and VUR. Approximately 50% of patients with PUV will have VUR. Vesicoureteral reflux and dysplasia (VURD) syndrome is characterized by high-grade VUR into a poorly

functioning kidney with a contralateral preserved kidney. Although it was originally hypothesized these children would have better long-term renal function, studies have demonstrated this not to be the case.[31]

Bloodwork Serum creatinine in the first year of life has been shown to be a strong predictor for future renal outcomes. A study by Mcleod and colleagues demonstrated that nadir creatinine in the first year of life can be used to risk stratify patients with PUV, with 0% of patients with a value <0.4 having ESRD after 10 years follow-up, while 100% of patients with >1.0 had ESRD.[32]

Treatment After stabilization of the patient, the most important aspect of treatment is relieving bladder obstruction. Stabilization is crucial in a neonate, where respiratory status may be compromised. This is initially accomplished by placement of a urethral catheter. It is important to remember that catheter placement may be challenging due to dilated posterior urethra and high bladder neck. Prophylactic antibiotics are commonly used to reduce incidence of UTIs during initial management.

Surgical resection of the valves via a cystoscope to restore urine flow and normal bladder cycling is the definitive treatment. The timing for this depends on the ability to pass the resectoscope through the urethra. If this is not possible, temporizing measures such as vesicostomy are performed. Although over half of patients with PUV have VUR, this resolves in over 60% of patients.[33] Circumcision is typically performed to reduce the risk of UTI. A study demonstrated a 20% risk of UTI in uncircumcised males and PUV versus 3% in circumcised males with PUV.[34]

Continued bladder management and monitoring of renal function is essential post operatively, as many patients will have lifelong abnormalities due to the changes of the composition of the bladder and concentrating ability of the upper tracts. Many infants and children will require intermittent catheterization and medications to assist in proper emptying and storage. The treatment should be individualized and in close conjunction with nephrology to monitor renal function.

Case study #3, urinary tract infection in a circumcised male

A 5-year-old male presented to the clinic with chief complaint of recurrent UTI over the last year. Symptoms included dysuria, urgency, and urinary leakage. Previous UC × 2 demonstrated >100K CFU/mL of *Staphylococcus*. Physical examination demonstrated circumcised phallus, no meatal stenosis, no testicular tenderness. Due to recurrent

Table 8
Online calculators to predict outcomes in patients with vesicoureteral reflux

Online Calculator	Components	Calculator Website
Vesicoureteral Reflux Index (VURx) *Emory University School of Medicine*	Predicts resolution of VUR in children • Gender -VUR timing (voiding, late filling early filling) • Ureteral anomalies (yes/no) • VUR grade	https://www.mdcalc.com/calc/10478/vesicoureteral-reflux-index-vurx
iReflux Risk Calculator *Childrens Hospital of Orange County*	Predicts the risk of breakthrough UTI • Age • Gender • Maximal VUR grade • Laterality • BBD or constipation (yes/no) • VUR diagnosed after (prenatal hydronephrosis, UTI, sibling screen) • Circumcision status	https://www.choc.org/programs-services/urology/ireflux-risk-calculator/
Vesicoureteral Reflux Prediction Model *University of Iowa*	Predicts if child will outgrow VUR in 2 y • Sex • Age • Presentation (febrile UTI, non-febrile UTI, antenatal hydronephrosis, other) • Laterality • Volume (as % of predicted bladder capacity) • Grade of reflux on each side • When reflux starts on each side • Duplication (yes/no) • Voiding dysfunction • Relative renal function in refluxing kidney • Renal scan (abnormal/normal)	http://pedsurocomp.lab.uiowa.edu/
VUR Resolution Calculator *Boston Children's Hospital*	Predicts child's chance of resolving VUR at a given year after diagnosis • Child category (boys with any or girls with unilateral, girls with bilateral) • Clinical presentation (prenatal hydro or sibling, UTI) • Age at presentation (<1 y, older than 1 y) • Ureter anatomy (single/duplication) • Time to resolution • Grade of VUR	https://apps.childrenshospital.org/externalForms/vurCalculator/

UTI, an RBUS was obtained which demonstrated concern for bladder diverticulum versus ureterocele. VCUG was then obtained which confirmed bladder diverticulum.

When evaluating pediatric males for UTI, circumcision status is crucial to evaluate. Uncircumcised infants have the highest risk for UTI. Circumcision in infant males results in an 85%

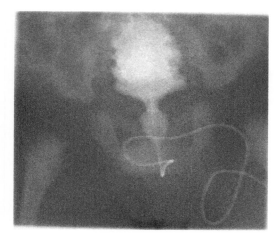

Fig. 3. VCUGdemonstrating trabeculated bladder and dilated posterior urethra.

reduction in the odds of UTI compared to uncircumcised males.[4] If an infant male presents with UTI and is uncircumcised, a discussion should be had for the potential treatment options in this population, which included steroid cream and circumcision.

Topical agents such as 0.1% betamethasone cream have been shown to decrease the risk of recurrent UTIs in patients with physiologic phimosis and normal renal US.[35] This may be an option where circumcision is undesirable due to parental preference or cultural reasons. Circumcision results in the greatest risk reduction of UTI in this population. Circumcision can also be

Table 9
Posterior urethral valves types described by Hugh Hampton Young (1919)[28]

Posterior Urethral Valves Type	Description
I (*Most frequently encountered*)	Originate at verumontanum and travel anteriorly to just proximal to the prostatomembranous junction
II (*Not reported since early literature*)	Originate at verumontanum and travel posteriorly and superiorly to the bladder neck Non obstructing
III	Annular ring at variable locations in posterior urethra

Mitchell M. Valve bladder syndrome. presented at: annual meeting of North Cental Section, American Urologic Association; 1980; Hamilton, Bermuda.

recommended to patients with VUR and PUV to decrease their risk for recurrent UTIs.

A recent study demonstrated that the prevalence of high-grade reflux and high-grade hydronephrosis was significantly higher in circumcised males.[36] Additionally, *Staphylococcus* UTI was associated with GU abnormalities such as bladder and paraureteral diverticula.[36] An RBUS/VCUG should be considered in this patient population to rule out GU abnormalities.

Case study #4, urinary tract infection in females with bladder and bowel dysfunction

A 7-year-old female with no past medical history presented for evaluation of 3 UTIs (2 febrile) in 8 months. Symptoms consisted of urgency, frequency, and dysuria. Previous imaging included RBUS (no hydronephrosis with mildly distended bladder and a mildly elevated PVR) and abdominal x-ray (moderate stool burden). The patient had small, hard bowel movements 2 to 3 times per week. She occasionally had daytime incontinence, related to her rushing to the bathroom to void. She exerted effort to void and complained of feelings of full bladder after voiding.

Bladder and bowel dysfunction (BBD) is a comprehensive term describing a combination of lower urinary tract dysfunction (LUTD) and bowel disturbances. The reference point used by International Children's Continence Society for LUTD is >5 years andfor functional bowel dysfunction is >4 years.[37] LUTD is common in children and adolescents, with studies demonstrating rates of 15% to 20% amongst school-aged children.[38] Recurrent UTI is commonly seen in BBD, especially in incomplete emptying, as in the earlier mentioned patient.

Diagnosis Voiding and bowel diaries should be utilized for initial evaluation of BBD. A 48-hour bladder and 7-day bowel diary are currently recommended. Standardized questionnaires, such as the Dysfunctional Voiding Scoring System can also be used to evaluate progress.

Imaging There is no standard imaging work up for BBD.[37] RBUS can be used to evaluate the upper tracts, particularly in patients with repeat infection, and evaluate the bladder (thickness, PVR). A rectal diameter can also often be measured with an RBUS, with over 4 cm being associated with BBD.[39] In patients with BBD and febrile UTIs, a VCUG should be obtained to rule out secondary reflux and anatomic anomalies, as patients with high-grade VUR and BBD are at highest risk for recurrent UTI.

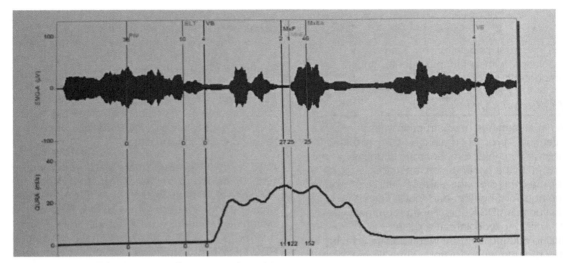

Fig. 4. Example uroflow tracing of interrupted voiding pattern.

Uroflow Uroflow, a non-invasive tool to assess flow patterns and voiding dynamics, is typically used during evaluation of BBD. Although not conclusive, patterns can be suggestive of certain pathologies (ie, interrupted flow in dysfunctional voiding, **Fig. 4**).

Treatment The treatment of UTI in patients with BBD focuses on bladder and bowel management and preventing infections. The standard initial first-line treatment includes education and behavioral modification (urotherapy), with the goal of normalizing voiding and bowel patterns.

Table 10
Bladder management for bladder and bowel dysfunction and lower urinary tract dysfunction

	Treatment Type	Details and Examples
1st line	Urotherapy	*Timed voiding-* child to void at a regular 2–3 h interval. *Reminder alarms-* to maintain regular voiding schedule. *Voiding techniques-* deep breathing, upright position, no holding maneuvers. *Voiding and bowel diaries-* to track progress.
2nd line	Pharmacotherapy **Off label for pediatric LUTD*	*Anticholinergics-*oxybutynin, tolterodine, and solifenacin approved for use in children >2 year old *Beta-agonists-*mirabegron approved in children >3 year old
	Physiotherapy	*Biofeedback-*assesses pelvic floor muscles interactions to direct therapy
3rd line	Intravesical Botox **Off label for pediatric LUTD* Neuromodulation **Use in pediatric LUTD controversial due to lack of controlled studies and understanding (AUA BBD)*	Requires repeat treatment with anesthesia at regular intervals Stimulation of peripheral or central nervous system to alter urinary function *Transcutaneous electrical nerve stimulation-*surface electrodes on sacrum to simulate S2–S3 nerve roots Most used option in pediatrics *Percutaneous tibial nerve stimulation-* needle electrode on medial malleolus to stimulate posterior tibial nerve *Sacral nerve modulation-* implantable electrode on S3 nerve root

Second-line and third-line therapies are used as an adjunct to the primary treatment. These include medication, pelvic floor physiotherapy, and neuromodulation (**Table 10**). Education is aimed at encouraging proper diet, fluid intake, and voiding habits. Behavioral modifications consist of timed voiding, reminder alarms, improving voiding posture, and decreasing holding maneuvers.[40]

Correcting constipation is paramount in reducing UTIs in BBD. The first step is to address diet and fluid intake. Measures such as increasing hydration, adding juices high in sorbitol (prune or pear), and pureed produce have been shown to improve constipation.[41] Often, patients will require the addition of laxatives such as polyethylene glycol to manage the symptoms. Treatment of constipation has been shown to result in up to a 50% reduction of voiding symptoms and UTIs in children.[42]

SUMMARY

UTIs are one of the most common bacterial illnesses amongst children, with high annual health care costs. High index of suspicion is required in the younger population, as signs and symptoms can be atypical. Urine culture is the gold standard for diagnosing UTIs. Procalcitonin can be a helpful evaluation tool in the acute setting to diagnose pyelonephritis. Treatment should be based on culture and local antibiotic susceptibility data. International guidelines differ on the recommended imaging test following UTI treatment. RBUS is recommended for initial evaluation after the first UTI by the AAP and AUA to detect potential anatomic abnormalities. VCUG is used to diagnosis VUR and PUV and is recommended by AAP after second febrile UTI or with abnormality on RBUS. DMSA scan may be used with RBUS and VCUG to aid in diagnosis in the acute setting or to evaluate renal scarring.

The acute management of UTI centers around urine culture results and local antibiotics sensitivities. VUR is a common finding after a pediatric UTI, present into up to 40% of patients presenting for evaluation of UTI. PUV may be diagnosed prenatally, or after an acute UTI episode. After surgical resection, continued renal monitoring and bladder management is necessary as many of these patients have lifelong urologic and nephrological issues. Circumcision status is important to consider during evaluation, as circumcised males with a UTI are more likely to have an anatomic abnormality. Patients with BBD are at an increased risk for recurrent UTIs with patient education, bladder management, and treatment of constipation as the first line of treatment.

CLINICS CARE POINTS

- AAP recommends UA/UC in all febrile infants aged 2 to 24 months prior to administration of antibiotics.
- Bagged urine specimen is not recommended due to high rates of contamination.
- AAP recommends VCUG after the second febrile UTI in patients 2 to 24 month old, unless abnormality on previous RBUS.
- AUA states a physician should consider RBUS in all children under <5 year old and all females regardless of age with febrile or recurrent UTIs.
- Trimethoprim-sulfamethoxazole has been highly prescribed as initial treatment in the past but has high resistance patterns; first-generation cephalosporins are now first line.
- The treatment of VUR is highly individualized and relies on many factors such as family preference, grade, and history of UTIs.
- PUV may be diagnosed prenatally or postnatally, and urinary drainage should be established promptly after patient stabilization.
- Physiologic phimosis can be treated with betamethasone cream to reduce risk of recurrent UTI.
- Circumcised boys with UTI have higher rates of GU abnormalities than uncircumcised boys with UTI.
- First-line treatment for BBD is education and behavioral modification, including dietary changes, timed voiding, and constipation management. First-line treatment should be continued when escalating to second-line or third-line treatments.

DISCLOSURE

The authors have nothing to disclose.

REFERENCES

1. Copp H, Shapiro D, Hersh A. National ambulatory antibiotic prescribing patterns for pediatric urinary tract infection, 1998-2007. Pediatrics 2011;127(6): 1027–33.
2. Freedman A. Urologic diseases in North America Project: trends in resource utilization for urinary tract infections in children. J Urol 2005;173(3):949–54.
3. Shaikh N, Morone N, Bost J, et al. Prevalence of urinary tract infection in childhood: a meta-analysis. Pediatr Infect Dis J 2008;27(4):302–8.

4. Singh-Grewal D, Macdessi J, Craig J. Circumcision for the prevention of urinary tract infection in boys: a systematic review of randomised trials and observational studies. Arch Dis Child 2005;90(8):853–8.

5. Chen L, Baker MD. Racial and ethnic differences in the rates of urinary tract infections in febrile infants in the emergency department. Pediatr Emerg Care 2006;22(7):485–7.

6. Craig J, Williams G, Jones M, et al. The accuracy of clinical symptoms and signs for the diagnosis of serious bacterial infection in young febrile children: prospective cohort study of 15 781 febrile illnesses. BMJ 2010;340:1594.

7. Roberts K. Urinary Tract Infection: Clinical Practice Guideline for the Diagnosis and Management of the Initial UTI in Febrile Infants and Children 2 to 24 Months. Pediatrics 2011;128(3):595–610.

8. Brandstrom P, Hansson S. Urinary tract infection in children. Pediatric Clinics of North America 2022; 69:1099–114.

9. Millner R, Becknell B. Urinary Tract Infections. Pediatric Clinics of North America 2019;66:1–13.

10. Robinson J, Finlay J, Long ME, et al. Urinary tract infection in infants and children: Diagnosis and management. Paediatr Child Health 2014;19(6):315–9.

11. Urinary tract infection in under 16s: diagnosis and management. London: National Institute for Health and Care Excellence; 2022.

12. 't Hoen LA, Bogaert G, Radmayr C, et al. Update of the EAU/ESPU guidelines on urinary tract infections in children. J Pediatr Urol 2021;17(2):200–7.

13. Simon L, Gauvin F, Amre D, et al. Serum procalcitonin and C-reactive protein levels as markers of bacterial infection: a systematic review and meta-analysis. Clin Infect Dis 2004;39(2):206–17.

14. Leroy S, Fernandez-Lopez A, Nikfar R, et al. Association of procalcitonin with acute pyelonephritis and renal scars in pediatric UTI. Pediatrics 2013; 131(5):870–9.

15. Nelson C, Johnson E, Logvinenko T, et al. Ultrasound as a screening test for genitalurinary anomalies in chilren with UTI. Pediatrics 2014;133(3):394–403.

16. Lebowitz R. The detection and characterization of vesicoureteral reflux in the child. J Urol 1992;148(5 Pt 2):1640–2.

17. Majd M, Nussbaum Blask A, Markle B, et al. Acute pyelonephritis: comparison of diagnosis with 99mTc-DMSA, SPECT, spiral CT, MR imaging, and power Doppler US in an experimental pig model. Radiology 2001;218(1):101–8.

18. Zhang X, Xu H, Zhou L, et al. Accuracy of Early DMSA Scan for VUR in Young Children With Febrile UTI. Pediatrics 2014;133(1):e30–8. https://doi.org/10.1542/peds.2012-2650.

19. Edin R, Shapiro D, Hersh A, et al. Antibiotic resistance patterns of outpatient pediatric urinary tract infections. J Urol 2013;190(1):222–7.

20. Practice parameter: the diagnosis, treatment, and evaluation of the initial urinary tract infection in febrile infants and young children. American Academy of PEdiatrics. Committee of Quality Improvement. Subcommittee on Urinary Tract Infections. Pediatrics 1999;103:843.

21. Veauthier B, Miller M. Urinary tract infections in young children and infants: common questions and answers. Am Fam Physician 2020;102(5):278–85.

22. Stephens F, Lenaghan D. The anatomical basis and dynamics of vesicoureteral reflux. J Urol 1962;87:669–80.

23. Medical versus surgical treatment of primary vesicoureteral reflux: report of the International Reflux Study Committee. Pediatrics 1981;67(3):392–400.

24. Cooper C, Austin J. Vesicoureteral reflux: who benefits from surgery? Urol Clin 2004;31(3):535–41.

25. Elder J, Peters C, Arant BJ. Pediatric Vesicoureteral Reflux Guideline Panel summary report on the management of primary vesicoureteral reflux in children. J Urol 1997;157(5):1846–51.

26. Khondker A, Kwong J, Yadav P, et al. A quantitative analysis of voiding cystourethrogram features confirms the association between high-grade vesicoureteral reflux with male sex, younger age, and hydronephrosis. Can Urol Assoc J 2023;17(8): 243–6.

27. Pulido J, Furth S, Zderic S, et al. Renal parenchymal area and risk of ESRD in boys with posterior urethral valves. Clin J Am Soc Nephrol 2014;9:499–505.

28. Mitchell M. Valve bladder syndrome. presented at: annual meeting of North Cental Section. Hamilton, Bermuda: American Urologic Association; 1980.

29. Malin G, Tonks A, Morris R, et al. Congenital lower urinary tract obstruction: a population-based epidemiological study. BJOG 2012;119(12):1455–64.

30. Young H, Frontz W, Baldwin J. Congenital obstruction of the posterior urethra. J Urol 1919;3:289.

31. Cuckow P, Dinneen M, Risdon R, et al. Long-term renal function in the posterior urethral valves, unilateral reflux, and renal dysplasia syndrome. J Urol 1997;158:1004.

32. McLeod D, Syzmanski K, Gong E, et al. Renal replacement therapy and intermittent catheterization risk in posterior urethral valves. Pediatrics 2019; 143(3):e20182656.

33. Tourchi A, Kajbafzadeh A, Aryan Z, et al. The management of vesicoureteral reflux in the setting of posterior urethral valves with emphasis on bladder function and renal outcomes: a single center cohort study. Urology 2014;83:199–205.

34. Harper L, Blanc T, Peycelon M, et al. Circumcision and Risk of Febrile Urinary Tract Infection in Boys with Posterior Urethral Valves: Result of the CIRCUP Randomized Trial. Eur Urol 2021;81(1):64–72.

35. Chen C, Satyanarayan A, Schlomer B. The use of steroid cream for physiologic phimosis in male infants with a history of UTI and normal renal

ultrasound is associated with decreased risk of recurrent UTI. J Pediatr Urol 2019;15(5):472.e1–6.

36. Holzman S, Grant C, Zee R, et al. High incidence of abnormal imaging findings in circumcised boys diagnosed with urinary tract infections. J Pediatr Urol 2020;16:560–5.

37. Austin P, Bauer S, Bower W, et al. The standardization of terminology of the lower urinary tract function in children and adolescents: update report from the Standardization Committee of the International Children's Continence Society. J Urol 2014;191:1863.

38. Vaz G, Vasconcelos M, Oliveira E, et al. Prevelence of lower urinary tract symptoms in school-age children. Pediatr Nephrol 2012;27:597–603.

39. Watanabe Y, Ikeda H, Onuki Y, et al. Fecal impaction detected by imaging predicts recurrent urinary tract infection. Pediatr Int 2022;64(1): e15171.

40. Schafer S, Niemczyk J, Gontard A, et al. Standard urotherapy as first-line intervention for daytime incontinence: a meta-analysis. Eur Child Adolesc Psychiatr 2018;27(8):949–64.

41. Medina-Centeno R. Medications for constipation in 2020. Curr Opin Pediatr 2020;32(5):668–73.

42. Loening-Baucke V. Urinary incontinence and urinary tract infection and their resolution with treatment of chronic constipation of childhood. Pediatrics 1997; 100(2):228–32.

Urinary Tract Infection and Neuropathic Bladder

Sherry S. Ross, MD[a],*, Catherine S. Forster, MD, MS[b], Kristy Borawski, MD[c]

KEYWORDS

- Urinary tract infection • Neurogenic bladder • Urobiome

KEY POINTS

- Urinary tract infections (UTIs) are the most common infection in patients with neurogenic bladder (NGB).
- Diagnostic criteria for UTI in patients with NGB variers.
- UTIs can result in major morbidity for patients with NGB so prompt diagnosis and treatment is important.

INTRODUCTION

Patients with insults to the central and peripheral nervous system are likely to have an impact on normal bladder function with resulting neurogenic bladder (NGB). Etiology varies and includes spinal cord injury (SCI), multiple sclerosis (MS), spina bifida (SB), cerebral palsy, and Parkinson disease.[1] Urinary tract infection (UTI) is the most common infection in people with NGB with an estimated overall rate of 2.5 UTI episodes per patient year.[2] As a result, UTIs result in a tremendous burden on the health care system.

PATHOGENESIS

The pathogenesis of the increased risk of UTI in people with NGB is complex and multifactorial (**Fig. 1**). Abnormal bladder function can result in increased post-void residuals, urinary stasis, and secondary vesicoureteral reflux (VUR), decreased bladder compliance with high bladder pressures and a potential dysfunctional immune response.[3] Normal bladder emptying is important in eliminating bacteria, which suggest that incomplete bladder emptying with high post-void residuals may increase risk of UTI.[4] Elevated intravesical pressures may impact perfusion of the bladder and decrease movement of inflammatory cells and antibiotics to the bladder, and result in secondary VUR, increasing the risk of pyelonephritis.[5] High pressure bladders may alter bladder anatomy, impacting urine flow and increase the risk of UTI.[4] The glycosaminoglycan (GAG layer) acts as a protective barrier to bacterial invasions and may be disrupted in the NGB.[6] Immunoglobulin A, which is responsible for agglutinating bacteria and preventing bacterial adherence, may be reduced in the setting of NGB.[4] Finally, there are studies that suggest immunity in the NGB differs from the normally functioning bladder: Animal studies have shown the immune response in the SCI rat model is dysregulated with elevations of proinflammatory markers prior to infection, which decrease after infection introduction.[3,7] Research is needed to better understand the correlation of these factors and the increased risk of UTI in the NGB populations.

DIAGNOSIS

Defining Urinary Tract Infection

Prompt diagnosis of a UTI has been shown to both improve outcomes and prevent UTI-associated

a Department of Urology, The University of North Carolina at Chapel Hill, Campus Box 7235, Chapel Hill, NC 27599, USA; b Department of Pediatrics, UPMC Children's Hospital of Pittsburgh, 4401 Penn Avenue, Pittsburgh, PA 15224-1334, USA; c Department of Urology, The University of North Carolina at Chapel Hill, Campus Box 7235, Chapel Hill, NC 27599, USA
* Corresponding author.
E-mail address: Sherry_Ross@med.unc.edu

Urol Clin N Am 51 (2024) 551–559
https://doi.org/10.1016/j.ucl.2024.06.009
0094-0143/24/© 2024 Elsevier Inc. All rights reserved, including those for text and data mining, AI training, and similar technologies.

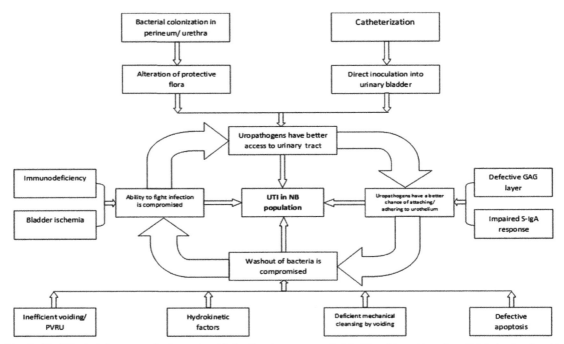

Fig. 1. Multifactorial causes of urinary tract infection in neurogenic bladder. (*From* Vasudeva P, Madersbacher H. Factors implicated in pathogenesis of urinary tract infections in neurogenic bladders: Some revered, few forgotten, others ignored. Neurourol Urodyn 2014;33(1):95 to 100; with permission.)

sequela.[8] However, accurate diagnosis of UTI is challenging since there is no global consensus on the definition of UTI. A 2013 systematic review of UTI in pediatric SB patients found that only one-third of studies reported a definition for UTI, most of which were variable.[9] A 2021 follow-up study found some improvement in UTI definition, although with notable continued variation.[10] Both the National Institute on Disability and Rehabilitation Research (NIDRR) Consensus Statement and the Infectious Disease Society of America (IDSA) have provided guidelines for diagnosis of UTI in complex patients. The NIDDR defines UTI in indwelling catheterization (IC), clean intermittent catheterization (CIC) and condom-catheter patients as any detectable concentration of bacteria greater than 10 2 and 104, respectively (NIDDR 1992). The IDSA definition is based on catheter-associated UTI (CA-UTI), which is then extrapolated to patients with NGB. In patients, who perform CIC or have an indwelling urethral or suprapubic catheter, an UTI is diagnosed when there are signs or symptoms of UTI with 103 colony forming units (CFU) of 1 or more bacteria cultured from urine collected via a mid-stream void or a single catherized urine specimen, assuming the catheter source has been removed within 48 hours.[11,12] The United States (US)

Centers for Disease Control and Prevention: National Health Safety Network defines CA-UTI as the presence of a fever, suprapubic tenderness, or costovertebral angle pain, along with a colony count greater than 100000 CFU/mL with no more than 2 different organisms.[13] Finally, guidelines for the Care of People with SB defines a UTI as a positive urine analysis (>10 white blood cells per high-powered field (wbc/hpf) in uncentrifuged urine or greater than 5 wbc/hpf centrifuged urine) and positive urine culture (>50,000 CFUs/mL in a urine specimen obtained by catheterization or suprapubic aspirate or >100000 CFUs/mL in a clean voided specimen) with symptoms such as fever (100.4 F/38C), new leakage with CIC, and back or pelvic pain.[14] There remains no gold standard definition of UTI in patients with NGB and additional research is desperately needed.

Symptoms of Urinary Tract Infection

In the NGB population, usual UTI symptoms are often absent due to impairment of sensation, which can complicate the decision to evaluate for infection. While symptoms may also vary based on the diagnosis resulting in NGB, in general fever, back or pelvic pain, pain with catheterization, or changes in continence should prompt UTI evaluation. For patients with SCI, dysuria, spasticity, lethargy or uneasy feeling, malaise, cloudy or malodorous urine, or autonomic dysreflexia (AD) are also important symptoms.[15] When considering UTI, patient symptoms should be included in the decision tree.

Bladder Colonization

The diagnosis of UTI is also complicated by bladder colonization or asymptomatic bacteriuria (ASB). The use of CIC and IC results in colonization of the urine, which can result in an abnormal urinalysis. Studies in both SCI patients and patients with SB report elevated WBCs, positive nitrites, and cultures without symptoms of UTI.[16,17] In the absence of urinary symptoms, no treatment for ASB is recommended.[2,12] The only exception is select populations such as those on immunosuppression, pregnant women, or patients undergoing urologic procedures.[12,18]

Urine Collection

The collection of a urine specimen should always precede the initiation of antibiotic treatment. The method of urine collection is important to ensure an accurate interpretation of the results. Bagged urine specimens are only helpful if urinalysis and urine culture is negative. For patients who can void, urine should be collected by voiding into a sterile container. For people who are unable to void, sterile catheterization and suprapubic aspiration remain the optimal urine collection technique. If patients have an IC present for more than 2 weeks, the ISDA recommends removal of the old catheter and placement of a clean catheter with urine specimen obtained with catheter exchange. Specimens should be sent for urine microanalysis and urine culture. Laboratories suggestive of UTI include elevated serum inflammatory markers, urinalysis with elevated WBCs, plus/minus nitrite positivity with guideline-based colony forming unit positivity. Treatment should be initiated when UTI is suspected, with consideration of hospitalization for ill or unstable patients (**Fig. 2**).

TREATMENT

Treatment of UTI in patients with NGB requires additional considerations relative to the general population. Studies have shown variations in bacterial species and resistance. *Escherichia coli* (*E. coli*), the most common uropathogen in non-NGB UTI, accounts for only 18% of symptomatic UTIs.[19] One study of patients with SB reported that *E. coli* accounted for 41% of UTIs, followed by *Klebsiella* (17%), *Proteus* (6%), and *Enterococcus* (6%) with multi-drug resistant (MDR) bacteria comprising 21% of UTI episodes.[20] Studies in the SCI population have reported high levels of resistant bacteria with up to 50% of strains resistant to multiple antibiotics.[21,22] In the MS population studies report the most common organisms are *E. coli* (23%) followed by *Pseudomonas* (22%) and *Klebsiella* (12%), with increased antibiotic resistance especially in patients with a history of multiple infections.[23]

There is a lack of data to support optimal route or duration of antibiotics for patients with NGB and UTI. Antibiotic treatment should be based on previous cultures if available, or local antibiograms. Broad spectrum antibiotics should be initiated for ill-appearing patients, with addition of anti-pseudomonal antibiotics for patients with ICs. Antibiotic treatment should be narrowed and implemented for the shortest duration of treatment that is clinically safe.[2] Overall, a 7 to 10 day treatment is recommended for UTI without a fever and 14 days if a fever is present.[24] If the patient has developed urosepsis, treatment duration may be extended.

SEQUELA OF URINARY TRACT INFECTION
Urosepsis

Urosepsis is defined as sepsis causes by an infection in the urogenital tract and accounts for 20% to 30% of all sepsis cases. Urosepsis has a high mortality rate ranging from 20% to 40% with severe infections.[25] Patients infected with MDR organisms have worse outcomes and a higher mortality when compared to patients infected with a more susceptible organism.[26] Given the challenges with accurate diagnosis of UTI coupled with a higher rate of MDR organisms, urosepsis is more common and often more lethal in the NGB population. Ortiz and colleagues reported a 10-fold increase in urosepsis in children with SB with 57% of events caused by MDR organisms.[20] In one study of 147 veterans with SCI, death due to urosepsis was second only to pneumonia.[27] Given the complexity of UTI in this population, pre-antibiotic urine cultures, prompt treatment and careful monitoring is important in preventing urosepsis, septic shock, and death.

Renal Scarring

Patients with NGB are at high risk for renal injury due to poor bladder function resulting in high pressure uninhibited bladder contractions and detrusor-sphincter dyssynergia, which may lead to VUR, hydronephrosis, and urinary stasis, thus, increasing the risk of pyelonephritis and renal

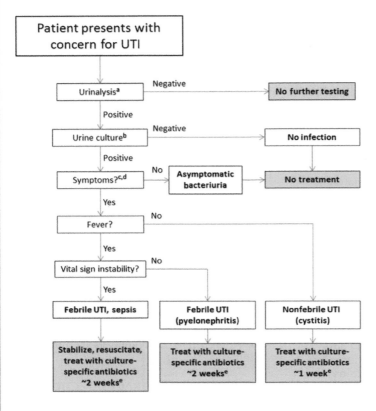

Fig. 2. Management algorithm for patients with neurogenic bladder and suspected urinary tract infection. [a] Positive urinalysis: greater than 10 WBC/HPF on microscopy (not validated end point). [b] Positive urine culture: greater than 10^2 CFU/mL from intermittent catheterized specimen, greater than 10^4 CFU/mL from condom catheter, and any value from indwelling and suprapubic catheters (not validated). [c] Symptoms include 2 or more of: fever greater than 38C, abdominal pain, new back pain, new or worse incontinence, pain with catheterization or urination, and malodorous or cloudy urine. [d] Urine culture should not be performed in the absence of symptoms, but often is, thus, is included in this algorithm. [e] Treatment duration may vary based on other considerations. (*Data from* Madden-Fuentes RJ, Ross SS. Urinary tract infections in the spina bifida population. Novel Insights into Urinary Tract Infections and Their Management 2014:61; and Everaert K, Lumen N, Kerckhaert W, et al. Urinary tract infections in spinal cord injury: prevention and treatment guidelines. Acta Clin Belg 2009;64(4): 335–40.)

scarring. In one study, renal scarring was present in 32% of SB patient with higher rates of hypertension (46%) and chronic renal disease (18%).[28] In a similar study of patients with SCI, 59% of patients had renal scarring.[29] Since UTIs can accelerate renal damage, it is important to promptly diagnose and treat UTIs effectively.

Co-morbidity Exacerbation

Patients with NGB often have medical issues that may be exacerbated in the presence of infection. MS patients may be immunocompromised so there is pressing need for prompt diagnosis and treatment of UTI to prevent progression of infection.[30] Further, any infection in patients with MS may increase the risk of relapse of their MS symptoms, which can be more severe and sustained after infection.[31,32]

Patients with SCI above T6 are susceptible to AD. UTIs are a common inciting event for AD. Since there is a 300% to 400% increased risk of stroke in the setting of AD, it is important to recognize the signs of impending onset, which include severe headache, hypertension, diaphoresis, flushing, and piloerection above the level of injury, cool and pale

skin, visual changes, nasal stuffiness, anxiety, nausea, vomiting, and dizziness.[33]

URINARY TRACT INFECTION PREVENTION IN THE NEUROGENIC BLADDER
Catheter Management

Management of the NGB with some form of bladder drainage is a key to prevent UTI and renal failure. While there are no randomized studies comparing drainage options, one prospective study, which compared various methods of bladder management in patients with SCI and reported the lowest incidence of UTI was in the CIC group, which is the preferred method of bladder management if patients have the dexterity, mobility, and body habitus to catheterize on regular intervals.[5] Condom catheters are appropriate NGB patients if bladder storage pressures are low and bladder emptying is possible. UTI rates appear to be similar to CIC.[2] For patients with intraurethral catheter or suprapubic catheter, a closed drainage system is the most important measure against UTI. Drainage bag and tubing should be placed below the level of the bladder to allow urine to drain from the bladder to the bag and prevent bagged urine backflow.[12] Catheter change intervals may vary by provider but generally are changed on a monthly basis to prevent biofilms and encrustation. A recent Cochran review reported insufficient evidence to support one catheter technique, strategy, or design over another interms of UTI prevention.[34]

Overnight Bladder Drainage

Overnight bladder drainage allows the bladder to drain continuously overnight via an IC, which is removed in the morning with resumption of CIC during the day. This allows the bladder to remain decompressed while the patient is sleeping. Studies have reported fewer UTIs in children with NGB after implementing overnight bladder drainage.[35,36] Larger, controlled studies are needed to determine the efficacy of this intervention.

Bowel Management

Patients with NGB often have neurogenic bowel resulting in constipation and possible encopresis. While it is unclear how optimizing bowel management reduces the frequency of UTI, it appears to have some impact. In one study of children with NGB and bowel, reducing rectal diameter with aggressive treatment significantly reduced UTIs ($P<.00$).[37] In a study of SCI patients, bowel management resulted in a 29% reduction of UTIs.[38,39] Neurogenic bowel should be addressed in this population, especially if UTIs are recurrent.

Antibiotic Prophylaxis

Antibiotic prophylaxis in patients with NGB is a controversial subject, with ongoing debates that weigh long-term efficacy against concern for development of antibiotic resistance. A recent metanalysis evaluating continuous antibiotic prophylaxis in children with SB did not recommend prophylaxis for NGB.[40] For some patients who have frequent or severe infections, alternating antibiotic prophylaxis with antimicrobials targeting various bacterial mechanisms may challenge bacterial flora, thus, reducing resistance. In one study of patients with SCI, alternating 2 different antibiotics on a weekly basis reduced the rate of symptomatic UTIs from 9.4 per year to 1.8 per year.[41] While these methods may impact the rate of symptomatic UTI there are concerns about the long-term effectiveness of antibiotics coupled with selection pressure, and a global increase of MDR organisms.[42]

Bladder Irrigation or Instillation

Bladder irrigation has been considered as a potential method to prevent UTI in the NGB bladder population. The most frequently used irrigate are those with antimicrobial properties. In a recent study, gentamycin instillation was reportedly effective in both the treatment and prevention of UTIs in children with complex bladder abnormalities that included NGB, with no adverse reactions or increase in serum gentamycin levels.[43] However, other studies evaluating gentamycin irrigation have found no significant difference in the rate of symptomatic UTIs or UTIs requiring hospital admission.[44] A recent study looked at the use of povidone-iodine bladder irrigation and reported a greater than 99% reduction in recurrent UTI.[45] While these studies appear to suggest some benefit, they are all limited by a small number of patients.

Recently, studies have focused on repair of the bladder GAG layer with intravesical instillation of hyaluronic acid and chondroitin sulfate (HA/CS). Studies have reported reductions in UTI with HA/CS instillation.[46,47] More studies are needed to better understand the use of this option.

Cranberry and D-Mannose

D-Mannose and cranberry work to inhibit bacterial binding and invasion into uroepithelial cells. In one small study of patients with MS, D-Mannose demonstrated promising results regarding UTI prevention.[48] A 2008 Cochran Review concluded that routine use of cranberry in patients with NGB managed with CIC was not beneficial.[49] However, 2 different cross-over randomized control trials in children with NGB due to SB or SCI, reported significant decreases in recurrent UTIs with cranberry use.[50,51]

Probiotics

Probiotics have been studied as a potential non-antibiotic option to prevent UTIs in both non-complicated and complicated bladder populations. A randomized double-blind factorial-design placebo-controlled trial, which included 207 patients with SCI and stable NGB found a combination of oral *Lactobacillus* species or *Lactobacillus* + *Bifidobacterium* species had no impact on UTI prevention in this patient population.[52] A recent study that evaluated self-instillation of intravesical *Lactobacillus* species in both adults (N = 96) and children (N = 7) with SCI, SB, or MS found this approach may be effective at reducing urinary symptoms in adults.[53] More studies are needed to evaluate the efficacy of both oral and intravesical probiotics in reducing recurrent UTIs in people with NGB.[54]

Bacterial Interference

Bacterial interference utilizes inoculation and colonization of the bladder with benign microorganisms to limit the growth of uropathogenic bacteria. Three prospective blinded randomized control trials reported that interference with non-uropathogenic *E. coli* significantly decreased the rate of UTI in patients with NGB.[55,56] There are currently no commercially available therapies, limiting the use of the option.

Immunotherapy

Immunotherapy to prevent UTI is based on the introduction of substances that stimulate an immune response that subsequently prevents infection. There is some evidence that oral immunotherapy may be beneficial in people with NGB.[57] Ongoing studies are important to better understand how immunotherapy may prevent UTIs in this population.

Future Strategies

Microbiome

The human microbiome is defined as the organisms that live on and in the human body, with variation in components of the respective microbiota based on anatomic location. Historically, the urine was considered sterile. However, studies have identified a urinary microbiome (urobiome) with increasing amounts of evidence to suggest the relevance of the urobiome in various pathologies of the urinary tract.[58,59] Perturbations in the urobiome (referred to as "dysbiosis") have been reported in multiple disease states.[60–62] The early data on the urobiome of people with NGB has shown that it is distinct from the urobiome of people without NGB.[63,64] Further, data from a cohort of children with SB suggests there are additional differences in the urobiome among people with NGB based on bladder management technique.[65]

The evidence base around the urobiome in people with NGB and UTI is mainly limited to cross-sectional studies, thus, limiting the applicability of this data. Early urobiome data in a cohort of adults with IC found that those who had recurrent UTIs had lower diversity of the urobiome compared to people without recurrent UTIs.[66] Other work, which did include longitudinal samples from a small number of people with SCI that had UTIs, reported changes in the urinary microbiome prior to UTI with return to microbiota after treatment.[67] The data in people without NGB has suggested that the urobiome may have utility in distinguishing between UTI and ASB.[68,69] While using the urobiome to distinguish UTIs from ASB in people with NGB is of great interest, there are limited published data demonstrating the role of the urobiome in this area.[65] The other application of the urobiome in the management of UTIs in people with NGB is within the realm of therapeutics.

While the use of oral probiotics has not shown to prevent UTIs in people with SCI,[52] ongoing research is centered on using intravesical probiotics as a means to restore the urobiome and decrease symptom burden in people with NGB.[70–73] Using the urobiome to differentiate UTI from ASB in people with NGB, as well as restoring the urobiome to a non-dysbiotic state, remain areas of active research.

Surgery for prevention of urinary tract infection

Surgical intervention may alter NGB function thus, decreasing UTI risk. Botox is an effective treatment for NGB. Studies have reported that Botox may decrease symptomatic UTIs.[74] Sacral neuromodulation has been used to treat detrusor overactivity and neurogenic detrusor. There have been some studies that suggest use of sacral neuromodulation may prevent UTI in people with NGB.[75] Finally, augmentation cystoplasty increases bladder capacity, decreases bladder pressures and often resolves secondary VUR.[76] However, recurrent UTI remains a common problem but may be improved with aggressive bladder irrigation and irrigation with gentamycin.[77,78] More studies are needed to better understand how surgical intervention may impact symptomatic UTI in people with NGB.

SUMMARY

UTI in the NGB is complex. There are multiple potential etiologies for increased risk of UTI. The diagnosis of UTI remains complex, given variations in how to define UTI in this population. Prompt treatment is necessary, and given the increased in MDR bacteria, use of urinalysis and culture should drive antibiotic administration. Prevention of UTI is the best option to prevent morbidity and mortality. A better understanding of the urinary microbiome with likely is the key to future management of UTIs in people with NGB.

CLINIC CARE POINTS

- UTI in the NGB may result in renal injury and urosepsis. Providers should be suspicious of UTI if patients present with fever, back pain, pain with catheterization, new urinary incontinence, or other suspicious symptoms.
- UTI may exacerbate co-morbidities in patients with NGB. It is important to be aware of symptoms for problems such as automatic dysreflexia and promptly treat when symptoms arise.

- Methods to prevent UTI vary but often include catheter management and bowel management at baseline. It is important to consider prevention techniques such as bladder irrigation or probiotics in patients with recurrent infection. Other techniques such as immunotherapy are currently being studies so familiarity with current literature is important for those caring for the NGB population.

DISCLOSURE

Drs S. S. Ross, C. S. Förster and K. M. Borawski have no disclosures.

REFERENCES

1. Dorsher PT, McIntosh PM. Neurogenic bladder. Adv Urol 2012;2012:816274.
2. Siroky MB. Pathogenesis of bacteriuria and infection in the spinal cord injured patient. Am J Med 2002; 113(Suppl 1A):67S–79S.
3. Chaudhry R, Madden-Fuentes RJ, Ortiz TK, et al. Inflammatory response to Escherichia coli urinary tract infection in the neurogenic bladder of the spinal cord injured host. J Urol 2014;191(5):1454–61.
4. Vasudeva P, Madersbacher H. Factors implicated in pathogenesis of urinary tract infections in neurogenic bladders: some revered, few forgotten, others ignored. Neurourol Urodyn 2014;33(1):95–100.
5. Esclarín De Ruz A, García Leoni E, Herruzo Cabrera R. Epidemiology and risk factors for urinary tract infection in patients with spinal cord injury. J Urol 2000;164(4):1285–9.
6. Parsons CL, Greenspan C, Moore SW, et al. Role of surface mucin in primary antibacterial defense of bladder. Urology 1977;9(1):48–52.
7. Balsara ZR, Ross SS, Dolber PC, et al. Enhanced susceptibility to urinary tract infection in the spinal cord-injured host with neurogenic bladder. Infect Immun 2013;81(8):3018–26.
8. Dik P, Klijn AJ, van Gool JD, et al. Early start to therapy preserves kidney function in spina bifida patients. Eur Urol 2006;49(5):908–13.
9. Madden-Fuentes RJ, McNamara ER, Lloyd JC, et al. Variation in definitions of urinary tract infections in spina bifida patients: a systematic review. Pediatrics 2013;132(1):132–9.
10. Forster CS, Kowalewski NN, Atienza M, et al. Defining Urinary Tract Infections in Children With Spina Bifida: A Systematic Review. Hosp Pediatr 2021;11(11):1280–7.
11. The prevention and management of urinary tract infections among people with spinal cord injuries. National Institute on Disability and Rehabilitation Research Consensus Statement. January 27-29, 1992. J Am ParaplegiaSoc 1992;15(3):194–204.
12. Hooton TM, Bradley SF, Cardenas DD, et al. Diagnosis, prevention, and treatment of catheter-associated urinary tract infection in adults: 2009 International Clinical Practice Guidelines from the Infectious Diseases Society of America. Clin Infect Dis 2010;50(5):625–63.
13. Neelakanta A, Sharma S, Kesani VP, et al. Impact of changes in the NHSN catheter-associated urinary tract infection (CAUTI) surveillance criteria on the frequency and epidemiology of CAUTI in intensive care units (ICUs). Infect Control Hosp Epidemiol 2015;36(3):346–9.
14. Spina Bifida Association. Guidelines for the Care of People with Spina Bifida 2018. 2024. Available at: http://www.spinabifidaassociation.org/guidelines/.
15. Goetz LL, Cardenas DD, Kennelly M, et al. International spinal cord injury urinary tract infection basic data set. Spinal Cord 2013;51(9):700–4.
16. Jayawardena V, Midha M. Significance of bacteriuria in neurogenic bladder. J Spinal Cord Med. 2004; 27(2):102–5.
17. Ben-David R, Carroll F, Kornitzer E, et al. Asymptomatic bacteriuria and antibiotic resistance profile in children with neurogenic bladder who require clean intermittent catheterization. Spinal Cord 2022;60(3): 256–60.
18. Mahadeva A, Tanasescu R, Gran B. Urinary tract infections in multiple sclerosis: under-diagnosed and under-treated? A clinical audit at a large University Hospital. Am J Clin Exp Immunol 2014;3(1):57–67.
19. Hooton TM. Clinical practice. Uncomplicated urinary tract infection. N Engl J Med 2012;366(11):1028–37.
20. Ortiz TK, Velazquez N, Ding L, et al. Predominant bacteria and patterns of antibiotic susceptibility in urinary tract infection in children with spina bifida. J Pediatr Urol 2018;14(5):444.e1–8.
21. Togan T, Azap OK, Durukan E, et al. The prevalence, etiologic agents and risk factors for urinary tract infection among spinal cord injury patients. Jundishapur J Microbiol 2014;7(1):e8905.
22. Yoon SB, Lee BS, Lee KD, et al. Comparison of bacterial strains and antibiotic susceptibilities in urinary isolates of spinal cord injury patients from the community and hospital. Spinal Cord 2014;52(4):298–301.
23. Li V, Barker N, Curtis C, et al. The prevention and management of hospital admissions for urinary tract infection in patients with multiple sclerosis. Mult Scler Relat Disord 2020;45:102432.
24. Everaert K, Lumen N, Kerckhaert W, et al. Urinary tract infections in spinal cord injury: prevention and treatment guidelines. Acta Clin Belg 2009;64(4): 335–40.
25. Dreger NM, Degener S, Ahmad-Nejad P, et al. Urosepsis–etiology, diagnosis, and treatment. Dtsch Arztebl Int 2015;112(49):837–48.

26. Vardakas KZ, Rafailidis PI, Konstantelias AA, et al. Predictors of mortality in patients with infections due to multi-drug resistant Gram negative bacteria: the study, the patient, the bug or the drug? J Infect 2013;66(5):401–14.

27. Rabadi MH, Mayanna SK, Vincent AS. Predictors of mortality in veterans with traumatic spinal cord injury. Spinal Cord 2013;51(10):784–8.

28. Imamura M, Hayashi C, Kim WJ, et al. Renal scarring on DMSA scan is associated with hypertension and decreased estimated glomerular filtration rate in spina bifida patients in the age of transition to adulthood. J Pediatr Urol 2018;14(4):317.e1–5.

29. Edhem I, Harrison SC. Renal scarring in spinal cord injury: a progressive process? Spinal Cord 2006;44(3):170–3.

30. Rakusa M, Murphy O, McIntyre L, et al. Testing for urinary tract colonization before high-dose corticosteroid treatment in acute multiple sclerosis relapses: prospective algorithm validation. Eur J Neurol 2013;20(3):448–52.

31. Mackenzie IS, Morant SV, Bloomfield GA, et al. Incidence and prevalence of multiple sclerosis in the UK 1990-2010: a descriptive study in the General Practice Research Database. J Neurol Neurosurg Psychiatry 2014;85(1):76–84.

32. Tullman MJ, Oshinsky RJ, Lublin FD, et al. Clinical characteristics of progressive relapsing multiple sclerosis. Mult Scler 2004;10(4):451–4.

33. Allen KJ, Leslie SW. Autonomic dysreflexia. In: StatPearls. Treasure Island (FL). StatPearls Publishing; 2023.

34. Prieto JA, Murphy CL, Stewart F, et al. Intermittent catheter techniques, strategies and designs for managing long-term bladder conditions. Cochrane Database Syst Rev 2021;10(10):CD006008.

35. Koff SA, Gigax MR, Jayanthi VR. Nocturnal bladder emptying: a simple technique for reversing urinary tract deterioration in children with neurogenic bladder. J Urol 2005;174(4 Pt 2):1629–32.

36. Nguyen MT, Pavlock CL, Zderic SA, et al. Overnight catheter drainage in children with poorly compliant bladders improves post-obstructive diuresis and urinary incontinence. J Urol 2005;174(4 Pt 2):1633–6.

37. Eid AA, Badawy H, Elmissiry M, et al. Prospective evaluation of the management of bowel dysfunction in children with neuropathic lower urinary tract dysfunction and its effect on bladder dynamics. J Pediatr Surg 2019;54(4):805–8.

38. Christensen P, Bazzocchi G, Coggrave M, et al. A randomized, controlled trial of transanal irrigation versus conservative bowel management in spinal cord-injured patients. Gastroenterology 2006;131(3): 738–47.

39. Emmanuel A, Kumar G, Christensen P, et al. Long-term cost-effectiveness of transanal irrigation in patients with neurogenic bowel dysfunction. PLoS One 2016;11(8):e0159394. Published 2016 Aug 24.

40. Autore G, Bernardi L, Ghidini F, et al. Antibiotic prophylaxis for the prevention of urinary tract infections in children: guideline and recommendations from the emilia-romagna pediatric urinary tract infections (UTI-Ped-ER) study group. Antibiotics 2023;12(6): 1040.

41. Salomon J, Denys P, Merle C, et al. Prevention of urinary tract infection in spinal cord-injured patients: safety and efficacy of a weekly oral cyclic antibiotic (WOCA) programme with a 2 year follow-up–an observational prospective study. J Antimicrob Chemother 2006;57(4):784–8.

42. Johnson JR, Johnston B, Clabots C, et al. Escherichia coli sequence type ST131 as the major cause of serious multidrug-resistant E. coli infections in the United States. Clin Infect Dis 2010;51(3):286–94.

43. Marei MM, Jackson R, Keene DJB. Intravesical gentamicin instillation for the treatment and prevention of urinary tract infections in complex paediatric urology patients: evidence for safety and efficacy. J Pediatr Urol 2021;17(1):65.e1–11.

44. Mouhssine M, Al Ani D, Al Shibli A, et al. Intravesical gentamicin instillation in the prevention of recurrent urinary tract infections in children with neurogenic bladder- a single-center retrospective observational study. J Pediatr Urol 2023;19(1):64.e1–7.

45. Moussa M, Chakra MA, Papatsoris AG, et al. Bladder irrigation with povidone-iodine prevent recurrent urinary tract infections in neurogenic bladder patients on clean intermittent catheterization. Neurourol Urodyn 2021;40(2):672–9.

46. King GK, Goodes LM, Hartshorn C, et al. Intravesical hyaluronic acid with chondroitin sulphate to prevent urinary tract infection after spinal cord injury. J Spinal Cord Med. 2023;46(5):830–6.

47. Cicek N, Yildiz N, Alpay H. Intravesical hyaluronic acid treatment in recurrent urinary tract infections in children with spina bifida and neurogenic bladder. J Pediatr Urol 2020;16(3):366.e1–5.

48. Phé V, Pakzad M, Haslam C, et al. Open label feasibility study evaluating D-mannose combined with home-based monitoring of suspected urinary tract infections in patients with multiple sclerosis. Neurourol Urodyn 2017;36(7):1770–5.

49. Jepson RG, Williams G, Craig JC. Cranberries for preventing urinary tract infections. Cochrane Database Syst Rev 2012;10(10):CD001321.

50. Mutlu H, Ekinci Z. Urinary tract infection prophylaxis in children with neurogenic bladder with cranberry capsules: randomized controlled trial. ISRN Pediatr 2012;2012:317280.

51. Hess MJ, Hess PE, Sullivan MR, et al. Evaluation of cranberry tablets for the prevention of urinary tract infections in spinal cord injured patients with neurogenic bladder. Spinal Cord 2008;46(9):622–6.

52. Toh SL, Lee BB, Ryan S, et al. Probiotics [LGG-BB12 or RC14-GR1] versus placebo as prophylaxis for

urinary tract infection in persons with spinal cord injury [ProSCIUTTU]: a randomised controlled trial. Spinal Cord 2019;57(7):550–61.

53. Groah S, Ljungberg I, Tractenberg R, et al. Self-management of urinary symptoms using a probiotic in people with spinal cord Injuries, spina bifida, and multiple sclerosis. Washington (DC): Patient-Centered Outcomes Research Institute (PCORI); 2020.

54. Darouiche RO, Green BG, Donovan WH, et al. Multicenter randomized controlled trial of bacterial interference for prevention of urinary tract infection in patients with neurogenic bladder. Urology 2011; 78(2):341–6.

55. Darouiche RO, Thornby JI, Cerra-Stewart C, et al. Bacterial interference for prevention of urinary tract infection: a prospective, randomized, placebo-controlled, double-blind pilot trial. Clin Infect Dis 2005;41(10):1531–4.

56. Sundén F, Håkansson L, Ljunggren E, et al. Escherichia coli 83972 bacteriuria protects against recurrent lower urinary tract infections in patients with incomplete bladder emptying. J Urol 2010;184(1):179–85.

57. Hachen HJ. Oral immunotherapy in paraplegic patients with chronic urinary tract infections: a double-blind, placebo-controlled trial. J Urol 1990;143(4):759–63.

58. Hilt EE, McKinley K, Pearce MM, et al. Urine is not sterile: use of enhanced urine culture techniques to detect resident bacterial flora in the adult female bladder. J Clin Microbiol 2014;52(3):871–6.

59. Price TK, Dune T, Hilt EE, et al. The clinical urine culture: enhanced techniques improve detection of clinically relevant microorganisms. J Clin Microbiol 2016;54(5):1216–22.

60. Halverson T, Mueller ER, Brubaker L, et al. Urobiome changes differ based on OAB treatment in adult females. Int Urogynecol J 2023;34(6):1271–7.

61. Hong SY, Yang YY, Xu JZ, et al. The renal pelvis urobiome in the unilateral kidney stone patients revealed by 2bRAD-M. J Transl Med 2022;20(1):431.

62. Zeng J, Zhang G, Chen C, et al. Alterations in urobiome in patients with bladder cancer and implications for clinical outcome: a single-institution study. Front Cell Infect Microbiol 2020;10:555508. Published 2020 Dec 15.

63. Groah SL, Pérez-Losada M, Caldovic L, et al. Redefining healthy urine: a cross-sectional exploratory metagenomic study of people with and without bladder dysfunction. J Urol 2016;196(2):579–87.

64. Fouts DE, Pieper R, Szpakowski S, et al. Integrated next-generation sequencing of 16S rDNA and metaproteomics differentiate the healthy urine microbiome from asymptomatic bacteriuria in neuropathic bladder associated with spinal cord injury. J Transl Med 2012;10:174.

65. Forster CS, Panchapakesan K, Stroud C, et al. A cross-sectional analysis of the urine microbiome of children with neuropathic bladders. J Pediatr Urol 2020;16(5):593.e1–8.

66. Horwitz D, McCue T, Mapes AC, et al. Decreased microbiota diversity associated with urinary tract infection in a trial of bacterial interference. J Infect 2015;71(3):358–67.

67. Bossa L, Kline K, McDougald D, et al. Urinary catheter-associated microbiota change in accordance with treatment and infection status. PLoS One 2017;12(6):e0177633.

68. Marshall CW, Kurs-Lasky M, McElheny CL, et al. Performance of conventional urine culture compared to 16s rrna gene amplicon sequencing in children with suspected urinary tract infection. Microbiol Spectr 2021;9(3):e0186121.

69. Shaikh N, Lee S, Krumbeck JA, et al. Support for the use of a new cutoff to define a positive urine culture in young Children. Pediatrics 2023;152(4). e2023061931.

70. Tractenberg RE, Groah SL, Frost JK, et al. Effects of Intravesical Lactobacillus Rhamnosus GG on urinary symptom burden in people with neurogenic lower urinary tract dysfunction. Pharm Manag PM R 2021;13(7):695–706.

71. Groah SL, Rounds AK, Ljungberg IH, et al. Intravesical *Lactobacillus rhamnosus GG* is safe and well tolerated in adults and children with neurogenic lower urinary tract dysfunction: first-in-human trial. Ther Adv Urol 2019;11. 1756287219875594.

72. Groah SL, Rounds AK, Pérez-Losada M. Intravesical *Lactobacillus rhamnosus GG* alters urobiome composition and diversity among people with neurogenic lower urinary tract dysfunction. Top Spinal Cord Inj Rehabil 2023;29(3):44–57.

73. Forster CS, Hsieh MH, Pérez-Losada M, et al. A single intravesical instillation of *Lactobacillus rhamnosus* GG is safe in children and adults with neuropathic bladder: A phase Ia clinical trial. J Spinal Cord Med. 2021;44(1): 62–9.

74. Jia C, Liao LM, Chen G, et al. Detrusor botulinum toxin A injection significantly decreased urinary tract infection in patients with traumatic spinal cord injury. Spinal Cord 2013;51(6):487–90.

75. Darouiche RO, Al Mohajer M, Siddiq DM, et al. Short versus long course of antibiotics for catheter-associated urinary tract infections in patients with spinal cord injury: a randomized controlled noninferiority trial. Arch Phys Med Rehabil 2014;95(2):290–6.

76. Zhang HC, Yang J, Ye X, et al. Augmentation enterocystoplasty without reimplantation for patients with neurogenic bladder and vesicoureteral reflux. Kaohsiung J Med Sci 2016;32(6):323–6.

77. Husmann DA. Long-term complications following bladder augmentations in patients with spina bifida: bladder calculi, perforation of the augmented bladder and upper tract deterioration. Transl Androl Urol 2016; 5(1):3–11.

78. Cox L, He C, Bevins J, et al. Gentamicin bladder instillations decrease symptomatic urinary tract infections in neurogenic bladder patients on intermittent catheterization. Can Urol Assoc J. 2017;11(9):E350–4.

Management of Asymptomatic Bacteriuria in Non-Catheterized Adults

Allison Grant, MD[1],*, Zoë Cohen, MD[1], Kimberly L. Cooper, MD

KEYWORDS

- Asymptomatic bacteriuria • Urinary tract infection • Screening • Antibiotics

KEY POINTS

- Asymptomatic bacteriuria (ASB), or the presence of the same bacterial species in a quantity greater than or equal to 100,000 colony forming units, has a prevalence that ranges based on sex, age, and place of living. Risk factors for ASB include increasing age, female sex, living in long-term care facilities, menopause, diabetes, and catheterization.
- Historically, there was a concern that untreated ASB may lead to the development of multiple sequelae including urinary tract infection (UTI); however, a 2012 comparative study determined that the presence of ASB was not predictive of future UTI.
- Guidelines recommend against screening for and treating ASB in most populations, excluding pregnant women and patients who are undergoing urologic procedures in which transmucosal bleeding is anticipated.
- While there is still much to learn about the urinary microbiome, research into the prevention of UTI with the use of avirulent bacteria as "bacterial interference" has emerged over the last several years.

INTRODUCTION AND BACKGROUND

Asymptomatic bacteriuria (ASB) is the presence of bacteria in a noncontaminated urine sample in a person with no signs or symptoms of a urinary tract infection (UTI). In women, the diagnosis of ASB requires the identification of the same bacterial species in a quantity greater than or equal to 100,000 colony forming units (CFUs) on 2 consecutive non-contaminated voiding samples. In men, diagnosis only requires one clean-catch voided sample positive for a bacterial species in a quantity greater than or equal to 100,000 CFUs. Alternatively, ASB can be diagnosed in men or women when one *catheterized* urine sample is positive for a bacterial species in a quantity greater than or equal to 100,000 CFUs[1] (**Box 1**). ASB is commonly identified in healthy female individuals, elderly, and those with underlying urologic abnormalities. Screening and treatment guidelines for all populations have evolved over time. Herein, we provide an up-to-date review of the literature and report the prevalence, screening, and treatment guidelines for ASB across different patient populations.

Prevalence and Risk Factors

The prevalence of ASB (**Table 1**) varies depending on age, sex, and comorbidities. The prevalence of ASB increases with age, with only 1% of school-age girls testing positive compared to greater than 20% of healthy women aged over 80 years living in the community.[2] Age as a risk factor for ASB is also observed in men; while ASB is uncommon in young men, rates among male community dwellers aged over 75 years are estimated to be

Department of Urology, Columbia University Irving Medical Center, 161 Fort Washington Avenue, 11th Floor, New York, NY 10032, USA
[1] These 2 authors share the first authorship.
* Corresponding author.
E-mail address: alg2247@cumc.columbia.edu

Urol Clin N Am 51 (2024) 561–570
https://doi.org/10.1016/j.ucl.2024.06.010
0094-0143/24/© 2024 Elsevier Inc. All rights reserved, including those for text and data mining, AI training, and similar technologies.

between 6% and 15%.[2,3] Prevalence of ASB in both men and women community dwellers differs dramatically from the rates of ASB in those living in long-term care facilities, which is estimated at 25% to 50% for women and 15% to 40% of men.[4]

Menopause also increases the risk of ASB with a prevalence of 2.8% to 8.6% in healthy postmenopausal women aged between 50 and 70 years compared to just 1% to 5% in healthy premenopausal women.[2] Moreover, sexual activity is a risk factor for the development of ASB. Indeed, sexually active premenopausal, married women saw higher rates of ASB (4.6%) compared to age-matched nuns (0.7%) who were sexually inactive.[5]

Diabetes is an important risk factor for ASB, given the prevalence of diabetes in our country. An increasing prevalence of ASB is associated with longer duration of diabetes as well as poorly controlled disease.[6]

Unsurprisingly, the prevalence of ASB is higher among patients with indwelling catheters and in patients with spinal cord injury (SCI) who perform clean intermiteent catheterization (CIC). For those with chronic indwelling catheters, the prevalence of ASB is 100%. Further, for those who perform CIC, the rate of ASB has been documented anywhere from 23% to 89%.[7,8] As such, risk factors

for ASB include increasing age, female sex, living in long-term care facilities, menopause, diabetes, and catheterization.[9]

Common Pathogens

Common pathogens responsible for ASB vary based on the sex, catheter status, and place of living of the patient. In the community, the predominant pathogen isolated in older women with ASB was *Escherichia coli*, which Linhares and colleagues[10] found to make up 51.4% of samples. Interestingly, the strains of *E coli* responsible for ASB were found to have fewer virulence factors that those that cause symptomatic UTIs.[11] For men, however, the most common pathogens identified in the urine are gram-negative bacilli, enterococci, and coagulase-negative staphylococci.[12,13] For those adults living in long-term care facilities, and those with indwelling catheters, polymicrobial bacteriuria with *Pseudomonas aeruginosa*, *Morganella morganii*, and *Providencia stuartii* is most common.[1,14]

Relationship Between Asymptomatic Bacteriuria and Recurrent Urinary Tract Infection

A historical concern that untreated ASB may lead to long-term sequelae including hypertension, renal insufficiency, and development of urinary tract cancer has been repudiated.[15,16] Interestingly, a 2012 comparative study[17] determined that the presence of ASB was not predictive of future UTI. Furthermore, as antibiotic treatment of ASB can increase the risk of subsequent symptomatic UTI and carries the risk of adverse effects from antibiotics, as well as breed antibiotic resistance, studies have established that treating ASB indiscriminately is potentially harmful.[18,19]

DISCUSSION
Screening and Treatment Recommendations

The Infectious Disease Society of America (IDSA) guidelines for the management of ASB in various populations were updated in 2019, and they provide a strong framework for providers to reference when managing patients with ASB.[20]

The initial version of guidelines recommends against treating ASB in most cases including in the following populations: premenopausal, nonpregnant women, women with diabetes, older community dwellers, elderly institutionalized patients, patients with SCI, and patients with indwelling catheters. The 2019 guidelines recommend against the treatment of ASB in the following additional populations: infants and children, men with diabetes, renal

Table 1
Prevalence of asymptomatic bacteriuria in selected populations as seen in Campbell-Walsh-Wein 12th edition section on asymptomatic bacteriuria

Population	Prevalence (%)	References
Healthy, premenopausal women	1.0–5.0	Nicolle,[2] 2003
Pregnant women	1.9–9.5	Nicolle,[2] 2003
Postmenopausal women aged 50–70 y	2.8–8.6	Nicolle,[2] 2003
Patients with diabetes		
Women	9.0–27	Zhanel et al,[71] 1991a
Men	0.7–11	Zhanel et al,[71] 1991a
Elderly persons in the community		
Women	10.8–16	Nicolle,[2] 2003
Men	3.6–19	Nicolle,[2] 2003
Elderly persons in a long-term care facility		
Women	25–50	Nicolle,[4] 1997
Men	14–50	Nicolle,[4] 1997
Patients with spinal cord injuries		
Intermittent catheter use	23–89	Bakke & Digranes,[7] 1991
Sphincterotomy and condom catheter in place	57	Waites et al,[49] 1993b
Patients undergoing hemodialysis	28	Chaudhry et al,[72] 1993
Patients with indwelling catheter use		
Short-term	9–23	Stamm,[73] 1991
Long-term	100	Warren,[8] 1982

Data from Nicolle LE, Bradley S, Colgan R, et al.: Infectious Diseases Society of America guidelines for the diagnosis and treatment of asymptomatic bacteriuria in adults. *Clin Infect Dis* 40:643–654, 2005.

transplant recipients who received their transplant more than 1 month prior, patients with solid (nonrenal) organ transplants, and those undergoing nonurologic surgeries.[20]

It is critical to know which specific populations with ASB should always be treated. These populations include pregnant women and patients who are undergoing urologic procedures in which transmucosal bleeding is anticipated.[20] There is no consensus regarding whether to treat ASB in patients with neutropenia.[20]

The US Preventive Services Task Force 2019 update on ASB was consistent with the IDSA guidelines, recommending against screening for ASB in all groups except for in pregnant women.[21,22]

Furthermore, a 2015 Cochrane review[23] assessing the safety and effectiveness of antibiotic treatment in adults with ASB examined 9 randomized or "quasi" randomized controlled studies including a total of 1614 subjects. The review excluded studies examining pregnant women, those who either had indwelling catheters or performed CIC, those who had indwelling stents or nephrostomy tubes, transplant recipients, those with bacteriuria related to recent urologic procedures, patients with SCI, or hospitalized patients. The review

concluded that symptomatic UTI, complications, and death were similar across subjects treated with antibiotics and those who were not. While bacteriuria resolved in the treated subjects, these subjects also saw more adverse effects. Overall, the authors concluded that treating ASB in this adult population does not provide a clinical benefit.

Healthy Nonpregnant Women

The IDSA recommends against screening for or treating ASB in healthy nonpregnant women. Studies show that ASB in healthy nonpregnant women is not associated with hypertension, development of chronic kidney disease, or mortality.[1] Though women with ASB may be at an increased risk of symptomatic UTI, there is no evidence currently that attributes symptomatic UTI to the ASB.[24] Moreover, there is evidence that highlights an absence of a predictive relationship between ASB and UTI.[17] Treatment with antibiotics can be harmful due to resulting in adverse effects, increased antibiotic resistance, and increasing medical costs.[25]

Available evidence also suggests that treatment with antibiotics may, in fact, increase the risk of symptomatic UTI and antibiotic resistance in this specific population.[18,19,24] In a 2012 randomized clinical trial (RCT), Cai and colleagues[18] prospectively examined 673 women with ASB and compared rates of recurrent UTI between the treatment (those who were treated for ASB) and control (those who were not treated for ASB) groups. The researchers found higher rates of symptomatic UTI recurrence in those who were treated for ASB compared to those who were not treated at 6 month and 12 month follow-ups (P<.0001). In 2015, Cai and colleagues[19] did a follow-up study to investigate the impact that antibiotic treatment of ASB had on antibiotic resistance in this patient population. They found higher antibiotic resistance to amoxicillin-clavulanic acid, trimethoprim-sulfamethoxazole, and ciprofloxacin in those who were treated for ASB compared to those who were not.

Pregnant Women

Screening and treatment of ASB is recommended for pregnant women according to the IDSA. Rates of ASB in pregnant women range from 2% to 7%.[1,26] The recommendation to screen and treat this population is based on prospective randomized studies from the 1960s to 1980s. These studies reported a decreased incidence of pyelonephritis in pregnant women with ASB from 20% to 35% if untreated to 1% to 4% if treated.[1] Historically, studies suggested that the treatment of ASB in this population may also reduce the risk of preterm labor.[27,28]

Treatment with antibiotics is recommended for 4 to 7 days depending on the antibiotic used.[29,30] A Cochrane review from 2015 comparing multidose antibiotic regimens with single-dose regimens found a trend toward lower rates of clearance of bacteriuria with single-dose regimens; however, this finding was not statistically significant (1.28 [95% CI, .87–1.88]; low quality).[30] One moderate-quality study included in the review found that a 7 day course of nitrofurantoin was more effective in preventing low birth weight when compared to a single-dose of nitrofurantoin (relative risk, 1.65 [95% CI, 1.06–2.57]).[31]

Of note, recommendations for the screening and treatment of ASB in pregnant women are based on trials conducted several decades ago. More recent evidence calls into question whether treatment of ASB in pregnancy is needed. An RCT published in 2015 compared outcomes between pregnant women with ASB who were treated with antibiotics and those who were treated with a placebo.[28] The authors found no difference in rates of preterm birth between the treatment and placebo groups.

They did, however, find higher rates of pyelonephritis in women with ASB who received placebo or were untreated compared to those who were treated with antibiotics, but an absolute risk of pyelonephritis in women with ASB was low (2.4%).[28] Nonetheless, the recommendation of the IDSA remains to screen and to treat ASB in pregnant women.

Elderly Persons

It is neither recommended to screen for or to treat ASB in functionally impaired elderly persons nor in elderly persons living in long-term care facilities. This recommendation is based on evidence from decades of randomized trials and cohort studies with years of follow-up.[32–36]

Fortunately, ASB in the elderly rarely progresses to symptomatic infection even when antibiotics are not initiated.[37] As such, the treatment of bacteriuria in older persons who are residing in long-term care facilities should be based on the presence of clinical symptoms.[38] In other words, patients with a positive urine culture and pyuria warrant treatment of symptomatic UTI when they report 2 of the following clinical criteria: fever, increased urinary urgency or frequency, dysuria, suprapubic tenderness, or costovertebral tenderness.

Unfortunately, inappropriate treatment of ASB in the elderly who do not meet minimum clinical criteria is particularly common.[39] One study of elderly persons with advanced dementia found that 75% of residents with bacteriuria were treated with antibiotics when only 16% of them met the above minimum criteria for treatment.[40] Notably, inappropriate treatment of elderly patients with ASB with antibiotics not only bred antibiotic resistance but has also been associated with an increased morbidity. In their retrospective study, Rotjanapan and colleagues[41] reported an 8.5 times higher likelihood of developing a *Clostridioides difficile* infection in those who were inappropriately treated for bacteriuria compared to those with bacteriuria who were not treated.

Differentiating Asymptomatic Bacteriuria from Symptomatic Urinary Tract Infection in Older Functionally Impaired or Cognitively Impaired Patients

Differentiating between symptomatic UTI and ASB in the older functionally and cognitively impaired population is challenging, yet critical. Due to high rates of ASB among the elderly, urine testing will often yield a positive urinalysis or urine culture. However, in the absence of systemic signs or local genitourinary symptoms, older functionally or cognitively impaired patients with ASB presenting with delirium or after a fall should *not* be indiscriminately treated with antibiotics. Instead, they should be carefully observed, and a thorough workup should ensue.

A review by Mody and colleagues[42] published in 2014 proposes a clinical algorithm to guide the decision to send urine tests for this patient population (**Fig. 1**). For patients who have or who develop UTI-specific symptoms such as acute dysuria, new or worsening frequency or urgency, new incontinence, gross hematuria, urine tests are recommended. Patients with nonspecific symptoms (chronic frequency, urgency, or incontinence) should not have routine urine testing and rather, should undergo evaluation for other etiologies, such as dehydration and adverse effects from medications. The evaluation of clinical resolution for these patients is based on symptomatic improvement and not based on subsequent negative urine culture testing. Specifically for the cognitively impaired patients, urine studies are indicated when there is a persistent change in mental status and a change in urine quality that does not improve with hydration.

Patients with Diabetes

It is not recommended to screen for or to treat ASB in patients with diabetes. This recommendation is based on data from 1 RCT[6] and 2 prospective cohort studies.[43,44] In the randomized trial, there was no significant difference in rates of symptomatic UTI (40% vs 42% over 36 months) between those who were treated with antibiotics and those who were not. Rates of pyelonephritis were also not significantly different between treatment and placebo groups. Of note, these studies did not further stratify participants based on glycosylated hemoglobin values.

Kidney Transplant Patients

Renal transplant recipients who are greater than 1 month out from transplant surgery should not

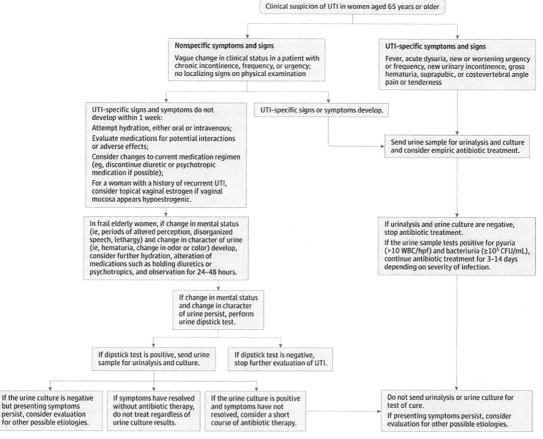

Fig. 1. Clinical algorithm guiding the decision to send urine tests for older cognitively impaired population. (*Reproduced with permission from* JAMA. Feb 26 2014;311(8):844-54. doi:10.1001/jama.2014.303. Copyright © 2014 American Medical Association. All rights reserved, including those for text and data mining, AI training, and similar technologies.)

be screened or treated for ASB.[29] It does not appear that the treatment of ASB greater than 1 month after transplant prevents pyelonephritis or graft rejection.[45,46] Treatment of ASB in this population promotes resistance to antimicrobials, which can compromise response to treatment of symptomatic UTI and other nonurologic infections in these patients.

Solid Organ Transplant Patients (Nonrenal)

Nonrenal solid organ transplant (NRSOT) patients should not be screened for ASB.[29] This recommendation is based on the overall low risk of symptomatic UTI in this population. Reports from a prospective data registry support this notion by presenting low incidence of symptomatic UTI per 1000 patient-days in NRSOT patients with at least 1 year follow-up: 0.06 for 1507 liver transplants, 0.07 for 404 heart transplants, and 0.02 for 303 lung transplants.[47]

Spinal Cord Injury and Neurogenic Bladder Patients with Impaired Voiding

Patients with SCI and lower urinary tract dysfunction (both those with and without indwelling catheters) should not be screened for or treated for ASB, as this population has high prevalence of bacteriuria, and antimicrobial treatment has not been documented to improve outcomes.[29,48] Moreover, research has identified early recurrence of bacteriuria in patients treated with antibiotics for ASB. Unsurprisingly, the recurring uropathogens often carry higher antimicrobial resistance.[49] Together, these findings support the recommendation against screening for and treating ASB in this patient population. Furthermore, there are RCT data to suggest that nonpathogenic E coli bacteriuria is protective against symptomatic UTI in patients with neurogenic bladder, again supporting the recommendation against treating ASB and eradicating what may serve as protective bacteria.[50,51]

Due to impaired or heightened sensation, and frequent genitourinary symptoms at baseline in patients with neurogenic bladder/SCI, distinguishing between ASB and UTI is challenging, and these patients are often misdiagnosed.[29,52] A retrospective cohort study published in 2024[53] evaluated ASB and UTI management in 291 patients with neurogenic bladder and described factors associated with inappropriate treatment. The researchers found that nearly half of the patient encounters were managed inappropriately, mostly due to false UTI diagnoses in patients with ASB. Of note, SCI patients with *symptomatic* UTI may present with typical or atypical symptoms including fever, malaise, lethargy, new or worsening leaking around an indwelling catheter or urinary incontinence, spasticity, cloudy or malodorous urine, back pain, dysuria, or autonomic dysreflexia.[29,54] It is important to consider these symptoms when differentiating between ASB and symptomatic UTI in this patient population, as inappropriate treatment with antibiotics is not without consequence.

Patients Undergoing Elective Nonurologic Surgery

Patients undergoing nonurologic elective surgery should not be screened or treated for ASB. Over the last several decades, research has concluded that preoperative ASB is not a risk factor for postoperative complications, including surgical site infections.[55–57]

In particular, the impact of ASB on surgical site and joint infections after orthopedic implant surgery is widely studied. Specifically, a multicenter, multinational study by Sousa and colleagues[58] not only reported the prevalence of ASB among 2497 hip and knee arthroplasty patients but also evaluated the association between ASB and joint infection and assessed whether preoperative antibiotics reduced the risk of postoperative joint infection.

The study found a significantly higher joint infection rate in the group with preoperative ASB (4.3%) compared to those without bacteriuria (1.4%); however, the treatment of ASB did not significantly alter the development of postoperative joint infections. Specifically, a nonrandomized cohort of the ASB group was treated preoperatively with antibiotics, and postoperative joint infections were compared. Interestingly, the rate of joint infection between the treated (3.9%) and nontreated (4.7%) groups was not statistically significant, highlighting that preoperative antimicrobial treatment of ASB did not mitigate the risk of postoperative joint infection. Notably, the pathogens isolated from the postoperative implant infections differed from the pathogens found in the preoperative urine culture, raising suspicion for a nonurinary source for the infection.[58,59] The investigators postulate that these patients with ASB and postop joint infections are, at baseline, at a higher risk of developing infection than the perioperative patients without ASB. In other words, ASB may serve as a surrogate marker for having bacteria colonized elsewhere. As such, the recommendation is to *not* treat ASB prior to joint surgery.[58]

Furthermore, a 2017 study by Lamb and colleagues[60] found that the presence of ASB was not associated with the incidence of prosthetic joint infections and as such, preoperative urine cultures prior to orthopedic implant surgery were unnecessary. This study also found a potential savings of approximately US$20,000 per year for the health care system if preoperative urine cultures were not processed for these patients.[61]

Patients Undergoing Endourological Procedures

ASB in patients undergoing endoscopic urologic procedures associated with mucosal trauma should be treated prior to surgery. Preoperative urine should be collected and urine cultures should be performed, and culture-specific antibiotics should be administered, given that ASB is an established risk factor for infection in urologic procedures. Interestingly, infection risk varies based on the type of procedure performed.[62,63] Specifically, procedures in which the mucosa is violated carry a high risk of infectious complications and, thus, warrant antibiotic treatment. On the other hand, diagnostic or simple urologic procedures such as a catheter exchange, diagnostic cystoscopy, or urodynamics carry a low risk of infectious complications and do not require antimicrobial treatment.[62–64]

Findings from RCTs from the 1980s provide the foundation for the recommendation to treat ASB in patients prior to endoscopic urologic procedures associated with mucosal trauma. Grabe and colleagues[65] reported rates of elimination of ASB and rates of postoperative upper UTI for patients undergoing a transurethral resection of the prostate. Higher rates of elimination of ASB and lower rates of upper UTI were seen in patients treated with antibiotics compared to controls.

More recent evidence suggests that single-dose preoperative treatment of ASB is likely effective and associated with fewer adverse effects, shorter length of stay, and decreased patient anxiety compared to a multiple-dose regimen. An RCT published in 2012[66] evaluated the outcomes for 59 patients undergoing urothelium disrupting urologic procedures receiving long-term antibiotics (beginning 3 days prior to procedure and continuing for 15 days after procedure) or one preoperative antibiotic dose. Patients in the single-dose group were given a second dose if a catheter was placed postoperatively. Interestingly, no participants developed postoperative sepsis or upper UTI, regardless of antibiotic treatment status. Furthermore, a single dose of antibiotics was associated with decreased length of stay, decreased cost of antibiotic therapy, and subsequent isolation of fewer resistant microorganisms when compared to the longer course.[66]

Another RCT published in 2015[67] compared rates of postoperative UTI among patients with SCI undergoing elective endourologic proceudres. The subjects were randomized to a group receiving a single dose of pre procedural antibiotics 30 minutes prior to procedure (35 patients) or to a group that was given 3 to 5 days of preprocedural antibiotic treatment (25 patients). The frequency of post procedural UTI between groups was not significantly different. However, the authors found that the single dose antibiotic group was associated with lower cost to the patient, and lower pre-procedural anxiety, when compared to the 3 to 5 day antibiotic group.

SUMMARY AND FUTURE DIRECTIONS

In summary, ASB, defined as a noncontaminated urine sample with greater than 100,000 CFUs in the absence of illness or symptoms, is common in healthy women, the elderly, patients with neurogenic bladder or SCI, and patients with genitourinary tract abnormalities. Generally, ASB should not be treated, unless the affected person is a pregnant woman, or a patient undergoing a urologic procedure where the urothelium will be violated. When indicated, ASB should be treated with urine culture-specific antibiotics. Critically, inappropriate treatment of ASB can foster antibiotic resistance, increase health care costs, and may even predispose patients to future symptomatic UTI.

Screening and treatment guidelines pertaining to ASB have evolved over time. What was once a presumed pathologic condition warranting treatment, later became a benign variation of normal, requiring no treatment (except in certain high-risk populations). Now, we find ourselves researching ways that ASB may be protective against future infections. While there is still much to learn about the urinary microbiome, research into prevention of UTI with the use of avirulent bacteria as "bacterial interference" has emerged over the last several years.[68–70] This is an area of research that has the potential to move the field of UTIs and ASB forward and help our urologic patients with these conditions.

CLINICS CARE POINTS

- ASB is the presence of greater than 100,000 CFUs of bacteria in a noncontaminated urine culture in a person with no signs or symptoms of a UTI.
- Risk factors for ASB include increasing age, female sex, living in long-term care facilities, menopause, diabetes, and catheterization.[9]

- Common pathogens responsible for ASB vary based on the sex, catheter status, and place of living of the patient. In the community, the predominant pathogen isolated in older women with ASB was *E coli*. For men, however, the most common pathogens identified in the urine are gram-negative bacilli, enterococci, and coagulase-negative staphylococci.[12,13] For those adults living in long-term care facilities, and those with indwelling catheters, polymicrobial bacteriuria with *P aeruginosa, M morganii*, and *P stuartii* is most common.[1,14]

- Historically, there was a concern that untreated ASB may lead to the development of multiple sequelae including UTI, however a 2012 comparative study[17] determined that the presence of ASB was not predictive of future UTI.

- Guidelines recommend against screening for and treating ASB in most populations, excluding pregnant women and patients who are undergoing urologic procedures in which transmucosal bleeding is anticipated.[20]

- A review by Mody and colleagues[42] published in 2014 proposes a clinical algorithm to guide the decision to send urine tests for the older functionally/cognitively impaired patient population (see **Fig. 1**).

- Renal transplant recipients who are greater than 1 month out from transplant surgery should not be screened or treated for ASB.[29] It does not appear that the treatment of ASB greater than 1 month after transplant prevents pyelonephritis or graft rejection.[45,46]

- Patients undergoing nonurologic elective surgery should not be screened or treated for ASB. Over the last several decades, research has concluded that preoperative ASB is not a risk factor for postoperative complications, including surgical site infections.[55–57]

- Patients with SCI and lower urinary tract dysfunction (both those with and without indwelling catheters) should not be screened for or treated for ASB, as this population has high prevalence of bacteriuria, and antimicrobial treatment has not been documented to improve outcomes.[29,48]

- Patients with ASB and postorthopedic surgery joint infections are, at baseline, at a higher risk of developing infection than the perioperative patients without ASB. ASB may serve as a surrogate marker for having bacteria colonized elsewhere. As such, the recommendation is to *not* treat ASB prior to joint surgery.[58]

- ASB in patients undergoing endoscopic urologic procedures associated with mucosal trauma should be treated prior to surgery.

DISCLOSURE

None.
    There are no conflicts of interest or funding.

REFERENCES

1. Nicolle LE, Bradley S, Colgan R, et al. Infectious Diseases Society of America guidelines for the diagnosis and treatment of asymptomatic bacteriuria in adults. Clin Infect Dis 2005;40(5):643–54.
2. Nicolle LE. Asymptomatic bacteriuria: when to screen and when to treat. Infect Dis Clin North Am 2003;17(2):367–94.
3. Lipsky BA. Urinary tract infections in men. epidemiology, pathophysiology, diagnosis, and treatment. Ann Intern Med 1989;110(2):138–50.
4. Nicolle LE. Asymptomatic bacteriuria in the elderly. Infect Dis Clin North Am 1997;11(3):647–62.
5. Kunin CM, McCormack RC. An epidemiologic study of bacteriuria and blood pressure among nuns and working women. N Engl J Med 1968;278(12):635–42.
6. Harding GKM, Zhanel GG, Nicolle LE, et al. Antimicrobial treatment in diabetic women with asymptomatic bacteriuria. N Engl J Med 2002;347(20):1576–83.
7. Bakke A, Digranes A. Bacteriuria in patients treated with clean intermittent catheterization. Scand J Infect Dis 1991;23(5):577–82.
8. Warren JW, Tenney JH, Hoopes JM, et al. A prospective microbiologic study of bacteriuria in patients with chronic indwelling urethral catheters. J Infect Dis 1982;146(6):719–23.
9. Colgan R, Nicolle LE, McGlone A, et al. Asymptomatic bacteriuria in adults. Am Fam Physician 2006;74(6):985–90.
10. Linhares I, Raposo T, Rodrigues A, et al. Frequency and antimicrobial resistance patterns of bacteria implicated in community urinary tract infections: a ten-year surveillance study (2000-2009). BMC Infect Dis 2013;13:19.
11. Svanborg C, Godaly G. Bacterial virulence in urinary tract infection. Infect Dis Clin North Am 1997;11(3):513–29.
12. Lipsky BA, Inui TS, Plorde JJ, et al. Is the clean-catch midstream void procedure necessary for obtaining urine culture specimens from men? Am J Med 1984;76(2):257–62.
13. Mims AD, Norman DC, Yamamura RH, et al. Clinically inapparent (asymptomatic) bacteriuria in ambulatory elderly men: epidemiological, clinical, and microbiological findings. J Am Geriatr Soc 1990;38(11):1209–14.
14. Nicolle LE. Urinary tract infections in long-term care facilities. Infect Control Hosp Epidemiol 1993;14(4):220–5.
15. Bengtsson C, Bengtsson U, Bjorkelund C, et al. Bacteriuria in a population sample of women: 24-

year follow-up study. Results from the prospective population-based study of women in Gothenburg, Sweden. Scand J Urol Nephrol 1998;32(4):284–9.

16. Tencer J. Asymptomatic bacteriuria–a long-term study. Scand J Urol Nephrol 1988;22(1):31–4.

17. Beerepoot MA, den Heijer CD, Penders J, et al. Predictive value of Escherichia coli susceptibility in strains causing asymptomatic bacteriuria for women with recurrent symptomatic urinary tract infections receiving prophylaxis. Clin Microbiol Infect 2012;18(4):E84–90.

18. Cai T, Mazzoli S, Mondaini N, et al. The role of asymptomatic bacteriuria in young women with recurrent urinary tract infections: to treat or not to treat? Clin Infect Dis 2012;55(6):771–7.

19. Cai T, Nesi G, Mazzoli S, et al. Asymptomatic bacteriuria treatment is associated with a higher prevalence of antibiotic resistant strains in women with urinary tract infections. Clin Infect Dis 2015;61(11):1655–61.

20. Nicolle LE. Updated guidelines for screening for asymptomatic bacteriuria. JAMA 2019;322(12):1152–4.

21. Lin K, Fajardo K, U.S. Preventive Services Task Force. Screening for asymptomatic bacteriuria in adults: evidence for the U.S. Preventive Services Task Force reaffirmation recommendation statement. Ann Intern Med 2008;149(1):W20–4.

22. Owens DK, Davidson KW, Krist AH, et al. Screening for asymptomatic bacteriuria in adults: us preventive services task force recommendation statement. JAMA 2019;322(12):1188–94.

23. Zalmanovici Trestioreanu A, Lador A, Sauerbrun-Cutler MT, et al. Antibiotics for asymptomatic bacteriuria. Cochrane Database Syst Rev 2015;4(4):CD009534.

24. Asscher AW, Sussman M, Waters WE, et al. Asymptomatic significant bacteriuria in the non-pregnant woman. II. response to treatment and follow-up. Br Med J 1969;1(5647):804–6.

25. Kemper KJ, Avner ED. The case against screening urinalyses for asymptomatic bacteriuria in children. Am J Dis Child 1992;146(3):343–6.

26. Patterson TF, Andriole VT. Detection, significance, and therapy of bacteriuria in pregnancy. update in the managed health care era. Infect Dis Clin North Am 1997;11(3):593–608.

27. Smaill FM, Vazquez JC. Antibiotics for asymptomatic bacteriuria in pregnancy. Cochrane Database Syst Rev 2015;(8):Cd000490.

28. Kazemier BM, Koningstein FN, Schneeberger C, et al. Maternal and neonatal consequences of treated and untreated asymptomatic bacteriuria in pregnancy: a prospective cohort study with an embedded randomised controlled trial. Lancet Infect Dis 2015;15(11):1324–33.

29. Nicolle LE, Gupta K, Bradley SF, et al. Clinical practice guideline for the management of asymptomatic bacteriuria: 2019 update by the infectious diseases society of America. Clin Infect Dis 2019;68(10):e83–110.

30. Widmer M, Lopez I, Gülmezoglu AM, et al. Duration of treatment for asymptomatic bacteriuria during pregnancy. Cochrane Database Syst Rev 2015;2015(11):Cd000491.

31. Lumbiganon P, Villar J, Laopaiboon M, et al. One-day compared with 7-day nitrofurantoin for asymptomatic bacteriuria in pregnancy: a randomized controlled trial. Obstet Gynecol 2009;113(2 Pt 1):339–45.

32. Nicolle LE, Mayhew WJ, Bryan L. Prospective randomized comparison of therapy and no therapy for asymptomatic bacteriuria in institutionalized elderly women. Am J Med 1987;83(1):27–33.

33. Nicolle LE, Bjornson J, Harding GK, et al. Bacteriuria in elderly institutionalized men. N Engl J Med 1983;309(23):1420–5.

34. Boscia JA, Kobasa WD, Knight RA, et al. Therapy vs no therapy for bacteriuria in elderly ambulatory nonhospitalized women. JAMA 1987;257(8):1067–71.

35. Abrutyn E, Mossey J, Berlin JA, et al. Does asymptomatic bacteriuria predict mortality and does antimicrobial treatment reduce mortality in elderly ambulatory women? Ann Intern Med 1994;120(10):827–33.

36. Ouslander JG, Schapira M, Schnelle JF, et al. Does eradicating bacteriuria affect the severity of chronic urinary incontinence in nursing home residents? Ann Intern Med 1995;122(10):749–54.

37. D'Agata E, Loeb MB, Mitchell SL. Challenges in assessing nursing home residents with advanced dementia for suspected urinary tract infections. J Am Geriatr Soc 2013;61(1):62–6.

38. Loeb M, Bentley DW, Bradley S, et al. Development of minimum criteria for the initiation of antibiotics in residents of long-term-care facilities: results of a consensus conference. Infect Control Hosp Epidemiol 2001;22(2):120–4.

39. Stone ND, Ashraf MS, Calder J, et al. Surveillance definitions of infections in long-term care facilities: revisiting the McGeer criteria. Infect Control Hosp Epidemiol 2012;33(10):965–77.

40. Dufour AB, Shaffer ML, D'Agata EM, et al. Survival after suspected urinary tract infection in individuals with advanced dementia. J Am Geriatr Soc 2015;63(12):2472–7.

41. Rotjanapan P, Dosa D, Thomas KS. Potentially inappropriate treatment of urinary tract infections in two Rhode Island nursing homes. Arch Intern Med 2011;171(5):438–43.

42. Mody L, Juthani-Mehta M. Urinary tract infections in older women: a clinical review. JAMA 2014;311(8):844–54.

43. Geerlings SE, Stolk RP, Camps MJ, et al. Consequences of asymptomatic bacteriuria in women with diabetes mellitus. Arch Intern Med 2001;161(11):1421–7.

44. Semetkowska-Jurkiewicz E, Horoszek-Maziarz S, Galiński J, et al. The clinical course of untreated asymptomatic bacteriuria in diabetic patients–14-year follow-up. Mater Med Pol 1995;27(3):91–5.

45. Moradi M, Abbasi M, Moradi A, et al. Effect of antibiotic therapy on asymptomatic bacteriuria in kidney transplant recipients. Urol J 2005;2(1):32–5.

46. Origüen J, López-Medrano F, Fernández-Ruiz M, et al. Should asymptomatic bacteriuria be systematically treated in kidney transplant recipients? results from a randomized controlled trial. Am J Transplant 2016; 16(10):2943–53.

47. Vidal E, Torre-Cisneros J, Blanes M, et al. Bacterial urinary tract infection after solid organ transplantation in the RESITRA cohort. Transpl Infect Dis 2012;14(6):595–603.

48. Luu T, Albarillo FS. Asymptomatic bacteriuria: prevalence, diagnosis, management, and current antimicrobial stewardship implementations. Am J Med 2022;135(8):e236–44.

49. Waites KB, Canupp KC, DeVivo MJ. Eradication of urinary tract infection following spinal cord injury. Paraplegia 1993;31(10):645–52.

50. Darouiche RO, Thornby JI, Cerra-Stewart C, et al. Bacterial interference for prevention of urinary tract infection: a prospective, randomized, placebo-controlled, double-blind pilot trial. Clin Infect Dis 2005;41(10): 1531–4.

51. Sundén F, Håkansson L, Ljunggren E, et al. Escherichia coli 83972 bacteriuria protects against recurrent lower urinary tract infections in patients with incomplete bladder emptying. J Urol 2010;184(1): 179–85.

52. Dinh A, Davido B, Duran C, et al. Urinary tract infections in patients with neurogenic bladder. Med Mal Infect 2019;49(7):495–504.

53. Fitzpatrick MA, Wirth M, Burns SP, et al. Management of asymptomatic bacteriuria and urinary tract infections in patients with neurogenic bladder and factors associated with inappropriate diagnosis and treatment. Arch Phys Med Rehabil 2024;105(1):112–9.

54. Goetz LL, Cardenas DD, Kennelly M, et al. International spinal cord injury urinary tract infection basic data set. Spinal Cord 2013;51(9):700–4.

55. Irvine R, Johnson BL Jr, Amstutz HC. The relationship of genitourinary tract procedures and deep sepsis after total hip replacements. Surg Gynecol Obstet 1974;139(5):701–6.

56. David TS, Vrahas MS. Perioperative lower urinary tract infections and deep sepsis in patients undergoing total joint arthroplasty. J Am Acad Orthop Surg 2000;8(1):66–74.

57. Ollivere BJ, Ellahee N, Logan K, et al. Asymptomatic urinary tract colonisation predisposes to superficial wound infection in elective orthopaedic surgery. Int Orthop 2009;33(3):847–50.

58. Sousa R, Muñoz-Mahamud E, Quayle J, et al. Is asymptomatic bacteriuria a risk factor for prosthetic joint infection? Clin Infect Dis 2014;59(1):41–7.

59. Drekonja DM, Zarmbinski B, Johnson JR. Preoperative urine cultures at a veterans affairs medical center. JAMA Intern Med 2013;173(1):71–2.

60. Lamb MJ, Baillie L, Pajak D, et al. Elimination of screening urine cultures prior to elective joint arthroplasty. Clin Infect Dis 2017;64(6):806–9.

61. Soltanzadeh M, Ebadi A. Is presence of bacteria in preoperative microscopic urinalysis of the patients scheduled for cardiac surgery a reason for cancellation of elective operation? Anesth Pain Med 2013; 2(4):174–7.

62. Grabe M. Antimicrobial agents in transurethral prostatic resection. J Urol 1987;138(2):245–52.

63. Rao PN, Dube DA, Weightman NC, et al. Prediction of septicemia following endourological manipulation for stones in the upper urinary tract. J Urol 1991; 146(4):955–60.

64. Lightner DJ, Wymer K, Sanchez J, et al. Best practice statement on urologic procedures and antimicrobial prophylaxis. J Urol 2020;203:351.

65. Grabe M, Forsgren A, Hellsten S. The effect of a short antibiotic course in transurethral prostatic resection. Scand J Urol Nephrol 1984;18(1):37–42.

66. Sayin Kutlu S, Aybek Z, Tekin K, et al. Is short course of antimicrobial therapy for asymptomatic bacteriuria before urologic surgical procedures sufficient? J Infect Dev Ctries 2012;6(2):143–7.

67. Chong JT, Klausner AP, Petrossian A, et al. Pre-procedural antibiotics for endoscopic urological procedures: Initial experience in individuals with spinal cord injury and asymptomatic bacteriuria. J Spinal Cord Med 2015;38(2):187–92.

68. Reid G, Howard J, Gan BS. Can bacterial interference prevent infection? Trends Microbiol 2001;9(9): 424–8.

69. Nicolle LE. The paradigm shift to non-treatment of asymptomatic bacteriuria. Pathogens 2016;5(2):38.

70. Darouiche RO, Hull RA. Bacterial interference for prevention of urinary tract infection. Clin Infect Dis 2012;55(10):1400–7.

71. Zhanel GG, Harding GK, Nicolle LE. Asymptomatic bacteriuria in patients with diabetes mellitus. Rev Infect Dis 1991;13(1):150–4.

72. Chaudhry A, Stone WJ, Breyer JA. Occurrence of pyuria and bacteriuria in asymptomatic hemodialysis patients. Am J Kidney Dis 1993;21(2):180–3.

73. Stamm WE. Catheter-associated urinary tract infections: epidemiology, pathogenesis, and prevention. Am J Med 1991;91(3B):65S–71S.

Advances in the Treatment of Urinary Tract Infection and Bacteriuria in Pregnancy

Allison Grant, MD*, Ketty Bai, BS, Gina M. Badalato, MD,
Matthew P. Rutman, MD

KEYWORDS

- Asymptomatic bacteriuria • Urinary tract infection • Pregnancy • Pyelonephritis
- Antibiotics in pregnancy

KEY POINTS

- In pregnant women, the prevalence of asymptomatic bacteriuria (ASB) is 2% to 10%, urinary tract infection (UTI) is 1% to 4%, and pyelonephritis is 1% to 4%, with *Escherichia coli* being responsible for a vast majority (49%–85%) of these UTIs.
- Midstream, clean-catch urine culture early in pregnancy is the gold standard for ASB screening, as well as the preferred test for UTI diagnosis (greater than 10^5 colony forming units/mL of urine).
- Maternal complications from ASB and UTI include pyelonephritis, preterm birth, and pre-eclampsia with some data challenging the notion that ASB specifically increases risk of preterm birth. Historically, maternal UTI and ASB in pregnancy were thought to put the fetus/newborn at a risk for intrauterine growth restriction and low birth weight. However, recent research has refuted this association.
- In general, the treatment course for cystitis and ASB is 5 to 7 days, whereas treatment for pyelonephritis warrants intravenous antibiotics and a 14 day course.

INTRODUCTION
Background

Urinary tract infection (UTI) is defined as a symptomatic infection of the urinary bladder and/or kidney, known as cystitis and pyelonephritis, respectively. Common symptoms include dysuria, urgency, frequency, suprapubic discomfort, and hematuria. Asymptomatic bacteriuria (ASB), on the other hand, refers to the presence of bacteria in urine without signs of infection or associated urinary symptoms.[1] UTIs in women usually occur due to an ascending infection of pathogenic bacteria naturally residing in the lower GI and genitourinary tract, most commonly *Escherichia coli* (*E. coli*).[2] Uncomplicated, or simple UTI, refers to cystitis in non-pregnant, afebrile, immunocompetent women with no anatomic or functional abnormalities of the genital tract. Complicated UTI refers to urinary infection of an individual with at least 1 factor that increases the risk of acquiring UTI, or decreases the efficacy of therapy, such as pregnancy, male gender, immunocompromized status, and anatomic or functional abnormalities of the genital tract.[3] As such, all UTIs in pregnancy are categorized as complicated.

During pregnancy, the urinary tract undergoes significant anatomic and physiologic changes as early as 7 weeks gestation, which may put these women at risk of developing ASB and/or UTI. Hormonal changes such as elevated progesterone lead to urothelial smooth muscle relaxation, resulting in decreased ureteral peristalsis and decreased bladder tone. The resulting ureteral dilation and increased bladder capacity may allow for urinary

Department of Urology, 161 Fort Washington Avenue, 11th floor, New York, NY 10032, USA
* Corresponding author.
E-mail address: ALG2247@cumc.columbia.edu

Urol Clin N Am 51 (2024) 571–583
https://doi.org/10.1016/j.ucl.2024.07.001
0094-0143/24/© 2024 Elsevier Inc. All rights are reserved, including those for text and data mining, AI training, and similar technologies.

stasis and create a pathway for bacteria to ascend the urinary tract.[1,4,5] Furthermore, as the gravid uterus grows, it displaces the bladder antero-superiorly and can mechanically obstruct the ureter(s) at the pelvic brim. This dextrorotated uterus can also result in right-sided physiologic hydronephrosis of pregnancy.[6] Collectively, these anatomic and physiologic changes may increase the risk of UTI pathogenesis or urinary colonization.

During prenatal care, screening for ASB and monitoring for UTIs are important, as untreated infections can have adverse implications for maternal and fetal health. Both of these conditions have specifically been linked to maternal pyelonephritis/urosepsis, preterm labor, low birth weight, prematurity, and neonatal sepsis.[7,8] While fetal complications often arise as a consequence of maternal pyelonephritis/urosepsis, it is noteworthy that literature has documented these complications may exist even in the absence of such maternal conditions.[9,10] Herein, we provide an up-to-date review of the presentation and diagnosis, complications, and management of asymptomatic bacteriuria and UTIs in pregnancy.

Epidemiology of Urinary Tract Infections and Bacteriuria in Pregnancy

Prevalence and incidence

Due to the anatomic and physiologic changes in pregnancy that facilitate bacterial growth and colonization in the urinary tract, the incidence and prevalence of UTIs tend to increase in pregnancy. Prevalence of ASB in the general population is found to be the highest in women, with 1% to 6% prevalence in pre-menopausal non-pregnant women compared to 2% to 10% prevalence in pregnant women. More recently, a 2023 systematic review and meta-analysis reviewed 27 studies involving 30,641 pregnant women, determining the prevalence of symptomatic and ASB in this population to be 23.9%.[11] Furthermore, pregnant women are less likely to have spontaneous resolution of bacteriuria and are more likely to progress to UTI.[12] The prevalence of acute cystitis is reported in the literature to range from 1% to 4% in pregnant women.[13–17]

When ASB is untreated in pregnancy, 15% to 45% of patients go on to develop pyelonephritis. Pyelonephritis occurs in 1% to 4% of all pregnancies and is the most common non-obstetric cause of hospitalization during pregnancy in the United States (US). Conversely, in non-pregnant, healthy individuals, ASB can frequently spontaneously resolve without any associated long-term adverse outcomes.[18,19]

Risk factors during pregnancy

Risk factors that propagate urinary pathogenesis in the general population have been well-documented in the literature. These variables include childhood infections, dehydration, constipation, and voiding dysfunction.[20–22] While pregnant women have many of the same risk factors as their non-pregnant counterparts, the physiologic changes seen in pregnancy can put pregnant patients at greater risk.[20,23] This is supported by evidence that pyelonephritis is most common in the third trimester when the urinary tract changes are most significant,[24] with an estimated 50% to 90% of pregnant women demonstrating physiologic hydronephrosis by this time.[4]

Studies have also found certain demographic characteristics to be associated with increased risk of UTI in pregnancy. Historically, it was believed that lower socioeconomic status, multiparity, diabetes mellitus, and sickle cell trait were associated with an increased risk of UTI in pregnancy.[25] However, a 2006 study found no difference in rates of cystitis and ASB in pregnant women with sickle cell trait when compared to those without.[26] Furthermore, studies report inconsistent conclusions when evaluating the association of multiparity and low socioeconomic status with UTIs in pregnancy.[1,27] A recent retrospective study using the data from the National Birth Defects Prevention Study found the prevalence of UTIs was highest among women younger than 19 years of age at conception, those who self-reported American Indian or Alaska Native ethnicity, had low educational attainment, and those with an annual household income less than $10,000.[2]

Another risk factor for ASB or UTI in pregnancy is gestational diabetes mellitus. Notably, a 2023 meta-analysis[28] of 16 studies involving over 1.5 million pregnant women with gestational diabetes and their healthy counterparts investigated the association of gestational diabetes with infections during pregnancy. The study concluded that there was a significant association between gestational diabetes mellitus and the development of UTIs during pregnancy.

Microbiology of Urinary Tract Infection and Bacteriuria in Pregnancy

Common causative microorganisms

Unsurprisingly, the organisms responsible for UTI and bacteriuria in pregnancy are the same uropathogens that often colonize the urine and/or cause infections in non-pregnant women (**Table 1**). The most common causative pathogen is E. coli. Other gram-negative species such as Klebsiella,

Table 1
Common causative microorganisms of urinary tract infection and bacteriuria in pregnancy

Type of Microbe	Microorganisms	Comments
Gram-negative	*Escherichia coli*	• Most common causative microorganism • Found in GI tract and fecal flora
	Klebsiella pneumoniae	• Increased risk of struvite kidney stones • Found in GI tract and fecal flora
	Proteus mirabilis	• Increased risk of struvite kidney stones
	Pseudomonas spp	• Increased risk of struvite kidney stones
Gram-positive	Group B *Streptococcus*	• Most common gram-positive causative microorganism • If untreated, may cause neonatal sepsis and obstetric complications (preterm labor, preterm delivery)
	Enterococcus spp	• Found in GI tract • Majority of infections due to *E. faecalis* and *E. faecium*
	Staphylococcus saprophyticus	• Common cause of uncomplicated UTIs in young, sexually active women • Found in normal genitourinary and GI tract flora
	Staphylococcus aureus	• Uncommon cause of UTI

Abbreviations: GI, gastrointestinal; UTI, urinary tract infection.

Proteus, and *Enterobacter* are also frequently isolated. Gram-positive species such as *Enterococcus*, *Staphylococcus*, and *Streptococcus* are less commonly identified in the urine.[1,16,29]

E. coli, a gram-negative organism originating in the GI tract and fecal flora, often colonizes the peri-urethral area. Herein, *E. coli* has ascending access into the genitourinary tract, making for a conducive environment for urinary colonization or infection. It is responsible for a vast majority of UTIs in pregnancy, ranging from 49% to 85%.[1,16,30–32]

Gram-positive organisms, most often group B *Streptococcus* (GBS), comprise roughly 10% of UTIs in pregnancy. Additional data reveal that substantial GBS titers are present in the urine of 7% of pregnant women.[1,33,34] GBS, like *E. coli*, is frequently detected in the GI flora. GBS may also be found in the reproductive tract of all females, serving as yet another source for GBS colonization. Moreover, a meta-analysis featured in *The Lancet Global Health* reported that, in the year 2020, an estimated 19.7 million pregnant women worldwide were identified as carriers of GBS.[33,35]

GBS identification in urine or rectovaginal flora peri-partum is critical, as GBS colonization can cause neonatal sepsis and is associated with several obstetric complications such as preterm rupture of membranes, preterm labor, and preterm delivery.[16] Neonatal GBS colonization or infection occurs when GBS is vertically transmitted from the mother to the baby as it passes through the vaginal canal during delivery, making screening for GBS colonization essential. The American College of Obstetricians and Gynecologists (ACOG) recommends GBS screening with a recto-vaginal swab between 36 weeks and 37 weeks 6 days gestation. Intrapartum antibiotic prophylaxis, most often penicillin or amoxicillin, unless an allergy is present, is given to reduce the risk of transmission to the baby at birth.[16,36] Antibiotic prophylaxis is indicated in mothers with GBS positive recto-vaginal swabs, GBS bacteriuria during the pregnancy, or history of neonate with invasive GBS disease. If a laboring patient has unknown GBS status, intrapartum prophylaxis is given in the presence of certain risk factors such as preterm labor, amniotic membrane rupture for more than 18 h, and intrapartum temperature greater than 100.4°F.[36]

Impact of nephrolithiasis on bacteriuria/urinary tract infection

Colonization or infection with urease-splitting bacteria such as *Klebsiella*, *Proteus*, *Pseudomonas*, or certain *Staphylococcus* species can cause urinary alkalization and struvite stone formation. Conversely, the presence of kidney stones in pregnancy has been associated with an increase in the risk of UTI and bacterial persistence and reinfection.[37,38] A systematic review and meta-analysis of 4.7 million pregnancies across North America, Europe, Asia, and Africa, determined the pooled incidence of renal stones in pregnancy to be

0.49%. The analysis revealed a significant association between renal stones and the development of preeclampsia and UTIs (ASB, cystitis, and pyelonephritis).[37] Moreover, contemporary studies have reported that approximately 33% to 50% of pregnant women with stones will suffer from UTIs.[38,39]

Clinical Presentation and Diagnosis

Signs and symptoms of urinary tract infections in pregnant women

The signs and symptoms of UTI in pregnant women are similar to those in non-pregnant women. Whereas ASB, by definition, presents without symptoms, acute cystitis most often presents with symptoms such as suprapubic discomfort, dysuria, urgency, frequency, nocturia, and hematuria. It is important to note that these symptoms may result from physiologic changes in pregnancy and therefore must be accompanied by a positive urine culture to qualify as an UTI.[13] Patients with acute cystitis are afebrile, with no signs of systemic illness. Acute pyelonephritis, on the other hand, may present with systemic symptoms such as fever, nausea, vomiting, and chills, as well as flank pain. In acute pyelonephritis, the symptoms of acute cystitis may or may not be present.[16]

Screening and diagnosis of urinary tract infections in pregnancy

The routine screening of ASB in pregnancy is recommended by major guidelines from North America, South America, Australia, and most of Europe. The Infectious Diseases Society of America,[40] US Preventive Services Task Force (USPSTF),[18] and ACOG[13] currently recommend a midstream, clean-catch urine culture early in pregnancy as the gold standard for ASB screening. Notably, the USPSTF downgraded its recommendation from A to B level in 2019 due to increasing concerns of antimicrobial resistance, potential adverse effects of antibiotics on the microbiome, and lack of recent clinical trials studying the use of updated antibiotic regimens.[18]

A quantitative urine culture is the test used to diagnose UTI,[41] with a threshold of 10^5 colony forming units (CFU) per mL of urine. In studying urinalysis as a screening tool, nitrites have been found to be the most specific dipstick finding for UTIs in pregnant women. However, a recent study found that among its cohort of pregnant women with significant bacteriuria, none had positive nitrites. It hypothesized that nitrites may better indicate ongoing UTI rather than ASB.[42]

Other patient-specific variables may affect the accuracy of urinary diagnostic testing. A study of pregnant women found that increased body mass index provided a significantly increased risk of contaminated urine samples; this same study found that, on multivariable analysis, maternal age, gestational stage, and parity did not significantly increase risk of contamination.[43]

DISCUSSION
Complications and Risks

The significance of UTI and ASB during pregnancy lies in their potential to give rise to complications for both the mother and the fetus/newborn.

Maternal complications

UTIs, as well as ASB, put pregnant women at risk for pyelonephritis, pre-eclampsia, preterm labor, and septic shock.[1,5,16,30]

Pyelonephritis

Acute pyelonephritis, an ascending bacterial UTI causing inflammation of the kidneys, most often presents with fever, flank pain, costovertebral angle tenderness, and urinary symptoms, with or without associated nausea and vomiting. Similar to the general population, pregnant women with pyelonephritis are at risk of developing sepsis and acute kidney injury. However, pregnant women with pyelonephritis are at an additional increased risk of developing disseminated intravascular coagulation, anemia, acute respiratory distress syndrome, and preterm birth.[5,19,30,44]

The incidence of acute pyelonephritis in pregnancy varies by source and ranges from 0.5% to 4%.[19,30,44,45] Women are most affected in the second or third trimesters, with first trimester infection comprising only 10% to 20% of cases.[30,44] Data show that pregnant women with untreated first trimester ASB are more likely to develop pyelonephritis, relative to their ASB negative counterparts. Specifically, a prospective cohort study with an embedded randomized control trial found the incidence of pyelonephritis to be 2.4% in the ASB group and 0.6% in the ASB negative group.[46] These findings support treating ASB in pregnant women. Furthermore, a 2014 18-year retrospective cohort study reported an association between pyelonephritis in pregnancy with Black race and Hispanic ethnicity, young age, lower education level, nulliparous status, delayed access to prenatal care, and history of smoking during pregnancy.[30]

Preterm labor

In the past, untreated ASB had a known association with preterm labor, likely due to the predisposition to developing pyelonephritis.[1,5,16,30] However, contemporary studies raise skepticism on this association. After the introduction of screening for ASB, the USPSTF systematically reviewed outcomes in pregnant women. Of the 6 studies that reported on differences in preterm birth between those treated and untreated for ASB, 3 reported a decrease in preterm births with antibiotic treatment, while 3 studies reported no significant difference in delivery outcomes.[47] Furthermore, a 2015 prospective cohort study/randomized controlled trial[46] found there was no significant change in preterm delivery at less than 34 weeks between the ASB positive and ASB negative group.

Unsurprisingly, data support that UTIs, rather than ASB, in pregnancy increase the likelihood of preterm labor.[1,5,16,31] A retrospective cohort study published in 2021 evaluated the risk of preterm (<37 weeks) and early term (37 and 38 weeks) birth among women seen in a hospital for UTI. The researchers found that pregnant women with an UTI diagnosis had a 1.4 times greater risk of preterm delivery.[48]

Clearly, the current data continue to support the notion that symptomatic UTI in pregnancy increases risk of preterm labor, upholding the indication to treat pregnant women in this scenario. On the contrary, contemporary data question the previously established belief that ASB increases risk of preterm labor. The treatment of ASB in pregnancy, as it relates to preterm birth, remains an active area of research.

Preeclampsia

Pre-eclampsia is a condition characterized by proteinuria and hypertension (blood pressure >140/90 mm Hg) after 20 weeks gestation. The diagnosis carries high maternal and fetal or newborn morbidity and has historically been associated with UTI and ASB in pregnancy. Recent research has found that women with pre-eclampsia are 6.8 and 7.7 times more likely to have significant bacteriuria than those without pre-eclampsia.[49,50] Furthermore, a 2018 meta-analysis[51] utilizing 19 observational studies on UTI (defined as a positive urine culture regardless of symptoms) and pre-eclampsia upheld prior literature findings. The meta-analysis found UTI to be a risk factor for development of pre-eclampsia, with a pooled odds ratio of 1.31.

Fetal and neonatal complications

In terms of risks to the fetus, UTI and ASB have been associated with prematurity, low birth weight, and neonatal sepsis. As discussed earlier, UTI and ASB predispose the mother and fetus to preterm birth, and therefore, any complication that may result from prematurity.

Low birth weight

Historically, maternal UTI and ASB in pregnancy were thought to put the fetus/newborn at risk for intrauterine growth restriction and low birth weight,[16,47,52] an association that has been called into question in recent years. A 2019 study by USPSTF[47] did in fact identify a reduction in the incidence of low birth weight with the implementation of ASB screening (pooled relative risk 0.64; 95% confidence interval, 0.46–0.90), which upholds the existing belief. However, other contemporary studies report the conflicting data. Some report no significant difference in birth weight between neonates of mothers with UTI or ASB and neonates of mothers without UTI or ASB.[9,31]

Neonatal sepsis

Neonatal sepsis, while uncommon, is a feared complication of maternal UTI or ASB in pregnancy. As discussed in an earlier section, newborns of a GBS colonized mother are at increased risk of neonatal sepsis with an incidence of roughly 0.2%.[53] A 2023 prospective cohort study[32] collected urine cultures from 4506 pregnant and non-pregnant women and, among other things, evaluated what factors put neonates at an increased risk for sepsis. Within the group of pregnant women with UTI, E. coli and Klebsiella were the isolated microorganisms. The authors found that the presence of E. coli was significantly associated with neonatal sepsis after cesarean section (C-section) compared to the presence of Klebsiella.[32]

Prevention and Management

Antenatal screening for asymptomatic bacteriuria

While UTIs often present with symptoms, and thus, prompt evaluation with urine culture, ASB is identified by routine screening practices in the absence of symptoms. Per ACOG 2023 guidelines, current practices involve screening with a urine culture just once early on in the pregnancy, with the exact optimal time for culture being unknown.[13,54] Urine culture continues to be the gold standard screening method, as the data have shown other rapid urine screening tests in pregnancy to have poor performance metrics.[54]

Screening for ASB is a widely accepted practice in the US, but it is worthwhile to note that internationally there is still some discrepancy on the topic. An international review of 13 guidelines on management of UTI in pregnancy from 4 continents revealed that 85% (11/13) of the guidelines agreed with this standard. This leaves 2 of the 13 guidelines that do not recommend systematic screening for ASB in pregnancy.[55]

Prevention

Efforts to prevent UTI and ASB in pregnancy are critical. Lowering the incidence of UTI will not only decrease maternal and fetal health risks associated with the uropathogens themselves, but also reduce the risk of antibiotic side effects and limit the contribution to antibiotic resistance.

Screening for ASB is a form of prevention of further development of symptomatic cystitis or pyelonephritis. While there is no robust research on behavioral modifications, such as pre/post coital voiding, front to back wiping, avoiding hot tubs/baths in prevention of UTI in pregnancy, a 2018 systematic review evaluated the utility of non-antibiotic preventive measures.[56] The paper identified 8 eligible articles and identified 5 safe non-antibiotic approaches to prevent UTI in pregnancy. The use of cranberry juice, hygienic measures, anti-bacterial immunization, Canephron (phytotherapeutic medicine comprised of 3 herbs), and ascorbic acid were reported to be safe and effective at preventing UTI in pregnancy, with hygiene behavior having the most reputable evidence. While the remaining 4 approaches did not have robust evidence with adequate power to recommend these practices in evidence-based guidelines, the initial findings suggest these practices may be protective against UTI in pregnancy and warrant further research.[56]

Treatment

Asymptomatic bacteriuria Once ASB is diagnosed, the patient should be treated with a 5 to 7 day course of culture-specific antibiotics. There is insufficient evidence to recommend for or against sending additional cultures following treatment to test for cure.[13]

The importance of treating ASB in pregnancy was highlighted in a Cochrane Library Systematic Review and Meta-Analysis published in 2019.[54] The authors synthesized data from 15 studies including over 2000 pregnant women with ASB to evaluate the effect of antibiotic treatment on the development of pyelonephritis, preterm birth, and low birth weight. The authors concluded that treatment with the antibiotics may be associated with reduction of incidence of preterm birth (3 studies), pyelonephritis (12 studies), low birth weight (6 studies), and persistent bacteriuria at delivery (4 studies). However, much of the evidence was of low certainty. Further, randomized studies have determined that a 5 to 7 day course of antibiotics is superior to a single dose in terms of cure rate and decreased incidence of low birth weight, but no difference in bacteriuria recurrence, pyelonephritis, or preterm birth.[13,57]

Urinary tract infection Similar to the treatment of ASB in pregnancy, UTI in pregnancy should be treated with a 5 to 7 day course of culture-specific antibiotic therapy. Repeat urine culture should only be sent if urinary symptoms recur 1 to 2 weeks following treatment. Clinicians may consider daily antimicrobial suppression throughout pregnancy for those patients with recurrent UTI. Furthermore, pregnant women with pyelonephritis should be treated in the inpatient setting with 14 days of intravenous antibiotics.[13]

While the 5 to 7 day course of antibiotics is widely accepted for the treatment of ASB and UTI, clinicians and researchers continue to investigate alternative treatment regimens in an effort to minimize antibiotic exposure and optimize treatment. In 2022 Schulz and colleagues[58] performed a systematic review and meta-analysis to compare single-dose antibiotic therapy with multi-dose therapy in lower UTIs in pregnancy. A total of 9 studies involving 1063 women were included. Antibiotics used in the single-dose regimens were fosfomycin, amoxicillin, ampicillin, and bactrim. Surprisingly, single-dose treatment, when compared to multiple day antibiotic regimens, had statistically similar results in clearing the urine culture of significant bacteria. This finding warrants further investigation, given that most guidelines recommend full multiple-day antibiotic regimens.

Antimicrobial therapy Antimicrobial safety profiles in pregnancy must be a foremost consideration when selecting a treatment regimen. Further, as with any other bacterial infection, the antibiotic choice is aimed at targeting the isolated pathogen.

Corrales and colleagues[55] nicely synthesized proposed antibiotic regimens for ASB, cystitis, and pyelonephritis in their 2022 review. They reported the first-line antibiotics: (1) for ASB to be nitrofurantoin, fosfomycin, and amoxicillin, (2) for cystitis to be nitrofurantoin, fosfomycin, trimethoprim, cephalexin, amoxicillin, and amoxicillin/clavulanate, and (3) for pyelonephritis to be ceftriaxone or cefuroxime ± gentamicin, ampicillin/gentamicin, or amoxicillin/gentamicin. These findings are similar to the antimicrobial recommendations put forth by ACOG 2023 guidelines.[13] ACOG; however, does not make a distinction between ASB and cystitis for antibiotic choice, recommending nitrofurantoin, cephalexin, trimethoprim-sulfamethoxazole, fosfomycin, amoxicillin, or amoxicillin-clavulanate. Pyelonephritis requires intravenous administration of antibiotics to improve tissue penetration. Recommended antibiotics are ampicillin/gentamicin, ceftriaxone, cefepime, and for those with a beta-lactam allergy, aztreonam.[13] The safety considerations of

Table 2
Recommended and contraindicated antimicrobials for treatment of asymptomatic bacteriuria, acute cystitis, and pyelonephritis during pregnancy

Indication	Antimicrobial	Dosage	Duration	Considerations

Asymptomatic Bacteriuria/Acute Cystitis	Nitrofurantoin	100 mg PO q12 h	5–7 d	• Can be used in all trimesters; however, risk of facial malformation in first trimester and hemolytic anemia in the third trimester
				• Commonly used for lower UTIs
				  ○ Achieves excellent therapeutic level in urine
				• Not used for pyelonephritis
				  ○ Poor tissue penetration
				• Bactericidal activity against common uropathogens with limited resistance

	Cephalexin	250–500 mg PO q6h	5–7 d	• No activity against *Proteus, Serratia, and Pseudomonas* • First generation Cephalosporin • Good safety profile
	Sulfamethoxazole-trimethoprim	800/160 mg q12 h	5–7 d	• Not first-line in pregnancy • *Avoid in first trimester due to teratogenic risk of neural tube defects* ○ If no alternative treatment use with folic acid 5 mg/24h • If taken in third trimester, risk of neonatal hyperbilirubinemia and kernicterus
	Fosfomycin	3 g PO	Single dose	• Phosphonic acid derivative with broad coverage including MDR organisms; ESBL, MRSA, and VRE • Maintains high concentrations in urine for 3 d • Multiple randomized studies found no adverse outcomes with single-dose use
	Amoxicillin	500 mg PO q8h 875 mg PO q12 h	5–7 d	• First-line in pregnancy for sensitive bacteria • High rates of resistance in *E. coli* • Penicillins are oldest group of antibiotics with safety profile in pregnancy
	Amoxicillin–clavulanate	500 mg PO q8h 875 mg PO q12 h	5–7 d	• Especially useful for treatment of *GBS* • Risk of necrotizing enterocolitis in neonates • Suitable option throughout pregnancy

(continued on next page)

Table 2
(continued)

Indication	Antimicrobial	Dosage	Duration	Considerations
Pyelonephritis	Ampicillin + gentamicin	2g IV q6h 1.5 mg/kg IV q8h 5 mg/kg IV q24 h	After clinical improvement, should be transitioned to appropriate oral antimicrobial based on culture sensitivities to complete 14-d course of antimicrobial therapy	• Theoretic risk of ototoxicity and nephrotoxicity in mother and fetus, although have not been documented in literature • Gentamicin is the preferred aminoglycoside in pregnancy due to higher safety profile
	Ceftriaxone	1g IV q24 h		• Third generation Cephalosporin with good gram-negative and gram-positive coverage • Can be used in mild penicillin allergy • Well-established safety profile in pregnancy • If patient unstable, consider adding Gentamicin
	Cefuroxime	500 mg q12 h		• Second generation Cephalosporin • See Ceftriaxone
	Cefepime	1g IV q12 h		• Fourth generation Cephalosporin • See Ceftriaxone
	Aztreonam	1g IV q8-12h		• Low cross reactivity with Penicillin allergy • No harmful effects on fetus seen in animal studies although well-designed studies in pregnant women are lacking
Contraindications	Streptomycin	N/a	N/a	• Aminoglycoside drug class • Irreversible bilateral deafness • FDA pregnancy category rating D
	Tetracycline Minocycline Doxycycline			• Tetracycline drug class • Contraindicated past the 5th week of gestation • Permanent tooth discoloration, bone anomalies • FDA pregnancy category rating D
	Ciprofloxacin Levofloxacin			• Fluoroquinolone drug class • Renal toxicity, cardiac defects, central nervous system toxicity in fetus • May be safe in first trimester, but generally not recommended • FDA pregnancy category rating C

Tigecycline	• Glycylcycline drug class
	• Fetal loss in animal studies, no human studies performed
	• FDA pregnancy category rating D
Sulfamethoxazole-trimethoprim	See ASB/Acute cystitis section
Nitrofurantoin	See ASB/Acute cystitis section

FDA Pregnancy Category Rating C: risk not ruled out. Animal studies show negative impacts on fetus, but no robust human studies. FDA Pregnancy Category Rating D: evidence of risk to human fetuses established through human studies.

Abbreviations: ASB, asymptomatic bacteriuria; ESBL, extended-spectrum beta-lactamases; FDA, Food and Drug Administration; GBS, group B *Streptococcus*; MDR, multi-drug-resistant; MRSA, methicillin-resistant *Staphylococcus aureus*; VRE, vancomycin-resistant *Enterococci*.

Data from Refs. [1,13,55,60]

these antimicrobials, including the trimesters in which certain antibiotics should be avoided, are outlined in **Table 2**.

It is important to note that the recommended dose and schedule of fosfomycin are 3 g orally 1 time. Fosfomycin has been proven to have equivalent clinical outcomes relative to multi-day antibiotic counterparts. As such, the use of fosfomycin is seen as an exception to the concept that multi day antibiotic regimens prevail over single-dose therapy.[13,59]

Careful antibiotic choice is critical when treating pregnant women for ASB or UTI, as certain antibiotics in pregnancy carry irreversible and devastating risks to the fetus. While some antimicrobials, such as streptomycin and the tetracyclines, are contraindicated throughout the entire pregnancy, other antibiotics, such as nitrofurantoin and sulfamethoxazole-trimethoprim are safe only during certain trimesters, and carry significant risk in other parts of the pregnancy.[60] A summary of recommended antibiotics and regimens, contraindicated antibiotics, and notable considerations, can be found in **Table 2**.

Antibiotic resistance patterns As with any bacteria, uropathogens in pregnancy are susceptible to developing resistance to antibiotics. For years there has been an increase in the prevalence of drug-resistant and multi-drug-resistant organisms.[1] A recent study revealed 92% of uropathogens to be resistant to at least 1 antibiotic, with the majority (80%) being resistant to 2 or more drugs.[61] Further literature has determined that the antibiotics with most uropathogen resistance are ampicillin, 2nd and 3rd generation cephalosporins, and trimethoprim-sulfamethoxazole, with *Proteus* and *Klebsiella* species having significant resistance to ciprofloxacin. Nitrofurantoin, carbapenems, and amikacin were the antibiotics with lowest rates of uropathogen resistance.[62,63] Interestingly, a 2023 prospective cohort study[32] collected urine cultures from 4506 pregnant and non-pregnant women and found that overall the uropathogens isolated from non-pregnant women had significantly more antibiotic resistance compared to the organisms isolated from pregnant women. The rising prevalence of antibiotic resistance, as well as the continued evolution of resistant patterns, highlights the importance of treating infections or ASB in pregnancy with culture-specific antibiotics, rather than empiric treatment.

FUTURE DIRECTIONS AND RESEARCH

Although there are well-established guidelines for screening and management of UTI and ASB in pregnancy, researchers and clinicians should not be dissuaded from engaging in research to further optimize urinary care for pregnant women. With constantly evolving microorganisms and antibiotic resistance patterns, research and antimicrobial stewardship are critical to improve our treatment regimens while protecting maternal and fetal health. Future research can focus on investigating novel prevention techniques and non-antibiotic management as seen in the Gouri and colleagues' study.[56] Additionally, an area that can be further explored is health care disparities and access to care amongst pregnant women, to better identify differences in, and barriers to, care that may contribute to worse outcomes in certain populations.

SUMMARY

UTIs in pregnancy can have significant adverse implications on maternal and fetal health. Physiologic changes during pregnancy, including hydro-ureteronephrosis and decreased bladder tone, cause an increased risk of UTI and ASB in pregnant women. The most common causative uropathogens in pregnant women are the same as those in their non-pregnant counterparts; however, pregnant women have GBS UTIs more commonly than non-pregnant women. All pregnant women should undergo an early pregnancy mid-stream urine culture screening test for ASB and diagnostic urine culture when presenting with urinary symptoms. A positive urine culture, regardless of symptoms, should be treated with appropriate antimicrobial therapy, as recommended by evidence based, published guidelines. Active and future research on non-antibiotic preventive measures, as well as on regimens to minimize antibiotic exposure for mother and fetus, continue to improve how we approach treating ASB and UTI in pregnancy, ultimately improving care for our patients.

CLINICS CARE POINTS

- In pregnant women, the prevalence of ASB is 2% to 10%, UTI is 1% to 4%, and pyelonephritis is 1% to 4%.[12,18]

- Prevalence of UTIs is highest among women less than 19 yearsof age at conception, self-reported American Indian or Alaska Native ethnicity, low educational attainment, and having an annual household income less than $10,000, in one study.[2]

- *E. coli* is responsible for a vast majority of UTIs in pregnancy ranging from 49% to 85%.[1,16,30–32]

- GBS, frequently detected in the female GI and reproductive tract, is the most commonly found gram-positive organism, comprising roughly 10% of UTIs in pregnancy. Substantial GBS titers are present in the urine of 7% of pregnant women.[1,33]

- Midstream, clean-catch urine culture early in pregnancy is the gold standard for ASB screening, as well as the preferred test for UTI diagnosis (greater than 10^5 CFU/mL of urine).[13]

- Maternal complications from ASB and UTI include pyelonephritis, preterm birth, and pre-eclampsia with some data challenging the notion that ASB specifically increases risk of preterm birth.

- Historically, maternal UTI and ASB in pregnancy were thought to put the fetus/newborn at a risk for intrauterine growth restriction and low birth weight.[16,47,52] However, recent research has refuted this association.[9,31]

- The presence of E coli was significantly associated with neonatal sepsis after C-section compared to Klebsiella.[32]

- The use of cranberry juice, hygienic measures, immunization, Canephron, and ascorbic acid were reported to be safe and effective at preventing UTI in pregnancy, with hygiene behavior having the most evidence.[56]

- In general, the treatment course for cystitis and ASB is 5 to 7 days and for pyelonephritis treatment course should be 14 days.

- Understanding the mechanism of action and side effect profiles of antibiotic agents is paramount to optimize responsible and safe prescribing patterns during pregnancy.

DISCLOSURE

The authors have nothing to disclose.

FUNDING

There was no funding involved in this research.

REFERENCES

1. Glaser AP, Schaeffer AJ. Urinary Tract Infection and Bacteriuria in Pregnancy. Urol Clin North Am 2015; 42(4):547–60. https://doi.org/10.1016/j.ucl.2015.05. 004.

2. Johnson CY, Rocheleau CM, Howley MM, et al. Characteristics of Women with Urinary Tract Infection in Pregnancy. J Womens Health (Larchmt) 2021;30(11):1556–64. https://doi.org/10.1089/jwh. 2020.8946.

3. Anger J, Lee U, Ackerman AL, et al. Recurrent Uncomplicated Urinary Tract Infections in Women: AUA/CUA/SUFU Guideline. J Urol 2019;202(2):282–9. https://doi.org/10.1097/ju.0000000000000296.

4. White J, Ory J, Lantz Powers AG, et al. Urological issues in pregnancy: A review for urologists. Can Urol Assoc J 2020;14(10):352–7. https://doi.org/10.5489/cuaj.6526.

5. Ansaldi Y, Martinez de Tejada Weber B. Urinary tract infections in pregnancy. Clin Microbiol Infect 2023; 29(10):1249–53. https://doi.org/10.1016/j.cmi.2022. 08.015.

6. Mandal D, Saha MM, Pal DK. Urological disorders and pregnancy: An overall experience. Urol Ann Jan-Mar 2017;9(1):32–6. https://doi.org/10.4103/0974-7796.198901.

7. Partin AW, Peters C, Kavoussi LR, et al. Campbell-walsh urology. 12th edition review 2020.

8. Field MJ, Harris DC, Pollock CA. Pregnancy and the kidney. In: Field DCH MJ, Pollock CA, editors. The renal system. 2nd edition. London, UK: Churchill Livingstone; 2010. p. 121–30.

9. Bilgin H, Yalinbas EE, Elifoglu I, et al. Maternal Urinary Tract Infection: Is It Associated With Neonatal Urinary Tract Infection? J Fam Reprod Health 2021;15(1): 8–12. https://doi.org/10.18502/jfrh.v15i1.6067.

10. Sheiner E, Mazor-Drey E, Levy A. Asymptomatic bacteriuria during pregnancy. J Matern Fetal Neonatal Med 2009;22(5):423–7. https://doi.org/10. 1080/14767050802360783.

11. Salari N, Khoshbakht Y, Hemmati M, et al. Global prevalence of urinary tract infection in pregnant mothers: a systematic review and meta-analysis. Publ Health 2023;224:58–65. https://doi.org/10. 1016/j.puhe.2023.08.016.

12. Sheppard M, Ibiebele I, Nippita T, et al. Asymptomatic bacteriuria in pregnancy. Aust N Z J Obstet Gynaecol 2023;63(5):696–701. https://doi.org/10.1111/ajo.13693.

13. Urinary Tract Infection in Pregnant Individuals. Clinical Consensus No 4. 435-445. Obstetrics gynecology 2023;142.

14. Gilstrap LC, Ramin SM. Urinary tract infections during pregnancy. Obstet Gynecol Clin N Am 2001;28(3): 581–91. https://doi.org/10.1016/s0889-8545(05)70219-9.

15. Sabharwal ER. Antibiotic susceptibility patterns of uropathogens in obstetric patients. N Am J Med Sci 2012;4(7):316–9. https://doi.org/10.4103/1947-2714.98591.

16. Delzell JE Jr, Lefevre ML. Urinary tract infections during pregnancy. Am Fam Physician 2000;61(3): 713–21.

17. Ferroni M, Taylor AK. Asymptomatic Bacteriuria in Non-catheterized Adults. Urol Clin North Am 2015;42(4): 537–45. https://doi.org/10.1016/j.ucl.2015.07.003.

18. Owens DK, Davidson KW, Krist AH, et al. Screening for Asymptomatic Bacteriuria in Adults: US

Preventive Services Task Force Recommendation Statement. JAMA 2019;322(12):1188–94. https://doi.org/10.1001/jama.2019.13069.

19. Hill JB, Sheffield JS, McIntire DD, et al. Acute pyelonephritis in pregnancy. Obstet Gynecol 2005;105(1):18–23. https://doi.org/10.1097/01.AOG.0000149154.96285.a0.

20. Storme O, Tirán Saucedo J, Garcia-Mora A, et al. Risk factors and predisposing conditions for urinary tract infection. Ther Adv Urol Jan-Dec 2019;11. https://doi.org/10.1177/1756287218814382.1756287218814382.

21. Beetz R. Mild dehydration: a risk factor of urinary tract infection? Eur J Clin Nutr 2003;57(Suppl 2):S52–8. https://doi.org/10.1038/sj.ejcn.1601902.

22. Carter D, Beer-Gabel M. Lower urinary tract symptoms in chronically constipated women. Int Urogynecol J 2012;23(12):1785–9. https://doi.org/10.1007/s00192-012-1812-1.

23. Jagtap S, Harikumar S, Vinayagamoorthy V, et al. Comprehensive assessment of holding urine as a behavioral risk factor for UTI in women and reasons for delayed voiding. BMC Infect Dis 2022;22(1):521. https://doi.org/10.1186/s12879-022-07501-4.

24. Cunningham FG, Lucas MJ. Urinary tract infections complicating pregnancy. Baillieres Clin Obstet Gynaecol 1994;8(2):353–73. https://doi.org/10.1016/s0950-3552(05)80325-6.

25. Stenqvist K, Dahlén-Nilsson I, Lidin-Janson G, et al. Bacteriuria in pregnancy. Frequency and risk of acquisition. Am J Epidemiol 1989;129(2):372–9. https://doi.org/10.1093/oxfordjournals.aje.a115140.

26. Thurman AR, Steed LL, Hulsey T, et al. Bacteriuria in pregnant women with sickle cell trait. Am J Obstet Gynecol 2006;194(5):1366–70. https://doi.org/10.1016/j.ajog.2005.11.022.

27. Haider G, Zehra N, Munir AA, et al. Risk factors of urinary tract infection in pregnancy. J Pak Med Assoc 2010;60(3):213–6.

28. Yefet E, Bejerano A, Iskander R, et al. The Association between Gestational Diabetes Mellitus and Infections in Pregnancy-Systematic Review and Meta-Analysis. Microorganisms 2023;11(8). https://doi.org/10.3390/microorganisms11081956.

29. Habak PJ, Griggs JRP. Urinary tract infection in pregnancy, StatPearls. Treasure Island, FL: StatPearls Publishing LLC; 2024. StatPearls Publishing Copyright © 2024.

30. Wing DA, Fassett MJ, Getahun D. Acute pyelonephritis in pregnancy: an 18-year retrospective analysis. Am J Obstet Gynecol 2014;210(3):219.e1–6. https://doi.org/10.1016/j.ajog.2013.10.006.

31. Balachandran L, Jacob L, Al Awadhi R, et al. Urinary Tract Infection in Pregnancy and Its Effects on Maternal and Perinatal Outcome: A Retrospective Study. Cureus 2022;14(1):e21500. https://doi.org/10.7759/cureus.21500.

32. Angulo-Zamudio UA, Flores-Villaseñor H, Leon-Sicairos N, et al. Virulence-associated genes and antimicrobial resistance patterns in bacteria isolated from pregnant and nonpregnant women with urinary tract infections: the risk of neonatal sepsis. Can J Microbiol 2023;69(12):488–500. https://doi.org/10.1139/cjm-2023-0046.

33. Muller AE, Oostvogel PM, Steegers EA, et al. Morbidity related to maternal group B streptococcal infections. Acta Obstet Gynecol Scand 2006;85(9):1027–37. https://doi.org/10.1080/00016340600780508.

34. Platte RRK. Urinary Tract Infections in Pregnancy. Drugs and Diseases Obstetrics & Gynecology 2023;. . [Accessed 13 July 2023].

35. Gonçalves BP, Procter SR, Paul P, et al. Group B streptococcus infection during pregnancy and infancy: estimates of regional and global burden. Lancet Glob Health 2022;10(6):e807–19. https://doi.org/10.1016/s2214-109x(22)00093-6.

36. Gynecologists TACoOa. Prevention of Group B Streptococcal early Disease in Newborns. Committee Opinion 2020(Number 797). Obstet Gynecol 2020;135(2):e51–72.

37. Kirubarajan A, Taheri C, Yau M, et al. Incidence of kidney stones in pregnancy and associations with adverse obstetrical outcomes: a systematic review and meta-analysis of 4.7 million pregnancies. J Matern Fetal Neonatal Med 2022;35(25):5282–90. https://doi.org/10.1080/14767058.2021.1878141.

38. He M, Lin X, Lei M, et al. The identification of pregnant women with renal colic who may need surgical intervention. BMC Urol 2022;22(1):30. https://doi.org/10.1186/s12894-022-00985-x.

39. Kuebker JM, Robles J, Kramer JJ, et al. Predictors of spontaneous ureteral stone passage in the presence of an indwelling ureteral stent. Urolithiasis 2019;47(4):395–400. https://doi.org/10.1007/s00240-018-1080-8.

40. Nicolle LE, Gupta K, Bradley SF, et al. Clinical Practice Guideline for the Management of Asymptomatic Bacteriuria: 2019 Update by the Infectious Diseases Society of America. Clin Infect Dis 2019;68(10):e83–110. https://doi.org/10.1093/cid/ciy1121.

41. McNair RD, MacDonald SR, Dooley SL, et al. Evaluation of the centrifuged and Gram-stained smear, urinalysis, and reagent strip testing to detect asymptomatic bacteriuria in obstetric patients. Am J Obstet Gynecol 2000;182(5):1076–9. https://doi.org/10.1067/mob.2000.105440.

42. O'Leary BD, Armstrong FM, Byrne S, et al. The prevalence of positive urine dipstick testing and urine culture in the asymptomatic pregnant woman: A cross-sectional study. Eur J Obstet Gynecol Reprod Biol 2020;253:103–7. https://doi.org/10.1016/j.ejogrb.2020.08.004.

43. Mignini L, Carroli G, Abalos E, et al. Accuracy of diagnostic tests to detect asymptomatic bacteriuria during

pregnancy. Obstet Gynecol 2009;113(2 Pt 1):346–52. https://doi.org/10.1097/AOG.0b013e318194f109.

44. Umeh CC, Okobi OE, Olawoye OI, et al. Pyelone-phritis in Pregnancy From the Lens of an Under-served Community. Cureus 2022;14(9):e29029. https://doi.org/10.7759/cureus.29029.

45. Sharma P, Thapa L. Acute pyelonephritis in preg-nancy: a retrospective study. Aust N Z J Obstet Gy-naecol 2007;47(4):313–5. https://doi.org/10.1111/j.1479-828X.2007.00752.x.

46. Kazemier BM, Koningstein FN, Schneeberger C, et al. Maternal and neonatal consequences of treated and untreated asymptomatic bacteriuria in pregnancy: a prospective cohort study with an embedded randomised controlled trial. Lancet Infect Dis 2015;15(11):1324–33. https://doi.org/10.1016/s1473-3099(15)00070-5.

47. Henderson JT, Webber EM, Bean SI. U.S. Preventive Services Task Force evidence syntheses, formerly systematic evidence reviews. Screening for asymp-tomatic bacteriuria in adults: an updated systematic review for the US preventive Services Task Force. Rockville, MD: Agency for Healthcare Research and Quality (US); 2019.

48. Baer RJ, Nidey N, Bandoli G, et al. Risk of Early Birth among Women with a Urinary Tract Infection: A Retrospective Cohort Study. AJP Rep 2021;11(1):e5–14. https://doi.org/10.1055/s-0040-1721668.

49. Rezavand N, Veisi F, Zangane M, et al. Association between Asymptomatic Bacteriuria and Pre-Eclampsia. Glob J Health Sci 2015;8(7):235–9. https://doi.org/10.5539/gjhs.v8n7p235.

50. Kaduma J, Seni J, Chuma C, et al. Urinary Tract In-fections and Preeclampsia among Pregnant Women Attending Two Hospitals in Mwanza City, Tanzania: A 1:2 Matched Case-Control Study. BioMed Res Int 2019;2019:3937812. https://doi.org/10.1155/2019/3937812.

51. Yan L, Jin Y, Hang H, et al. The association between uri-nary tract infection during pregnancy and preeclampsia: A meta-analysis. Medicine (Baltim) 2018;97(36):e12192. https://doi.org/10.1097/md.0000000000012192.

52. AUA. Medical Student Curriculum: Core Content Updated 2022. 2023. Available at: https://www.auanet.org/meetings-and-education/for-medical-students/medical-students-curriculum-x18427.

53. Heath PT, Jardine LA. Neonatal infections: group B streptococcus. BMJ Clin Evid 2014;2014.

54. Smaill FM, Vazquez JC. Antibiotics for asymptomatic bacteriuria in pregnancy. Cochrane Database Syst Rev 2019;(11):2019. https://doi.org/10.1002/14651858.CD000490.pub4.

55. Corrales M, Corrales-Acosta E, Corrales-Riveros JG. Which Antibiotic for Urinary Tract Infections in Preg-nancy? A Literature Review of International Guide-lines. J Clin Med 2022;11(23). https://doi.org/10.3390/jcm11237226.

56. Ghouri F, Hollywood A, Ryan K. A systematic review of non-antibiotic measures for the prevention of uri-nary tract infections in pregnancy. BMC Pregnancy Childbirth 2018;18(1):99. https://doi.org/10.1186/s12884-018-1732-2.

57. Widmer M, Lopez I, Gülmezoglu AM, et al. Duration of treatment for asymptomatic bacteriuria during pregnancy. Cochrane Database Syst Rev 2015;2015(11):Cd000491. https://doi.org/10.1002/14651858.CD000491.pub3.

58. Schulz GS, Schütz F, Spielmann FVJ, et al. Single-dose antibiotic therapy for urinary infections during preg-nancy: A systematic review and meta-analysis of ran-domized clinical trials. Int J Gynaecol Obstet 2022;159(1):56–64. https://doi.org/10.1002/ijgo.14087.

59. Wang T, Wu G, Wang J, et al. Comparison of single-dose fosfomycin tromethamine and other antibiotics for lower uncomplicated urinary tract infection in women and asymptomatic bacteriuria in pregnant women: A systematic review and meta-analysis. Int J Antimicrob Agents 2020;56(1):106018. https://doi.org/10.1016/j.ijantimicag.2020.106018.

60. Bookstaver PB, Bland CM, Griffin B, et al. A Review of Antibiotic Use in Pregnancy. Pharmacotherapy 2015;35(11):1052–62. https://doi.org/10.1002/phar.1649.

61. Ahmed SS, Shariq A, Alsalloom AA, et al. Uropatho-gens and their antimicrobial resistance patterns: Relationship with urinary tract infections. Int J Health Sci (Qassim) Mar-Apr 2019;13(2):48–55.

62. Kot B, Grużewska A, Szweda P, et al. Antibiotic Resistance of Uropathogens Isolated from Patients Hospitalized in District Hospital in Central Poland in 2020. Antibiotics (Basel) 2021;10(4). https://doi.org/10.3390/antibiotics10040447.

63. Demir M, Kazanasmaz H. Uropathogens and antibiotic resistance in the community and hospital-induced uri-nary tract infected children. J Glob Antimicrob Resist 2020;20:68–73. https://doi.org/10.1016/j.jgar.2019.07.019.

Management of Bacteriuria and Urinary Tract Infections in the Older Adult

Juan Teran Plasencia, MD[a],*, Muhammad Salman Ashraf, MBBS[a,b]

KEYWORDS

- Urinary tract infection • Bacteriuria • Older adult • Elderly

KEY POINTS

- Urinary tract infection (UTI) is one of the most frequent bacterial infections diagnosed in the older population and is the most common reason for antibiotic prescriptions in nursing homes.
- A systematic approach to diagnosis with a standard toolkit or algorithm is recommended in patients residing in post-acute and long-term care settings.
- Treatment of UTIs in the older adult is similar to that of the younger adult. Nitrofurantoin and trimethoprim-sulfamethoxazole remain as first-line agents for the treatment of acute simple cystitis for most patients while quinolones have been relegated to second-line given side effects and increasing resistance.
- A shorter duration of therapy has been proven safe and non-inferior in many situations in UTIs.
- Data support the use of vaginal estrogen therapy, methenamine hippurate, and continuous antibiotic prophylaxis in certain populations for the prevention of UTIs in those with recurrent infections. Continuous antibiotic use should only be used if all other measures have failed in carefully selected patients where the benefit of continuous antibiotic may outweigh the risks for resistance and other side effects.

INTRODUCTION

Urinary tract infection (UTI) is one the most common bacterial infections, which in 2007 led to an estimated 10.5 million office visits for UTI symptoms and 2 to 3 million visits to emergency departments.[1] The data from the Nationwide Inpatient Sample showed that in 2011 there were 400000 hospitalizations for UTI with an estimated cost of $2.8 billion. Patients admitted to the hospital had a mean age of 74.7 years and most of them were women (71.4%) with a mean length of stay of 4.24 days.[2]

In patients older than 65, the proportion of admissions with UTI due to isolates with antimicrobial resistance increased from 3.64% in 2009 to 6.88% in 2016 and they were more likely to be discharged to health care facilities compared to routine discharges (Odds ratio [OR]: 1.81. 95% confidence interval [CI], 1.75–1.86).[3]

A 1-day point prevalence survey cross-sectional analysis done in 2017 among nursing home residents within 10 states with an Emerging Infections Program showed that among 15275 nursing home residents, antimicrobial use prevalence was 8.2 per 100 residents (95% CI, 7.8–8.8) with 28.1%

[a] Division of Infectious Diseases, University of Nebraska Medical Center, 985400 Nebraska Medical Center, Omaha, NE 68198-5400, USA; [b] Division of Public Health, Nebraska Department of Health and Human Services, 301 Centennial Mall South, PO Box 95026, Lincoln, NE 68509, USA
* Corresponding author.
E-mail address: jteranplasencia@unmc.edu

Urol Clin N Am 51 (2024) 585–594
https://doi.org/10.1016/j.ucl.2024.07.002
0094-0143/24/© 2024 Elsevier Inc. All rights are reserved, including those for text and data mining, AI training, and similar technologies.

being used primarily for UTI and 18.2% for prophylaxis, most often for UTI prevention.[4]

Pathophysiology

The increased risk for UTI in the aging population is not completely understood and represents a complex interplay of changes in innate immunity, hormonal changes, chronic inflammation, and impaired mechanisms for the reduction of bacterial burden within the bladder.

Animal models have shed some light on some changes associated with aging. The lysosome is a critical structure for autophagy, cellular and protein turnover, cell signaling, and ion regulation. In the aging urothelium progressive accumulation of large endolysosomes has been seen with impaired luminal degradation and higher potential hydrogen (pH) when compared to younger controls.[5] The aged urothelium has also shown a higher level of reactive oxygen species with a blunted antioxidant response.[6] All these changes contribute to bladder dysfunction. Furthermore, an increased number of quiescent intracellular reservoirs of uropathogenic Escherichia coli (E. coli) have been found in the aging epithelium and have been associated with increased recurrence of infection.[6]

Hormonal changes have been associated with disruption of the normal vaginal flora. There is a notable reduction in the vaginal pH of the peri- and postmenopausal women,[7] which has been shown to lead to a loss of lactobacilli colonization and increased isolation of Enterobacterales from vaginal cultures.[8] Vaginal atrophy and uninhibited bladder contraction are also hypothesized to contribute to chronic inflammation in the aging uroepithelium.[9,10]

Microbiology

The prevalence of different pathogens and resistance patterns will largely depend on the population selected. In 2012, a survey of outpatient females from more than 200 institutions in the United States (US) showed that the most frequently identified bacteria were E. coli (64.9% of isolates), Klebsiella pneumoniae (10.1%), Proteus mirabilis (5.0%), Enterococcus faecalis (4.1%), and Pseudomonas aeruginosa (2.7%).[11]

The National Healthcare Surveillance Network in their 2018 to 2021 report showed that Enterococcus and Pseudomonas species were more common in those with catheter-associated UTIs. The top pathogens for long-term acute care hospitals were E. coli (22.8%), Pseudomonas species (22.7%), Klebsiella species (18.6%), Proteus species (8.7%), and Enterococcus faecalis (6.4%). For inpatient rehabilitation facilities the most common pathogens were E. coli (35.3%), Klebsiella species (17.2%), Pseudomonas species (15.9%), Enterococcus faecalis (6.7%), and Proteus species (6.1%).[12]

DIAGNOSTIC APPROACH
Asymptomatic Bacteriuria

The Infectious Diseases Society of America (IDSA) in their 2019 asymptomatic bacteriuria (ASB) guidelines define ASB as the presence of 1 or more species of bacteria growing in the urine at specified quantitative counts ($\geq 10^5$ colony-forming units [CFU]/mL or $\geq 10^8$ CFU/L) regardless of pyuria and in the absence of symptoms consistent with UTI. The guidelines recommend against screening older individuals; these recommendations hold both for healthy independent patients residing in the community and for functionally or cognitively impaired patients residing in long-term care. An exception is made for those planned to undergo invasive urologic procedures in which breakdown of the mucosa is expected.[13]

Symptomatic Urinary Tract Infection

Diagnosing UTI can be complex and varies according to the site of infection in the urinary tract (prostatitis, cystitis, and pyelonephritis), the presence or absence of an indwelling catheter, community versus post-acute and long-term care (PALTC) resident, host characteristics (immunocompromised, spinal cord injury, diabetes, etc.), and severity of infection.

In the cognitively intact older adult, the diagnosis of UTI is similar to that of the younger adult. Clinical diagnosis should be based on localizing signs and symptoms that include dysuria, frequency, urgency, new incontinence, gross hematuria, suprapubic pain, or costovertebral tenderness. However, chronic genitourinary symptoms are common in older adults, which may complicate the diagnosis and this population is also known to have an increased risk of UTI secondary to drug-resistant organisms.[3,14,15] Therefore, urinalysis and urine culture should be obtained in older adults before starting empiric antibiotics to further guide antibiotic treatment.

Making the diagnosis of UTI is more challenging when evaluating cognitively impaired older adults and PALTC residents who may not be able to verbalize their symptoms. AMDA – The Society for Post-Acute and Long-Term Care Medicine recommends adhering to a consensus criteria or validated clinical algorithm for the diagnosis and decision to initiate antibiotics for residents with suspected UTI and performing urinalysis and urine culture only for those who meet clinical criteria.[16]

Examples of consensus criteria and validated clinical algorithms include Loeb minimum criteria for initiating antibiotics,[17] the Agency for Healthcare Research and Quality toolkit,[18] an international Delphi consensus procedure for the empiric treatment of suspected UTI in frail older adults,[19] and the Improving Outcomes of UTI Management in Long-term Care Project Consensus Guidelines for the diagnosis of Uncomplicated Cystitis in nursing home residents.[20]

Approach to the Patient with Isolated Acute Delirium or Advanced Dementia

For patients with acute delirium and no localizing signs and symptoms of UTI, empirical antibiotic treatment for UTI should be avoided, and clinical observation while assessing other causes should be the primary approach. This is supported by a prospective study that followed patients aged 70 years or elder admitted to a medical unit and screened for delirium while being followed during their hospitalization. The primary outcome assessed the rate of poor functional recovery, which was a composite of death, new long-term care institutionalization, or decreased ability to perform activities of daily life. With a cohort of 343 patients, patients with delirium treated for UTI without urinary symptoms had a worse functional recovery compared to other patients with delirium with an RR of 1.30 (95% CI, 1.14–1.48). Similar results were seen when including patients with bacteriuria and delirium.[21]

Older individuals with advanced dementia represent a diagnostic challenge due to decreased communication capacity, frequent incontinence, and multiple comorbidities. Patients with advanced dementia are frequently misdiagnosed as having UTIs and are overly exposed to antibiotic therapy. In a prospective study from 25 nursing homes in the Boston area, change in mental status was the sole sign or symptom in 35.9% of suspected UTI events and only 16% met the clinical criteria for empirical use of antibiotic therapy. When stratified according to the presence of a urinary catheter, patients without an indwelling catheter were more likely to have mental status change reported on their chart (48.3% vs 13.3%) and less likely to have fever (33.3% vs 19%) and meet clinical criteria for empirical use of antibiotics (12.9% vs 40%). When considering both clinical and microbiological criteria, only 11.4% of suspected events met the criteria for UTI diagnosis but the vast majority received antimicrobial therapy (77.9%).[22]

These studies demonstrate that mental status change including acute delirium in the absence of other signs and symptoms of UTI may indicate alternative etiologies. Careful clinical evaluation and close observation are usually required before pursuing diagnostic workup for UTI in these cases. For PALTC residents with unequivocal delirium, AMDA's infection Advisory Committee consensus statement recommends that a UTI diagnosis should only be considered if there is no other cause identified for these acute, fluctuating symptoms. For those residents with mental status change who do not meet clinical criteria for UTI and do not have any warning signs (such as fevers, rigors, acute delirium, or unstable vital signs), they recommend "active monitoring", which includes observation of vital signs, hydration status, and repeated physical assessments by nursing staff.[16]

TREATMENT
Asymptomatic Bacteriuria

Many prospective studies in the 1980s and 1990s failed to show any clinical benefit in treating ASB. One of these studies performed in Canada evaluated 2 all-male long-term care facilities, which showed that ASB was a frequent finding among their residents ranging between 26% and 47%. Those who showed microbiological failure or relapse after a single dose of antibiotic therapy, they were randomized to either progressively longer courses of antibiotics if persistent failure or relapse or to no treatment at all. Ninety four percent of those in the treatment group had bacteriuria at the study termination versus 100% of those without treatment. There was no statistically significant difference in the number of infections or mortality between the 2 groups and those in the treatment arm showed subsequent bacteriuria with more resistant organisms.[23]

A group that has shown benefits from the treatment of ASB are those patients who will undergo endoscopic urologic procedures in which mucosal trauma is expected. Both the IDSA in their 2019 ASB guidelines and the American Urologic Association in their 2019 Best Practice Statement recommend one or two doses to be given right before the procedure.[13,24] Non-invasive procedures such as urodynamic studies and cystoscopy have not shown benefits from urine culture screening or antibiotic prophylaxis to prevent UTIs or bacteremia.[24,25]

Symptomatic Urinary Tract Infection

The older adult is at risk for adverse drug events and antibiotics should be selected with care and with appropriate monitoring. A good resource is the American Geriatric Society's Beers Criteria for Potentially Inappropriate Medication Use in

Older Adults, which in its most recent iteration from 2023 lists nitrofurantoin for its potential risk for pulmonary toxicity, hepatotoxicity, and peripheral neuropathy, especially with long-term use and recommends avoiding the medication when creatinine clearance is less than 30 mL per min. It lists trimethoprim-sulfamethoxazole for risk of worsening renal function and hyperkalemia with concurrent use of angiotensin-converting enzyme inhibitor, angiotensin receptor blocker, or angiotensin receptor-neprilysin inhibitor in presence of decreased creatinine clearance. It also recommends against the use of ciprofloxacin with creatinine clearance less than 30 mL per min due to its risk of central nervous system effects like seizure and confusion, as well as the risk of tendon rupture.[26]

Short courses of nitrofurantoin and trimethoprim-sulfamethoxazole remain as first-line treatment for acute simple cystitis for most patients (when there are no contraindications and drug-drug interactions) while quinolones have been relegated as second-line treatment due to their side effects and risk for *C. difficile*. Nitrofurantoin is not recommended for acute pyelonephritis or systemic infection.

Treatment of symptomatic UTI in the older adult does not vary significantly from the recommendations for younger adults. The importance of obtaining an adequate history to evaluate prior antibiotic exposure and review of prior cultures is paramount when deciding to start empiric antibiotic treatment; this was illustrated by the study of Talan and colleagues where patients admitted with a primary diagnosis of UTI were stratified according to infection with Enterobacterales with an extended-spectrum beta-lactamase (ESBL) versus those without ESBL, risk factors included exposure to antibiotics within the last 90 days (75% vs 45.2%), residing in long-term care within 90 days (24.4% vs 7.5%), having a prior history of a ceftriaxone-resistant isolate within the last year (41.6 vs 8.6%), having a prior history of a quinolone-resistant isolate within the last year (41.6 vs 14.7%).[27] Antibiotic choice should be adjusted as needed once culture result becomes available. The choice of empiric antibiotic will also depend on the UTI syndrome being treated (eg, acute simple cystitis vs acute pyelonephritis).

Classification

Classically, UTI has been classified in women as uncomplicated for acute simple cystitis (with infection limited to the bladder) and complicated for pyelonephritis or infection with underlying urologic abnormality (eg, obstructive uropathy).

Historically, in men all UTIs were considered complicated; however, there has been a movement away from this definition as men can also have acute simple cystitis (with infection limited to the bladder), and most recently a new classification for UTIs in men is to divide them into febrile versus non-febrile UTIs.

Uncomplicated or Simple Cystitis in Women

As with many other infectious conditions, there is a growing body of evidence showing that shorter courses of antibiotic therapy are not only effective but safer for patients. A Cochrane review from 2012 showed no significant difference in the number of persistent UTIs within the first 2 weeks of treatment between those who received a short course of antibiotics (3–6 days) compared to long course of treatment (7–14 days) with a RR: 0.85 (95% CI, 0.29–2.47) and no difference between the 2 groups at long-term follow-up with a RR: 0.85 (95% CI, 0.54–1.32).[28]

The 2010 International Clinical Practice Guidelines for the Treatment of Acute Uncomplicated Cystitis and Pyelonephritis in Women, endorsed by the European Society for Microbiology and Infectious Diseases (ESCMID) and the IDSA, gives the following options for the treatment of simple cystitis in women.[29]

- Nitrofurantoin monohydrate or macrocrystals 100 mg twice daily for 5 days.
- Trimethoprim-sulfamethoxazole 160 mg-800 mg twice daily for 3 days.
- Fosfomycin 3 g in a single dose.
- Pivmecillinam 400 mg twice daily for 3 to 7 days. The product is not available in the US.
- Fluoroquinolones for 3 days
- B-lactam agents including amoxicillin-clavulanate, cefaclor, and cefpodoxime for 3 to 7 days

If possible, quinolones should be avoided in UTIs given their risk for side effects including confusion, hypoglycemia, tendon rupture, QT prolongation, and *C difficile* infection.[26] Furthermore, increasing quinolone resistance has also been seen in North America with a systematic review showing that the rate of resistance in *E. coli* isolates from women with uncomplicated infections increased between 2008 and 2017 from 4% to 12%.[30] Similarly, a prospective study from 10 academic emergency departments in the US in patients with pyelonephritis showed that *E coli* isolates in uncomplicated versus complicated pyelonephritis had a quinolone resistance rate of 6.3% (range by site 0.0%– 23.1%) and 19.9% (0.0%–50.0%), respectively.[31]

Acute Pyelonephritis in Women

The 2010 International Clinical Practice Guidelines for the Treatment of Acute Uncomplicated Cystitis and Pyelonephritis in Women, endorsed by the ESCMID and the IDSA, gives the following options for the treatment of pyelonephritis in women.[29]

- Ciprofloxacin 500 mg twice daily for 7 days.
- Levofloxacin 750 mg once daily for 5 days.
- Trimethoprim-sulfamethoxazole 160 mg-800 mg twice daily for 7 to 14 days (depending on the rapidity of clinical response).
- Oral β-lactam for 10 to 14 days. If this option is used, then a dose of parenteral formulation like ceftriaxone is recommended.

Randomized clinical trials studying shorter durations for trimethoprim-sulfamethoxazole and oral β-lactams are limited. A study comparing 4 systematic reviews with a meta-analysis (which included studies using antibiotics like amoxicillin, cefixime, trimethoprim-sulfamethoxazole, and pivampicillin) showed results favoring a shorter course of antibiotics (≤7 days) when comparing them to longer courses with an RR of clinical failure of 0.70 (95% CI, 0.53–0.94) and no significant difference in the rate of microbiological failure with an RR of 1.06 (95%CI, 0.75–1.49).[32] With these findings, in patients with mild disease and good clinical response to antibiotic therapy, a shorter course of 7 to 10 days of trimethoprim-sulfamethoxazole or oral β-lactam (particularly those who received a dose of parenteral antibiotic) is probably adequate. Another important point to consider when considering the use of ciprofloxacin and levofloxacin for acute pyelonephritis is the increasing prevalence of resistance. In communities where prevalence of *E. coli* fluoroquinolone resistance is more than greater than 10%, a dose of long-acting parenteral antibiotic (such as ceftriaxone) should be administered before starting ciprofloxacin or levofloxacin and culture results should be followed to confirm antibiotic susceptibility. Similarly, when a patient has personal risk factors for having infection with multidrug resistant organisms (eg, recent hospitalization or antibiotic use or infection with multidrug resistant organism), administering a broader spectrum parenteral antibiotic may need to be considered while awaiting the culture results.

Non-febrile Urinary Tract Infection or Acute Simple Cystitis in Men

Men have not been included in the official 2010 guidelines by ESCMID and IDSA, but data support the use of the following.

- Nitrofurantoin monohydrate or macrocrystals 100 mg twice daily for 7 days.
- Trimethoprim-sulfamethoxazole 160 mg-800 mg twice daily for 7 days.
- Fluoroquinolones for 5 to 7 days.
- B-lactam agents like amoxicillin-clavulanate, cefaclor, or cefpodoxime for 7 days.

The use of trimethoprim-sulfamethoxazole and ciprofloxacin for 7 days is supported by a randomized clinical trial done at 2 Veterans Health Administration (VA) Medical Centers where 7 versus 14 days of therapy were compared for men with non-febrile UTI with the primary outcome measuring the proportion of patients reporting resolution of UTI symptoms by day 14 after the completion of the active treatment. With a study population of 272 and a median age of 69, it showed that the primary outcome occurred in 93.1% of the 7-day group versus 90.2% of the 14-day group with a difference of 2.9% (1-sided 97.5% CI of −5.2 to ∞) that was within the 10% non-inferiority margin.[33]

Data supporting shorter duration including additional classes of antibiotics could be seen in a retrospective study in men with non-febrile UTI treated mainly outpatient and selected from 3 specialty clinics and 2 urology private practices that included the use of the following antibiotic classes in descending order of frequency: quinolones, trimethoprim-sulfamethoxazole, nitrofurantoin, and β-lactam that had UTI recurrence as the outcome variable and measured treatment duration as the main exposure (≤7 days vs > 7 days). When controlling for multiple covariates (Charlson comorbidity index, type of antibiotic, diabetes, and age), in their cohort of 573 patients a longer duration of treatment was not associated with decreased rate of recurrence (OR: 1.95, 95% CI, 0.91–4.21).[34]

Febrile Urinary Tract Infection or Complicated Urinary Tract Infectionin Men

- Ciprofloxacin 500 mg twice daily for 7 days.
- Levofloxacin 750 mg once daily for 5 days.
- Trimethoprim-sulfamethoxazole 160 mg-800 mg 7 to 14 days (depending on the rapidity of clinical response).
- Oral β-lactam for 10 to 14 days. If this option is used, then a dose of parenteral formulation like ceftriaxone is recommended.

When selecting empiric antibiotic treatment, same considerations for antibiotic resistance and initial dose of long-acting parenteral agent apply as described earlier for complicated UTI in women. As far as duration is concerned, 2 randomized trials have given somewhat conflicting results. The first is a placebo-controlled, double-blind, non-inferiority trial from the Netherlands that enrolled women and men with febrile UTI and randomized them to 7 or 14 days of ciprofloxacin. The primary endpoint was clinical cure rate on post-treatment days 10 to 18 with a non-inferiority margin of 10%. A secondary endpoint also assessed clinical cure at 70 to 84 days post-treatment. With a cohort of 357 patients clinical cure occurred in 90% of the patients treated for 7 days and 95% of those treated for 14 days with a difference of −4.5% (90% CI, −10.7–1.7). Of note, the secondary outcome of clinical cure on long-term follow-up did not show a significant difference with clinical cure in 92% versus 91% with a difference of 1.6% (90% CI, −5.3–8.4).[35]

A multicenter, randomized, placebo-controlled trial from France comparing 7 to 14 days of ofloxacin for febrile UTI in men with a primary outcome of treatment success, which was defined as negative urine culture and absence of fever and subsequent antibiotic treatment between the end of treatment and 6 weeks after day 1. The study enrolled 240 participants and found treatment success in 55.7% of the patients in the 7-day group versus 77.6% in the 14-day group with a risk difference of −21.9% (95% CI, −33.3 to −10.1) showing inferiority. It is important to note that post-treatment culture or "test-of-cure" is not an endpoint that reflects common clinical practice as the recommendations are to avoid sending urinalyses or urine cultures in patients whose clinical symptoms are resolved.[36]

Given that the ideal duration of febrile UTI in men has not been clearly defined, a shorter duration of 7 to 10 days may be used in those with good clinical response who rapidly defervesced, while a longer duration of treatment of 10 to 14 days or more may need to be considered for those with a slow clinical response or additional complicating factors. Furthermore, no randomized clinical trials have been performed to define the duration for acute bacterial prostatitis and expert opinion still recommends a duration of therapy of up to 6 weeks.

PREVENTION
Local Estrogen Therapy

The use of vaginal estrogen therapy has been an underutilized tool for preventing UTIs in patients. In a large survey, up to 80% of postmenopausal women reported at least 1 symptom of vulvovaginal atrophy, 56% had never discussed vaginal symptoms with their health care providers, 20% were told that genitourinary symptoms were a normal part of aging, and only 23% were recommended the use of vaginal estrogen.[37]

Multiple randomized clinical trials have shown a decreased risk of symptomatic UTI in patients treated with vaginal estrogen therapy.[7,8,10,38,39] The largest of these studies from Šimunić and colleagues included 1612 patients with urogenital complaints who were randomized to micronized 17 β-estradiol versus placebo. When comparing UTI rates before treatment versus post-randomization, the estrogen therapy group showed a significant decrease from 23.7% to 6.2% (P-value 0.034) during the 12 months of treatment versus no significant difference in the placebo group from 21.1% to 16.4%. Additional benefits were shown in this trial including cystometric examination showing increased capacity and volume at which patient experienced urgency in the estrogen group while also showing less uninhibited detrusor contraction.[10]

Another notable finding was seen in the study of Raz and colleagues in which the cumulative likelihood of remaining UTI-free at 4 months for those receiving estriol cream was 95% versus 30% for those receiving placebo, it also showed that none of the postmenopausal women included in this trial had lactobacilli on vaginal cultures at enrollment but subsequent cultures showed increase colonization by lactobacilli while decreasing colonization by Enterobacterales.[8]

A recent meta-analysis pooled these 5 randomized trials showing an RR of 0.42 (95% CI, 0.30–0.59) for the recurrence of UTI in those patients treated with vaginal estrogen.[40] Given the robust clinical data available, the North American Menopause Society in their 2022 hormone therapy position statement recommends the use of low-dose vaginal estrogen for women with genitourinary syndrome of menopause not relieved with over-the-counter therapies and with no indication for systemic hormone therapy.[41]

Methenamine Hippurate

Methenamine hippurate is hydrolyzed to formaldehyde and ammonia in acidic environments, which has a bactericidal effect by denaturing proteins and nucleic acid. It has been described as an antibiotic-sparing option for those patients with recurrent UTIs. A 2012 Cochrane review could not provide major outcome measures due to the mixed quality of studies with significant underlying heterogeneity; however, subgroup analyses showed that it could be beneficial in preventing UTIs (RR 0.24, 95% CI 0.07–0.89) and ASB (RR 0.56, 95% CI 0.37–0.83) in patients without renal tract abnormalities.[42]

Since the publishing of that Cochrane review in 2012, 2 major randomized clinical trials have been published. The first is the ALTAR trial in 2022, which was a pragmatic, open-label, multicenter, randomized, non-inferiority trial based in the United Kingdom comparing methenamine hippurate to low-dose antibiotic therapy with a primary outcome measuring the incidence of symptomatic antibiotic-treated UTI. Of note, this trial included women aged 18 years or elder with recurrent UTIs and excluded those with correctible urinary tract abnormalities and those with neurogenic dysfunction. With 205 participants in the modified-intention-to-treat analysis, the incidence of UTI in the antibiotic group was 0.89 episodes per person-year and 1.38 episodes per person-year in the methenamine group with an absolute difference of 0.49 (90% CI 0.15–0.84), with a defined margin of 1 UTI episode per year; the study confirmed non-inferiority of methenamine when compared to low dose antibiotic prophylaxis.[43]

The second randomized trial was done in the US by Botros and colleagues. This was a single-center, open-label, randomized trial comparing methenamine to trimethoprim in women 18 or older with no urinary tract abnormalities. During the 12 months of follow-up, there was no statistically significant difference in the rate of UTIs, time to UTI, or number of UTIs. Both medications decreased the incidence of UTI from 4 to 1.5 UTI episodes per person-year in the trimethoprim group and from 3.7 to 1.6 episodes per person-year in the methenamine group.[44]

While the ALTAR trial did not specifically target older adults, approximately 60% of the patients were post-or-perimenopausal women. Similarly, the population in the trial by Botros and colleagues had a mean age of 71.9 and 93.4% were postmenopausal. Further research is needed to establish if there is a benefit from using methenamine hippurate in men, patients with urinary tract abnormalities, those with indwelling urinary catheters, and those with neurogenic bladder disorder. For the last group, the SINBA trial in 2006 failed to show improvement in time to recurrence when comparing methenamine to placebo in patients with spinal cord injury, many of whom had suprapubic catheters or had bladder management with clean intermittent self-catheterization.[45]

Continuous Antibiotic Prophylaxis

There has been no randomized clinical trial assessing the efficacy of continuous antibiotic prophylaxis in PALTC population. A randomized, double-blind, non-inferiority trial in the Netherlands comparing low-dose trimethoprim-sulfamethoxazole (single-strength tablet 80/400 mg once daily) to oral lactobacillus for postmenopausal women with recurrent UTIs showed that within their cohort of 252 women, those in the antibiotic group (n = 127), the rate of UTIs in the year before randomization was 7 episodes per year (standard deviation of 4.9) and during the 12 months of treatment the mean number of clinical recurrence was 2.9 (95% CI, 2.3–3.6) with a mean time to first recurrence of 6 months.[46]

A systematic review and meta-analysis published in 2017 assessed the efficacy of long-term antibiotic prophylaxis (duration of treatment in the intervention arms ranging from 6 to 12 months) to prevent recurrent UTIs in older patients (those 65 and older). A total of 3 randomized trials, none of them including men, compared antibiotic prophylaxis to lactobacillus, D-mannose, and vaginal estrogen, respectively. With a pooled cohort of 482 postmenopausal women, the use of antibiotics showed a 24% risk reduction for recurrent UTIs (RR: 0.76; 95% CI, 0.61–0.95) with a number needed to treat of 8.[47]

Continuous antibiotic prophylaxis, while effective, carries many risks including medication side effects in older patients,[26] increased risk for multi-drug resistant organisms,[27] and risk for C difficile colitis.[16] In the study performed in the Netherlands comparing trimethoprim-sulfamethoxazole to lactobacillus, after 1 month of antibiotic prophylaxis, the resistance to amoxicillin and trimethoprim-sulfamethoxazole from commensal E. coli in urine and feces increased from 20% to 40% to 80% to 95%. After 12 months of antibiotic therapy, all urinary isolates were resistant to trimethoprim-sulfamethoxazole and 38.5% of women had ASB. AMDA – Infection Advisory Committee consensus statement for diagnosis, treatment and prevention of UTI in PALTC residents acknowledge that even though continuous antibiotics may reduce the risk of recurrent, uncomplicated UTIs, the potential harms associated with long-term use, coupled with the prevalence of multidrug-resistant organisms among this patient group argues against long-term antibiotic prophylaxis. Similar risk exists for older patient in community settings too. Therefore, continuous antibiotic use should only be used if all other measures have failed in carefully selected patients where benefit of continuous antibiotic may outweigh the risks for resistance and other side effects. Continuous antibiotic prophylaxis is generally not recommended in patients with indwelling urinary catheters because of even higher risk of resistance.

Therapies with Inconclusive Evidence for the Prevention of Urinary Tract Infection

Probiotic therapy relies on the rationale that loss of vaginal lactobacilli in women has been shown to increase the incidence of gram-negative colonization and increased risk for UTI.[8] A 2015 Cochrane review found no reduction in recurrent UTI when comparing probiotic therapy to placebo (RR: 0.82 [95% CI, 0.60–1.12]) and no reduction when comparing probiotic to antibiotic therapy (RR: 1.12 [95% CI, 0.95–1.33]).[48] It is important to mention that the studies included in the Cochrane review had small sample sizes and insufficient methodologic details, which could lead to equivocal findings. Promising results were found in a recent randomized clinical trial from a tertiary care teaching hospital in India with a factorial design that compared the incidence rate of UTI between patients treated with placebo, oral probiotic, vaginal probiotic, and a combination of oral and vaginal probiotic with symptomatic UTI at 4 months reported as 70.4%, 61.3%, 40.9%, and 31.8%, respectively. There was a significant reduction in both the incidence of UTI and time-to-first symptomatic UTI in the vaginal and combination probiotic group when compared to the placebo and oral probiotic group.[49] More robust data are needed to assess the efficacy of probiotics in preventing UTIs.

D-mannose is a sugar that mimics the host's uroepithelial receptor and competitively binds to the uropathogen decreasing bacterial attachment to the mucosa. A 2022 Cochrane review could not perform a meta-analysis given the lack of comparable groups among the different studies.[50] Currently, further research with high-quality randomized clinical trials is needed to support the use of D-mannose.

Cranberry may decrease the adherence of uropathogens to the uroepithelial cells. There have been multiple randomized clinical trials exploring the use of cranberry for decreasing the risk of UTIs. A Cochrane review was recently updated with 26 new studies. Overall, cranberry seems to decrease the risk of UTIs with a RR of 0.70 (95% CI, 0.58–0.84; I^2: 69%); however, when subgroup analyses were performed, the risk in elderly institutionalized men and women showed no benefit with a RR of 0.93 (95% CI, 0.67–1.30; I^2: 9%).[51]

GOALS OF CARE IN THE PATIENT NEAR THE END OF LIFE

A careful balance should be achieved in the care of the older patient near the end of life. Every antibiotic exposure could be complicated by adverse drug events including *C difficile* infection and colonization or infection by multi-drug resistant organism.[27] Additionally, while overly conservative management may feel appropriate in frail patients near the end of life, antibiotic treatment is not always associated with improved outcomes. In a large cohort from 35 nursing homes in the Boston area, those adults aged 65 years or elder with advanced dementia and suspected UTI in whom antibiotics were used (oral, intramuscular, or intravenous), an adjusted Cox proportional hazards regression showed that antibiotic treatment was not associated with mortality.[52] This study shows that overutilization of antibiotic therapy and attributing non-specific symptoms to UTI is not an infrequent occurrence in older patients.

While being near the end of life or being enrolled in hospice is not a contraindication to receiving antibiotic therapy, having a systematic approach for the diagnosis of UTI, including using active monitoring in those with unclear presentation, will help avoid unnecessary use of antimicrobials. Finally, in cases where UTI is suspected, having a conversation regarding the goals of care and explaining the risks and benefits of antibiotic therapy will aid the provider in how to best approach management while honoring the patient's wishes.

CLINICS CARE POINTS

- Screening and treatment for asymptomatic bacteriuria is not recommended unless the patient is planned for a urological procedure in which injury to the mucosa is expected.

- For PALTC residents with mental status change who do not meet clinical criteria for UTI and do not have any warning signs (such as fevers, rigors, acute delirium, or unstable vital signs), active monitoring while investigating alternative causes should be the primary approach.

- Obtaining an adequate history to evaluate prior antibiotic exposure and review prior cultures is paramount when selecting an empiric antibiotic treatment.

- The use of vaginal estrogen is an underutilized tool for the prevention of UTIs in peri and post-menopausal women. Multiple randomized clinical trials have shown a decreased risk of symptomatic UTI with its use.

DISCLOSURES

J. Teran Plasencia has no disclosures to report. M.S. Ashraf has received support from Merck & Co., Inc, United States for a research project focused on studying the impact of training consultant pharmacists to promote antimicrobial stewardship in long-term care facilities. No conflict of interest for writing or reviewing this article.

REFERENCES

1. Flores-Mireles AL, Walker JN, Caparon M, et al. Urinary tract infections: epidemiology, mechanisms of infection and treatment options. Nat Rev Microbiol 2015;13(5):269–84.
2. Simmering JE, Tang F, Cavanaugh JE, et al. The increase in hospitalizations for urinary tract infections and the associated costs in the United States, 1998–2011. Open Forum Infect Dis 2017;4(1): ofw281.
3. Nguyen HQ, Nguyen NTQ, Hughes CM, et al. Trends and impact of antimicrobial resistance on older inpatients with urinary tract infections (UTIs): A national retrospective observational study. PLoS One 2019; 14(10):e0223409.
4. Thompson ND, Stone ND, Brown CJ, et al. Antimicrobial use in a cohort of US nursing homes, 2017. JAMA 2021;325(13):1286–95.
5. Truschel ST, Clayton DR, Beckel JM, et al. Age-related endolysosome dysfunction in the rat urothelium. PLoS One 2018;13(6):e0198817.
6. Joshi CS, Salazar AM, Wang C, et al. D-Mannose reduces cellular senescence and NLRP3/GasderminD/IL-1β-driven pyroptotic uroepithelial cell shedding in the murine bladder. Dev Cell 2024; 59(1):33–47.e5.
7. Eriksen BC. A randomized, open, parallel-group study on the preventive effect of an estradiol-releasing vaginal ring (Estring) on recurrent urinary tract infections in postmenopausal women. Am J Obstet Gynecol 1999;180(5):1072–9.
8. Raz R, Stamm WE. A controlled trial of intravaginal estriol in postmenopausal women with recurrent urinary tract infections. N Engl J Med 1993;329(11): 753–6.
9. Ligon MM, Joshi CS, Fashemi BE, et al. Effects of aging on urinary tract epithelial homeostasis and immunity. Dev Biol 2023;493:29–39.
10. Šimunić V, Banović I, Ciglar S, et al. Local estrogen treatment in patients with urogenital symptoms. Int J Gynecol Obstet 2003;82(2):187–97.
11. Sanchez GV, Babiker A, Master RN, et al. Antibiotic resistance among urinary isolates from female outpatients in the United States in 2003 and 2012. Antimicrob Agents Chemother 2016;60(5):2680–3.
12. Centers for Disease Control and Prevention. HAI Pathogens and Antimicrobial Resistance Report, 2018 – 2021. U.S. Department of Health and Human Services, CDC; Atlanta, GA, 2023. Available at: https://www.cdc.gov/nhsn/hai-report/index.html Accessed 15 March 2024.
13. Nicolle LE, Gupta K, Bradley SF, et al. Clinical practice guideline for the management of asymptomatic bacteriuria: 2019 update by the infectious diseases society of Americaa. Clin Infect Dis 2019;68(10): e83–110.
14. Nicolle LE. Asymptomatic bacteriuria in the elderly. Infect Dis Clin North Am 1997;11(3):647–62.
15. Lob SH, Nicolle LE, Hoban DJ, et al. Susceptibility patterns and ESBL rates of Escherichia coli from urinary tract infections in Canada and the United States, SMART 2010–2014. Diagn Microbiol Infect Dis 2016;85(4):459–65.
16. Ashraf MS, Gaur S, Bushen OY, et al. Diagnosis, treatment, and prevention of urinary tract infections in post-acute and long-term care settings: a consensus statement from AMDA's infection advisory subcommittee. J Am Med Dir Assoc 2020;21(1):12–24.e2.
17. Bentley DW, Bradley S, Crossley K, et al. Development of minimum criteria for the initiation of antibiotics in residents of long-term–care facilities: results of a consensus conference. Infect Control Hosp Epidemiol 2001;22(2):120–4.
18. Best Practices in the Diagnosis and Treatment of Asymptomatic Bacteriuria and Urinary Tract Infections. 2022. Agency for Healthcare Research and Quality; Rockville, MD. Available at: https://www.ahrq.gov/antibiotic-use/ambulatory-care/best-practices/uti.html Accessed 15 March 2024.
19. van Buul LW, Vreeken HL, Bradley SF, et al. The development of a decision tool for the empiric treatment of suspected urinary tract infection in frail older adults: a delphi consensus procedure. J Am Med Dir Assoc 2018;19(9):757–64.
20. Nace DA, Perera SK, Hanlon JT, et al. The improving outcomes of UTI management in long-term care project (IOU) consensus guidelines for the diagnosis of uncomplicated cystitis in nursing home residents. J Am Med Dir Assoc 2018;19(9):765–9.e3.
21. Dasgupta M, Brymer C, Elsayed S. Treatment of asymptomatic UTI in older delirious medical inpatients: a prospective cohort study. Arch Gerontol Geriatr 2017;72:127–34.
22. Agata ED, Loeb MB, Mitchell SL. Challenges in assessing nursing home residents with advanced dementia for suspected urinary tract infections. J Am Geriatr Soc 2013;61(1):62–6.
23. Nicolle LE, Bjornson J, Harding GKM, et al. Bacteriuria in elderly institutionalized men. N Engl J Med 1983;309(23):1420–5.
24. Lightner DJ, Wymer K, Sanchez J, et al. Best practice statement on urologic procedures and antimicrobial prophylaxis. J Urol 2020;203(2):351–6.
25. Chavarriaga J, Villanueva J, Varela D, et al. Do we need a urine culture before cystoscopy? time to shift away from routine testing. Urology 2023;172:13–7.
26. By the 2023 American Geriatrics Society Beers Criteria® Update Expert Panel. American geriatrics society 2023 updated AGS beers criteria® for potentially inappropriate medication use in older adults. J Am Geriatr Soc 2023;71(7):2052–81.
27. Talan DA, Takhar SS, Krishnadasan A, et al. Emergence of extended-spectrum β-lactamase urinary

tract infections among hospitalized emergency department patients in the United States. Ann Emerg Med 2021;77(1):32–43.

28. Lutters M, Vogt-Ferrier NB. Antibiotic duration for treating uncomplicated, symptomatic lower urinary tract infections in elderly women. Cochrane Database Syst Rev 2008;(3):CD001535.

29. Gupta K, Hooton TM, Naber KG, et al. International clinical practice guidelines for the treatment of acute uncomplicated cystitis and pyelonephritis in women: a 2010 update by the infectious diseases society of america and the european society for microbiology and infectious diseases. Clin Infect Dis 2011;52(5): e103–20.

30. Stapleton AE, Wagenlehner FME, Mulgirigama A, et al. Escherichia coli resistance to fluoroquinolones in community-acquired uncomplicated urinary tract infection in women: a systematic review. Antimicrob Agents Chemother 2020;64(10). 008622-e920.

31. Talan DA, Takhar SS, Krishnadasan A, et al. Fluoroquinolone-resistant and extended-spectrum β-lactamase–producing *Escherichia coli* infections in patients with pyelonephritis, United States1. Emerg Infect Dis 2016;22(9):1594–603.

32. Erba L, Furlan L, Monti A, et al. Short vs long-course antibiotic therapy in pyelonephritis: a comparison of systematic reviews and guidelines for the SIMI choosing wisely campaign. Internal and Emergency Medicine 2021;16(2):313–23.

33. Drekonja DM, Trautner B, Amundson C, et al. Effect of 7 vs 14 days of antibiotic therapy on resolution of symptoms among afebrile men with urinary tract infection: a randomized clinical trial. JAMA 2021; 326(4):324–31.

34. Germanos GJ, Trautner BW, Zoorob RJ, et al. No clinical benefit to treating male urinary tract infection longer than seven days: an outpatient database study. Open Forum Infect Dis 2019;6(6):ofz216.

35. van Nieuwkoop C, van der Starre WE, Stalenhoef JE, et al. Treatment duration of febrile urinary tract infection: a pragmatic randomized, double-blind, placebo-controlled non-inferiority trial in men and women. BMC Med 2017;15(1):70.

36. Lafaurie M, Chevret S, Fontaine J-P, et al. Antimicrobial for 7 or 14 days for febrile urinary tract infection in men: a multicenter noninferiority double-blind, placebo-controlled, randomized clinical trial. Clin Infect Dis 2023;76(12):2154–62.

37. Kingsberg SA, Krychman M, Graham S, et al. The women's EMPOWER survey: identifying women's perceptions on vulvar and vaginal atrophy and its treatment. J Sex Med 2017;14(3):413–24.

38. Dessole S, Rubattu G, Ambrosini G, et al. Efficacy of low-dose intravaginal estriol on urogenital aging in postmenopausal women. Menopause 2004;11(1): 49–56.

39. Ferrante KL, Wasenda EJ, Jung CE, et al. Vaginal estrogen for the prevention of recurrent urinary tract infection in postmenopausal women: a randomized clinical trial. Female Pelvic Med Reconstr Surg 2021;27(2):112–7.

40. Chen Y-Y, Su T-H, Lau H-H. Estrogen for the prevention of recurrent urinary tract infections in postmenopausal women: a meta-analysis of randomized controlled trials. Int Urogynecol J 2021;32(1):17–25.

41. The 2022 hormone therapy position statement of The North American Menopause Society. Menopause 2022;29(7):767–94.

42. Lee BS, Bhuta T, Simpson JM, et al. Methenamine hippurate for preventing urinary tract infections. Cochrane Database Syst Rev 2012;10(10):Cd003265.

43. Harding C, Mossop H, Homer T, et al. Alternative to prophylactic antibiotics for the treatment of recurrent urinary tract infections in women: multicentre, open label, randomised, non-inferiority trial. BMJ 2022; 376:e068229.

44. Botros C, Lozo S, Iyer S, et al. Methenamine hippurate compared with trimethoprim for the prevention of recurrent urinary tract infections: a randomized clinical trial. Int Urogynecol J 2022;33(3):571–80.

45. Lee BB, Haran MJ, Hunt LM, et al. Spinal-injured neuropathic bladder antisepsis (SINBA) trial. Spinal Cord 2007;45(8):542–50.

46. Beerepoot MAJ, ter Riet G, Nys S, et al. Lactobacilli vs antibiotics to prevent urinary tract infections: a randomized, double-blind, noninferiority trial in postmenopausal women. Arch Intern Med 2012;172(9): 704–12.

47. Ahmed H, Davies F, Francis N, et al. Long-term antibiotics for prevention of recurrent urinary tract infection in older adults: systematic review and meta-analysis of randomised trials. BMJ Open 2017;7(5):e015233.

48. Schwenger EM, Tejani AM, Loewen PS. Probiotics for preventing urinary tract infections in adults and children. Cochrane Database Syst Rev 2015;12: CD008772.

49. Gupta V, Mastromarino P, Garg R. Effectiveness of prophylactic oral and/or vaginal probiotic supplementation in the prevention of recurrent urinary tract infections: A randomized, double-blind, placebo-controlled trial. Clin Infect Dis 2023;78(5):1154–61.

50. Cooper TE, Teng C, Howell M, et al. D-mannose for preventing and treating urinary tract infections. Cochrane Database Syst Rev 2022;8(8):CD013608.

51. Williams G, Stothart CI, Hahn D, et al. Cranberries for preventing urinary tract infections. Cochrane Database Syst Rev 2023;11(11):CD001321.

52. Dufour AB, Shaffer ML, D'Agata EMC, et al. Survival after suspected urinary tract infection in individuals with advanced dementia. J Am Geriatr Soc 2015; 63(12):2472–7.

Statement of Ownership, Management, and Circulation
UNITED STATES POSTAL SERVICE® (All Periodicals Publications Except Requester Publications)

1. Publication Title	2. Publication Number	3. Filing Date
UROLOGIC CLINICS OF NORTH AMERICA	000 – 711	9/18/2024
4. Issue Frequency	5. Number of Issues Published Annually	6. Annual Subscription Price
FEB, MAY, AUG, NOV	4	$427.00

7. Complete Mailing Address of Known Office of Publication (Not printer) (Street, city, county, state, and ZIP+4®)

ELSEVIER INC.
230 Park Avenue, Suite 800
New York, NY 10169

Contact Person: Malathi Samayan
Telephone (include area code): 91-44-4299-4507

8. Complete Mailing Address of Headquarters or General Business Office of Publisher (Not printer)

ELSEVIER INC.
230 Park Avenue, Suite 800
New York, NY 10169

9. Full Names and Complete Mailing Addresses of Publisher, Editor, and Managing Editor (Do not leave blank)

Publisher (Name and complete mailing address)
Dolores Meloni, ELSEVIER INC.
1600 JOHN F KENNEDY BLVD. SUITE 1600
PHILADELPHIA, PA 19103-2899

Editor (Name and complete mailing address)
KERRY HOLLAND, ELSEVIER INC.
1600 JOHN F KENNEDY BLVD. SUITE 1600
PHILADELPHIA, PA 19103-2899

Managing Editor (Name and complete mailing address)
PATRICK MANLEY, ELSEVIER INC.
1600 JOHN F KENNEDY BLVD. SUITE 1600
PHILADELPHIA, PA 19103-2899

10. Owner (Do not leave blank. If the publication is owned by a corporation, give the name and address of the corporation immediately followed by the names and addresses of all stockholders owning or holding 1 percent or more of the total amount of stock. If not owned by a corporation, give the names and addresses of the individual owners. If owned by a partnership or other unincorporated firm, give its name and address as well as those of each individual owner. If the publication is published by a nonprofit organization, give its name and address.)

Full Name	Complete Mailing Address
WHOLLY OWNED SUBSIDIARY OF REED/ELSEVIER, US HOLDINGS	1600 JOHN F KENNEDY BLVD. SUITE 1600 PHILADELPHIA, PA 19103-2899

11. Known Bondholders, Mortgagees, and Other Security Holders Owning or Holding 1 Percent or More of Total Amount of Bonds, Mortgages, or Other Securities. If none, check box ► ☐ None

Full Name	Complete Mailing Address
N/A	

12. Tax Status (For completion by nonprofit organizations authorized to mail at nonprofit rates) (Check one)
The purpose, function, and nonprofit status of this organization and the exempt status for federal income tax purposes:
☒ Has Not Changed During Preceding 12 Months
☐ Has Changed During Preceding 12 Months (Publisher must submit explanation of change with this statement)

PS Form 3526, July 2014 [Page 1 of 4 (see instructions page 4)] PSN: 7530-01-000-9931 PRIVACY NOTICE: See our privacy policy on www.usps.com.

---

13. Publication Title	14. Issue Date for Circulation Data Below
UROLOGIC CLINICS OF NORTH AMERICA	AUGUST 2024

15. Extent and Nature of Circulation		Average No. Copies Each Issue During Preceding 12 Months	No. Copies of Single Issue Published Nearest to Filing Date
a. Total Number of Copies (Net press run)		143	138
b. Paid Circulation (By Mail and Outside the Mail)	(1) Mailed Outside-County Paid Subscriptions Stated on PS Form 3541 (Include paid distribution above nominal rate, advertiser's proof copies, and exchange copies)	74	53
	(2) Mailed In-County Paid Subscriptions Stated on PS Form 3541 (Include paid distribution above nominal rate, advertiser's proof copies, and exchange copies)	0	0
	(3) Paid Distribution Outside the Mails Including Sales Through Dealers and Carriers, Street Vendors, Counter Sales, and Other Paid Distribution Outside USPS®	56	69
	(4) Paid Distribution by Other Classes of Mail Through the USPS (e.g., First-Class Mail®)	10	13
c. Total Paid Distribution (Sum of 15b (1), (2), (3), and (4))	►	140	135
d. Free or Nominal Rate Distribution (By Mail and Outside the Mail)	(1) Free or Nominal Rate Outside-County Copies included on PS Form 3541	3	3
	(2) Free or Nominal Rate In-County Copies Included on PS Form 3541	0	0
	(3) Free or Nominal Rate Copies Mailed at Other Classes Through the USPS (e.g., First-Class Mail)	0	0
	(4) Free or Nominal Rate Distribution Outside the Mail (Carriers or other means)	0	0
e. Total Free or Nominal Rate Distribution (Sum of 15d (1), (2), (3) and (4))	►	3	3
f. Total Distribution (Sum of 15c and 15e)	►	143	138
g. Copies not Distributed (See instructions to Publishers #4 (page #3))	►	0	0
h. Total (Sum of 15f and g)	►	143	138
i. Percent Paid (15c divided by 15f times 100)		98.24%	97.83%

* If you are claiming electronic copies, go to line 16 on page 3. If you are not claiming electronic copies, skip to line 17 on page 3.

16. Electronic Copy Circulation	Average No. Copies Each Issue During Preceding 12 Months	No. Copies of Single Issue Published Nearest to Filing Date
a. Paid Electronic Copies ►		
b. Total Paid Print Copies (Line 15c) + Paid Electronic Copies (Line 16a) ►		
c. Total Print Distribution (Line 15f) + Paid Electronic Copies (Line 16a) ►		
d. Percent Paid (Both Print & Electronic Copies) (16b divided by 16c × 100) ►		

☒ I certify that 50% of all my distributed copies (electronic and print) are paid above a nominal price.

17. Publication of Statement of Ownership
☒ If the publication is a general publication, publication of this statement is required. Will be printed ☐ Publication not required.
in the NOVEMBER 2024 issue of this publication.

18. Signature and Title of Editor, Publisher, Business Manager, or Owner

Malathi Samayan Date 9/18/2024

Malathi Samayan - Distribution Controller

I certify that all information furnished on this form is true and complete. I understand that anyone who furnishes false or misleading information on this form or who omits material or information requested on the form may be subject to criminal sanctions (including fines and imprisonment) and/or civil sanctions (including civil penalties).

PS Form 3526, July 2014 (Page 2 of 4) PRIVACY NOTICE: See our privacy policy on www.usps.com.

Moving?

Make sure your subscription moves with you!

To notify us of your new address, find your **Clinics Account Number** (located on your mailing label above your name), and contact customer service at:

Email: journalscustomerservice-usa@elsevier.com

800-654-2452 (subscribers in the U.S. & Canada)
314-447-8871 (subscribers outside of the U.S. & Canada)

Fax number: 314-447-8029

Elsevier Health Sciences Division
Subscription Customer Service
3251 Riverport Lane
Maryland Heights, MO 63043

*To ensure uninterrupted delivery of your subscription, please notify us at least 4 weeks in advance of move.